PARASITIC INFECTIONS

CONTEMPORARY ISSUES in INFECTIOUS DISEASES VOL. 7

SERIES EDITORS

Merle A. Sande, M.D.

Richard K. Root, M.D.

Volumes Already Published

Vol. 1 New Dimensions in Antimicrobial Therapy
Richard K. Root, M.D. and Merle A. Sande, M.D., Editors

Vol. 2 Endocarditis
Merle A. Sande, M.D., Donald Kaye, M.D., and Richard K. Root, M.D., Editors

Vol. 3 Bacterial Meningitis
Merle A. Sande, M.D., Arnold L. Smith, M.D., and Richard K. Root, M.D., Editors

Vol. 4 Septic Shock
Richard K. Root, M.D. and Merle A. Sande, M.D., Editors

Vol. 5 Respiratory Infections
Merle A. Sande, M.D., Leonard D. Hudson, M.D., and Richard K. Root, M.D., Editors

Vol. 6 Infectious Diseases: New Surgical and Medical Approaches
Richard K. Root, M.D., Donald D. Trunkey, M.D., and Merle A. Sande, M.D., Editors

Forthcoming Volumes in the Series

Vol. 8 Immunization
Richard K. Root, M.D., Kenneth S. Warren, M.D., J. McLeod Griffiss, M.D., and Merle A. Sande, M.D., Editors

PARASITIC INFECTIONS

Edited by

James H. Leech, M.D.
Assistant Professor
Department of Medicine
University of California, San Francisco
School of Medicine
San Francisco, California

Merle A. Sande, M.D.
Professor and Vice Chairman
Department of Medicine
University of California, San Francisco
School of Medicine
Chief, Medical Service
San Francisco General Hospital
San Francisco, California

Richard K. Root, M.D.
Professor and Chairman
Department of Medicine
University of California, San Francisco
School of Medicine
San Francisco, California

Churchill Livingstone
New York, Edinburgh, London, Melbourne 1988

Library of Congress Cataloging-in-Publication Data

Parasitic infections.
(Contemporary issues in infectious diseases; vol. 7)
Includes bibliographies and index.
1. Parasitic diseases. I. Sande, Merle, A., date. II. Leech, James H. III. Root, Richard K. IV. Series. [DNLM: 1. Parasites. 2. Parasitic Diseases—diagnosis. 3. Parasitic Diseases—therapy.
W1 CO769MQV v.7 / WC 695 P2233]
RC119.P345 1988 616.9′6 88-20256
ISBN 0-443-08561-7

Distributed in the United Kingdom by Churchill Livingstone, Robert Stevenson House, 1–3 Baxter's Place, Leith Walk, Edinburgh EH1 3AF, and by associated companies, branches, and representatives throughout the world.

Accurate indications, adverse reactions, and dosage schedules for drugs are provided in this book, but it is possible that they may change. The reader is urged to review the package information data of the manufacturers of the medications mentioned.

The Publishers have made every effort to trace the copyright holders for borrowed material. If they have inadvertently overlooked any, they will be pleased to make the necessary arrangements at the first opportunity.

Acquisitions Editor: *Linda Panzarella*
Copy Editor: *Kathleen M. Carroll*
Production Designer: *Jill Little*
Production Supervisor: *Jocelyn Eckstein*

Printed in the United States of America

First published in 1988

Contributors

Nina Agabian, Ph.D. Professor, Department of Molecular Parasitology, University of California, Berkeley, School of Public Health, Berkeley, California; Professor, Department of Molecular Parasitology, University of California, San Francisco, School of Pharmacy, San Francisco, California

John C. Boothroyd, Ph.D. Assistant Professor, Department of Microbiology and Immunology, Stanford University School of Medicine, Stanford, California

J. Lawrence Burg, Ph.D. Postdoctoral Fellow, Department of Microbiology and Immunology, Stanford University School of Medicine, Stanford, California

Jeffrey D. Chulay, M.D. Chief, Division of Communicable Diseases and Immunology, Department of Immunology, Walter Reed Institute of Research, Washington, D.C.

William L. Current, Ph.D. Research Scientist, Department of Animal Health Research, Lilly Research Laboratories, A Division of Eli Lilly and Company, Greenfield, Indiana

J. Louise Gerberding, M.D. Fellow, Divisions of Clinical Pharmacology and Infectious Diseases, University of California, San Francisco, School of Medicine; Project Director, AIDS Health Care Worker Study, San Francisco General Hospital, San Francisco, California

Robert S. Goldsmith, M.D., D.T.M.H. Professor, Department of Epidemiology and International Health, University of California, San Francisco, School of Medicine, San Francisco, California

Terrence J. Hadley, M.D. Assistant Professor, Division of Oncology-Hematology, Department of Medicine, University of Louisville School of Medicine, Louisville, Kentucky

Donald Heyneman, Ph.D. Professor, Section of Parasitology, Department of Epidemiology and International Health, University of California, San

Francisco, School of Medicine, San Francisco, California; Professor and Chairman, University of California, Berkeley/University of California, San Francisco, Joint Medical Program, Berkeley, California

Robin C. Hightower, Ph.D. Postdoctoral Research Fellow, Departments of Biochemistry and Biophysics and Pharmaceutical Chemistry, University of California, San Francisco, School of Medicine, San Francisco, California

Philip C. Hopewell, M.D. Professor, Department of Medicine, University of California, San Francisco, School of Medicine; Associate Chief, Medical Service, San Francisco General Hospital, San Francisco, California

Joseph A. Kovacs, M.D. Senior Investigator, Critical Care Medicine Department, National Institutes of Health, Bethesda, Maryland

James H. Leech, M.D. Assistant Professor, Department of Medicine, University of California, San Francisco, School of Medicine, San Francisco, California

Henry Masur, M.D. Deputy Chief, Department of Critical Care Medicine, National Institutes of Health, Bethesda, Maryland

James H. McKerrow, M.D., Ph.D. Associate Professor, Department of Pathology, University of California, San Francisco, School of Medicine, San Francisco, California

Susana D. Nagel, Biochemist Graduate Student, Department of Microbiology and Immunology, Stanford University School of Medicine, Stanford, California

Theodore E. Nash, M.D. Senior Scientist, Laboratory of Parasitic Diseases, National Institute of Allergy and Infectious Diseases, National Institutes of Health, Bethesda, Maryland

Franklin A. Neva, M.D. Chief, Laboratory of Parasitic Diseases, National Institute of Allergy and Infectious Diseases, National Institutes of Health, Bethesda, Maryland

George R. Newport, Ph.D. Assistant Adjunct Professor, Department of Pharmaceutical Chemistry, University of California, San Francisco, School of Pharmacy, San Francisco, California

G. Richard Olds, M.D. Associate Professor, Program in Geographic Medicine, Brown University Program in Medicine; Director, Program in Geographic Medicine, Miriam Hospital, Providence, Rhode Island

Dalia Perelman, B.S. Technician, Department of Microbiology and Immunology, Stanford University School of Medicine, Stanford, California

Carolyn Petersen, M.D. Assistant Adjunct Professor, Department of Medicine, University of California, San Francisco, School of Medicine, San Francisco, California

Richard K. Root, M.D. Professor and Chairman, Department of Medicine, University of California, San Francisco, School of Medicine, San Francisco, California

Merle A. Sande, M.D. Professor and Vice Chairman, Department of Medicine, University of California, San Francisco, School of Medicine; Chief, Medical Service, San Francisco General Hospital, San Francisco, California

Daniel V. Santi, M.D., Ph.D. Professor, Departments of Biochemistry and Biophysics, Pharmaceutical Chemistry, University of California, San Francisco, School of Medicine, San Francisco, California

Richard S. Stephens, Ph.D. Assistant Adjunct Professor, Department of Pharmaceutical Chemistry, University of California, San Francisco, School of Pharmacy, San Francisco, California

Paul M. Sullam, M.D. Assistant Professor, Department of Medicine, University of California, San Francisco, School of Medicine; Member, Medical Service, Veterans Administration Medical Center, San Francisco, California

Joseph P. Sypek, Ph.D. Assistant Professor (Special & Scientific Staff), Department of Medicine, Division of Geographic Medicine and Infectious Diseases, Tufts University School of Medicine; Department of Geographic Medicine, New England Medical Center Hospitals, Boston, Massachusetts

Ching C. Wang, Ph.D. Professor, Department of Pharmaceutical Chemistry, University of California, San Francisco, School of Medicine, San Francisco, California

Kenneth S. Warren, M.D. Director, Division of Health Sciences, The Rockefeller Foundation, New York, New York

David J. Wyler, M.D. Professor, Department of Medicine, Division of Geographic Medicine and Infectious Diseases, Tufts University School of Medicine; Physician, Department of Geographic Medicine, New England Medical Center Hospitals, Boston, Massachusetts

Preface

Events of the last decade have increasingly brought parasitic diseases to the attention of scientists and clinicians. Scientists have been intrigued by the intricate relationships between parasites and their hosts, and their studies of the molecular details of host-parasite relationships are dramatically increasing our understanding of parasite biology and host biology as well. In addition, studies by basic scientists are increasing the prospects for the development of vaccines against parasitic diseases and for identifying new targets for chemotherapy. Clinicians in the industrialized countries are encountering more patients with parasitic diseases because of the influx of immigrants from the tropics and subtropics, increasing worldwide travel, and the epidemic of the human immunodeficiency virus, which is frequently complicated by parasitic disease.

The purpose of this book is to provide a sampling of recent advances in the biology and management of selected parasitic diseases. The topics were selected because of their medical importance or because they represent areas in which exciting advances in basic understanding are occurring. The format is somewhat unusual because the authors of the chapters are a mixture of basic scientists and clinicians. The chapters about parasite biology provide an in-depth analysis of specific research issues presented by investigators actively involved in researching these topics. In the clinical chapters, new information about the pathogenesis, diagnosis, and treatment of specific diseases is presented and analyzed. The authors have been encouraged to give their opinions in controversial areas. One of the premises of this book is that basic scientists and clinicians have important things to say to each other, and the book will have served its purpose if it can contribute to that dialogue.

James H. Leech, M.D.
Merle A. Sande, M.D.
Richard K. Root, M.D.

Contents

1 The Evolution of Parasitology

Kenneth S. Warren

Parasitology has been defined as the scientific study of parasites as noted by Paul Beaver,[1] who goes on to say:

> Here I should mention that while it is appropriate to classify bacteria and fungi as either freeliving or parasitic—and viruses too are parasitic—these forms generally are not included among the elements of parasitology. Thus it can be said that parasitology is the scientific study of parasitic protozoa, helminths, certain lesser groups of worms, parasitic arthropods, and the vectors of parasites, that is, parasitology is largely an amalgamation of protozoology, helminthology, entomology, and acarology.

Although Beaver considerably narrows the definition of parasitology it should be noted that he clearly implies that all infectious agents are parasites. The basic premise of a book that is essentially unique, T. W. M. Cameron's *Parasites and Parasitism,*[2] is that all infectious agents are parasites, including bacteria, fungi, spirochetes, protozoa, viruses, rickettsiae, helminths, and arthropods. Virtually all other major textbooks of parasitology in English deal only with protozoa, helminths, and arthropods.

The principal question posed in this study of the evolution of parasitology is why and how protozoa and helminths became separated from bacteria, viruses, and other infectious agents in the development of this scientific field. This is not a trivial question, as the dichotomy in the study of these groups of organisms—microbiology, covering bacteria and viruses, and parasitology, covering protozoa and helminths—has had enormous consequences. Microbiology is studied and taught in major departments in schools of medicine whereas parasitology has been relegated largely to schools of public health, veterinary medicine, and tropical medicine. Microbiology has not only nurtured the basic fields of immunology and molecular biology, which have had such broad applications in science and medicine, but it has been the home of the antibiotic "miracle drugs" and major vaccines against both bacterial and viral diseases. In contrast, there are no vaccines for any of the parasitic diseases of humans. Drugs for parasitic diseases are often relatively ineffective, many being highly toxic. Major means of control have been insecticides and molluscicides; either resistance has developed to these or their cost has escalated.

Before going on to the history of parasitology, it might be well to more clearly define the word *parasite*. The unabridged Oxford English Dictionary notes that the word stems from Greek and means literally "one who eats at the table at another's expense and repays him with flattery." Biologically it is defined as an animal or plant that lives in or upon another organism (technically called its *host*) from which it draws its nutriment directly. Even viruses, which would be difficult to classify as plants or animals, have been described as "parasites at the genetic level."[3]

Recently, the population biologists Roy Anderson and Robert May have suggested the following subdivision of parasites:

> Microparasites (viruses, bacteria, protozoa) are characterized by small size, short generation times, extremely high rates of direct reproduction within the host, and a tendency to induce immunity to reinfection in those hosts that survive the initial onslaught. The duration of infection is typically short in relation to the expected life span of a host, and therefore is of a transient nature . . . Macroparasites, which include parasitic helminths and arthropods, tend to have much longer generation times than the microparasites, and direct multiplication within the host is either absent or occurs at a low rate. The immune responses elicited by these metazoans generally depend on the number of parasites present in a given host, and tend to be of relatively short duration. Macroparasitic infections, therefore, tend to be of a persistent nature, with hosts being continually reinfected.[4]

In *Parasites and Parasitic Infection in Early Medicine and Science,* Rudolph Hoeppli observes that helminths are the first infectious agents known, as they were clearly visible to the human eye.[5] W. D. Foster in *A History of Parasitology,*[6] also begins with Hoeppli's investigations, pointing out further that in primitive tribes in Sarawack and North Borneo the majority of persons were familiar with intestinal worms. The first chapter, entitled "Parasitology from Ancient Times until the Middle of the Nineteenth Century," deals wholly with helminths, and the subsequent seven chapters describe specific helminths. The ninth chapter, entitled "The Parasitic Protozoa," begins in 1681 with Leeuwenhoek's observations in his own feces of "animalcules a-moving very prettily: some of 'em a bit bigger, others a bit less, than a blood globule . . . ."[6] For more than a hundred years after Leeuwenhoek's observations there was virtually no progress in the study of parasitic protozoa. The first human protozoan parasite of major importance to be described was the ameba of dysentery by Losch in 1875, but as late as 1886 no parasitic protozoan was generally accepted as the cause of any important human disease. Following a description of individual protozoa, Foster's five-page final chapter, "Parasitology Established," begins with the statement that the foundations of the science of parasitology were well laid by about the 1860s; the book ends in the first decade of the twentieth century with the field well established. It is quite remarkable that the author never discussed parasitology in the larger context of infectious diseases and never speculated on why and how helminths and protozoa were grouped together to constitute the field of parasitology.

For this reason the Rockefeller Foundation commissioned a study on the history of parasitology by Michael Worboys who had previously written an excellent article on the emergence of tropical medicine.[7] In his new paper,[8] Worboys starts the section entitled, "The Prehistory of Parasitology" with the books of Hoeppli and Foster. He notes that during the last quarter of the nineteenth century the biomedical sciences constituted a common or unspecialized scientific culture and involved biologists from a wide variety of different fields. Biomedical research was being pursued widely at this time, and what particularly stimulated research was the acceptance of the germ theory of disease. Interestingly, he concludes this section by stating that there is good evidence that suggests that the rapid acceptance of the germ theory was due to the ground work prepared for it by investigations on helminths in the mid-nineteenth century. In the next section, entitled "The Emergence of Parasitology," he claims that the field emerged in the period 1900–1918, the main impetus being the development of tropical medicine. Areas in the developing world were known as "the white man's grave," and it was generally perceived that disease was the major factor holding back development. Sir Patrick Manson, one of the great founders of tropical medicine, described the situation in the following way: "I now firmly believe in the possibility of tropical colonization by the white races. Heat and moisture are not in themselves the direct causes of any important tropical disease. The direct cause of 99 percent of these diseases are germs. . . . to kill them is simply a matter of knowledge and the application of this knowledge in sanitary science."[8] Manson himself played a major role in this research with, among many other things, the publication in 1878 of a seminal paper entitled, "The development of the *Filaria sanguinis-hominis* and the mosquito considered as a nurse," the first clear demonstration of disease transmission by mosquitoes.[9]

Laveran discovered the malaria parasite in Algeria in 1880. Bruce produced his magnificent studies of African trypanosomiasis from 1896 to 1902, and Chagas reported on American trypanosomiasis in 1908. The life cycle of *Schistosoma japonicum* was worked out in 1913 in Japan and that of *S. mansoni* and *S. haematobium* in Cairo soon thereafter. Two of the first ten Nobel prizes for physiology and medicine ([to] Ross and Laveran) were awarded for their work on malaria, and when Robert Koch and Paul Ehrlich received theirs in 1905 and 1907 respectively, both were working on problems related to tropical diseases.

Worboys's most startling statement relative to Foster's belief that parasitology was established between 1860 and 1910 appears in the next section entitled "The Establishment of Parasitology." He expresses the belief that its establishment occurred considerably later, during the period 1914–1940, "when scientists began to call themselves parasitologists, when parasitological institutes and associations were founded, when a parasitological education, usually post-graduate, became available, and when journals began to proliferate and were founded in the major scientific nations." The first journal in this field, *Parasitology,* initiated publication in 1908; its introductory statement mentions as appropriate subject matter "disease-transmitting insects, malaria, trypanosomiasis, spirochaetoses, piroplasmosis, and plague, as well as parasitic worms." The *Journal of Parasitology,* which first appeared in 1914, announced a major interest in "animal parasites" and elaborated by stating "emphasis will be laid on the morphology, life history and biology of zooparasites, and the relations of animals to disease."[10] In that context it is important to realize that the emerging field of parasitology was captured by zoologists, who considered the protozoa and helminths to be animals and thus called them animal parasites. It is amusing to note that Nuttall, one of the early parasitologists of note, called bacteria and viruses "vegetable parasites."

This confusion about the elements that comprise the field of parasitology was compounded by a failure to realize that while protozoa share many of the characteristics of bacteria and viruses, helminths are totally different types of organisms, as emphasized by their division into a separate group called macroparasites by Anderson and May.[4] Not only are the worms multicellular and all species of adult worms visible to the human eye, but they share the unique characteristic of not replicating directly (with rare exceptions) within the definitive human host. That this characteristic is not trivial is obvious because of its profound implications for transmission, host immunologic responses, treatment, and control, as described in an editorial by Warren.[11] Nevertheless, parasitologists, in contrast to microbiologists, who are clearly subdivided into bacteriologists and virologists, tend to move freely in their investigations between protozoa and helminths. Also, as Worboy's points out, "Scientifically, by 1918 the morphology and life cycles of most of the important tropical parasitic diseases were known; there were few prestigious discoveries left to be made. The problems were now more difficult, being related to the control of disease, pathogenicity, and epidemiology. In the laboratories parasitologists did not have the advantage of working with such cooperative organisms as bacteria. Certainly the cutting edge was very much in vector control, a trend that did much to advance the growth of entomology as an autonomous discipline."[8] This point of view was greatly strengthened by Sir Ronald Ross's belief that the future of disease control in the developing world lay in insect control and in the creation of better environments through water supplies, sanitation, and housing.[7]

Furthermore, there was a widespread belief that a major factor, if not the major factor, underlying all the infectious disease problems of the developing world was malnutrition. At a 1932 international conference of representatives of health services of African territories and British India, the following typical resolution was passed: "In an undernourished population . . . the mere treatment of disease, no matter how effective and widely carried out, will achieve negligible results. The first need is a continuous supply of sufficient and well balanced food for the nature to resist infection, and the next is the improvement of housing."[8] In more recent times Thomas McKeown has established the historical premise that in the developed world "the most acceptable explanation of the large reduction of mortality and growth of population which preceded advances in hygiene is an improvement in nutrition due to greater food supplies."[12] He went on to say, "These and other investigations show the enormous importance of nutrition in determining the outcome of infection, and the tragic synergistic relationship which exists between malnutrition and infectious disease." And he concludes, "There need be no disappointment with the conclusion that medical measures of immunization and treatment were relatively ineffective: they were also unnecessary." In his work McKeown extrapolates these interpretations of historical events in the developed world to the developing world at the present time.[12]

Going beyond McKeown is a large group of medical and social scientists who are concerned with health in the developing world and believe that radical health improvements will only come after a long period in which changes must occur both on the level of social, economic, and political structures and on the level of individual and community perceptions. These scientists suggest that the acceptance of this approach "precludes the acceptance of health programs based on medical and technological interventions."[13]

Worboys's conclusions on the historical aspects of parasitology was that the field "emerged to provide the zoological underpinning for tropical medicine. Its subject matter was defined on the one hand by the tropical medicine curriculum and on the other by the botany-zoology division and the way tropical parasites fitted neatly into the type-based zoological curriculum." He stressed that in the period of its emergence parasitology can be seen to have been at the forefront of a still highly mobile and largely interdisciplinary biomedical scientific community, the relative decline in the importance and standing of parasitology ironically coming with its institutionalization in the interwar period, when tropical disease problems lost their urgency, tropical medicine became routine, and research concentrated on vector control.[8] This situation was exacerbated by strong beliefs in the relative unimportance of infectious diseases per se and in the development of a luddite, antitechnology type of mentality among specialists in health care delivery in the developing world. Furthermore, the field of parasitology had become isolated in schools of public health, veterinary medicine, and tropical medicine and did not participate in the remarkable scientific advances going on in the medical schools and major research institutes. Finally, funding was meager: calculations made in 1977 revealed that global support for research on malaria, schistosomiasis, filariasis, amebiasis, and ascariasis—infections involving 2,200,000,000 people—amounted to not much more than $10 million while U.S. government support for research on cancer, an affliction of 10,000,000 people, cost $815 million.

The current status and future of parasitology were examined at a conference in New Orleans in 1980, sponsored jointly by the Josiah Macy, Jr. and Rockefeller foundations. With respect to the training of parasitologists, Paul Weinstein described a study done in 1978 by the American Society of Parasitologists, which surveyed 141 educational institutions in the United States and Puerto Rico. Of a total of 559 courses in various aspects of parasitology 4.7 percent were devoted to immunology, 3.6 percent to physiology and biochemistry, 0.7 percent to ultrastructure, and none to molecular biology.[14] An examination of the parasitology literature revealed that a total of 972 papers was published in 1979 in 19 major English language journals in the areas of general parasitology, specialty parasitology, tropical medicine, general medicine, specialty medicine, veterinary medicine, general science, and specialty sciences. In that year the *Journal of Immunology* alone published 960 papers.[10] With respect to subject matter in four major parasitology journals and three major tropical medicine journals, only 41 and 27 percent, respectively, of the articles dealt with the more modern scientific disciplines of immunology, biochemistry, physiology, and molecular biology.[10] In a further study of the scientific literature, presented at a 1982 conference entitled "Parasitology: A Global Perspective," a comparative study of journal citation analysis in parasitology, virology, and bacteriology revealed that the former is relatively isolated from the mainstream of modern biologic research. Moreover, there seems to have been little significant movement away from this isolation in the 1978 to 1980 period.[15] Furthermore, analysis of the subject matter in English language textbooks of parasitology[15] corroborated Paul Weinstein's concerns of 1980 that these textbooks have "been dominated by the traditional subject areas of morphology, biology and life cycles, pathogenicity and symptomatology, diagnosis and treatment, and epidemiology and control . . . Biology as a discipline, however, has undergone a revolutionary change in the past few decades, particularly molecular, cell, and developmental biology, and this has been accompanied at the organismal, population, and ecological levels by the synthesis of new and far reaching theoretical concepts."[14]

With respect to the status of major infectious diseases of the developing world, in the period 1977–1978 parasitic diseases still ranked exceedingly high, with malaria third after the diarrheal and respiratory infections, schistosomiasis fifth, and hookworm tenth, followed by Chagas' disease, onchocerciasis, amebiasis, ascariasis, etc.[16] Even today there are no vaccines for any of the protozoan or helminthic infections of man, and chemotherapeutic agents are largely deficient. Resistance to antimalarial drugs is creating a terrible problem globally. No significantly worthwhile drug is available for Chagas' disease; the drugs on the market for African sleeping sickness are exceedingly toxic, as are those for leishmaniasis; and the major drug used for amebiasis is putatively carcinogenic. Although good drugs are available for the intestinal helminthic infections, reinfection occurs exceedingly rapidly because the infectious forms are ubiquitous within tropical environments. Recently, however, excellent agents have become available for the filariases and for schistosomiasis.

In 1980, while the current status of parasitology looked bad, the future of parasitology as described by Joshua Lederberg at the Macy/Rockefeller conference looked very good indeed.

> The germ theory, and the basic techniques for the recognition and isolation of various species of pathogenic microorganisms in pure culture established by Louis Pasteur, Robert Koch, and Ferdinand Cohn, gave us a sweeping scientific principle looking for the appropriate questions to which it would be a solution. As far as I am aware this principle has had more important consequences for the improvement of public health than any other concept in the history of mankind. But today we are uneasy because we cannot so easily replicate that kind of comprehensive advance for our remaining health problems such as heart disease, cancer, and schizophrenia. . . . The introduction of the germ theory of disease led to a rapid penetration of one large set of public health problems. I hold the view that it is precisely in parasitic infection that we have the nearest analogue to that kind of opportunity. My major premise is that when our understanding of the eukaryotic agents of infection can be brought to a comparable level of depth and insight—complicated by the fact that parasites are indeed eukaryons, often intracellular in habitat, and resemble the metabolism of the host more closely than do bacterial parasites—we will see advances as sudden and as spectacular as were achieved for most of the bacterial infections . . . The assemblage of scientists at this conference is testimony to the capacity to mobilize a diverse set of experiences and intellectual resources. If the material resources could be made available, with the kind of nucleation represented here, very rapid progress, a veritable new wave of research would at this point be inevitable.[17]

With respect to resources, the Special Programme for Research and Training in Tropical Diseases was initiated by the World Health Organization in 1976 specifically to attack malaria, schistosomiasis, the filariases (including onchocerciasis), the trypanosomiases (both African sleeping sickness and the American form called Chagas' disease), the leishmaniases, and leprosy. The budget, which began at about $5 million per year, rose to a peak of about $25 million in 1980. In 1977 the Rockefeller Foundation began its program called The Great Neglected Diseases of Mankind. A research network was established at 14 major laboratories, including the Walter and Eliza Hall Institute in Melbourne, Mahidol University in Bangkok, the Weizmann Institute in Tel Aviv, the Biomedical Institute for Research on Infectious Diseases in Cairo, Oxford University, the Karolinska Institute in Stockholm, the Polytechnic Institute in Mexico City and, in the United States, the University of Washington in Seattle, Case Western Reserve University in Cleveland (units both in medicine and pharmacology), the University of Virginia, Tufts University, the Harvard School of Public Health, and Rockefeller University. The annual investment has been approximately $2 million. By the end of 1984 the Tropical Diseases Research Programme (TDR) had resulted in 3,817 publications and the Rockefeller Foundation program in 1,319. Hundreds of young scientists have been trained by both programs, and the TDR has developed a unique system of institutional strengthening in the developing world. During this period the Edna McConnell Clark Foundation developed a seminal program on schistosomiasis, in which a strategic plan was developed by a board of experts and carried out by research grants averaging more than $2 million per year. At the suggestion of Joshua Lederberg, the Clark and Rockefeller foundations helped to establish an annual course in the biology of parasitism at the Marine Biological Laboratories in Woods Hole, Massachusetts, which thus far has trained more than 100 young scientists in state-of-the-art methods, including monoclonal antibody production, genetic engineering, and fluorescent activated cell sorting. Finally, the John D. and Catherine T. MacArthur Foundation has developed a program in the biology of parasitic diseases, which is providing approximately $20 million over a 5-year period to 12 laboratories working at the state-of-the-art level in basic parasitologic research.

With the help of these relatively meager funding sources, which together provide little over 3 percent of the annual support now provided by the National Cancer Institute in the United States alone, progress on parasitic diseases has been quite remarkable in the last decade. The application of advanced techniques in ultrastructure, biochemistry, immunology, and molecular biology has led to striking developments in many fields. Progress towards vaccines for malaria has been particularly remarkable. With respect to the sporozoite stage with which the mosquito infects the human host, at least two vaccines are undergoing phase 1 clinical testing; one of these is genetically engineered and the other is a synthetic vaccine consisting of 12 amino acids attached to a protein carrier. Blood-stage vaccines are being developed, and one of the most promising ones is a protein of molecular weight 155,000, which was discovered almost simultaneously by groups in Stockholm and Melbourne. The Swedish group, which has obtained evidence from infected populations in Liberia that this may be a protective antigen, is focusing on a synthetic approach, while the Australian group is using genetic engineering and the vaccinia vector. New pharmacologic agents being developed for African sleeping sickness include allopurinol, (the drug for gout), and DL-α-difluoromethylornithine, an inhibitor of polyamine synthesis that offers great promise in treating advanced cerebral disease. Basic research has revealed that trypanosomes and leishmania contain trypanothione, a unique glutathione derivative, which is essential for detoxification within the organisms. Targeting of this substance for attack by pharmacologic agents could lead to a whole range of new drugs. Even in the area of the multicellular helminths there is significant progress. For instance, at least seven laboratories have protective monoclonal antibodies against schistosomes. Using these antibodies at least three laboratories have isolated protective antigens, and at least two of these antigens have been cloned by genetic engineering. One laboratory has produced an effective anti-idiotype vaccine for schistosomiasis in rats.

The enormous power of molecular biology to understand parasitic control mechanisms and to produce proteins that may function as vaccines is now being applied at a remarkable level. The African trypanosomes have become models for molecular biologists who are studying the remarkably complex genetic mechanisms of antigenic variation and the unique kinetoplast DNA. Consequently, the National Institute of Allergy and Infectious Diseases has recently provided more funds for research on these organisms, which cause the relatively rare though highly lethal African sleeping sickness, than for any of the vast diseases of hundreds of millions of people such as malaria and schistosomiasis. Furthermore, a MacArthur Foundation–University of California at Los Angeles symposium entitled Molecular Strategies of Parasitic Invasion, held in Utah in January 1986, attracted more than 400 participants. Keynote addresses were presented by Ruth and Victor Nussenzweig of New York University on the rational development of malaria vaccines and by Anthony Cerami of Rockefeller University on the cachexia associated with parasitic infections and the role of cachectin/TNF. Plenary sessions were on genome structure and plasticity, antigen structure, generation of antigenic diversity, functional aspects of parasite antigens, molecular recognition between host and parasite, developmental changes in the parasite life cycle, and RNA processing and catalytic RNA.

Parasitology has evolved in a most unusual way over the last century. Although all infectious agents—bacteria, viruses, fungi, protozoa, and helminths—are parasites, only the latter two comprise the field of parasitology. The field appears to have developed much later than had been previously believed and to have become relatively isolated from the rapidly advancing frontiers of biologic and medical research. In the last decade, however, all this began to change, and as stated in the foreword to the proceedings of the 1980 New Orleans conference on current status and future of parasitology, "a unique melding of the best of the classical and the modern biologies occurred that could lead to a veritable renaissance of parasitology. The benefits of such a rebirth could have enormous implications for the health of the people and domestic animals of this world."[18]

REFERENCES

1. Beaver PC: What is parasitology? p. 1. In Warren, KS, Purcell EF (eds): The Current Status and Future of Parasitology. Josiah Macy Jr Foundation, New York, 1981
2. Cameron TWM: Parasites and Parasitism. Methuen & Co, London, 1956
3. Watson JD: Molecular Biology of the Gene. 3rd Ed. Benjamin-Cummings Publishing Co., Menlo Park, CA 1975
4. Anderson RM, May RM: Population biology of infectious diseases: Part I. Nature 280:361, 1979
5. Hoeppli R: Parasites and Parasitic Infections in Early Medicine and Science. University of Malaya Press, Singapore. 1959
6. Foster WD: A History of Parasitology. E & S Livingstone Ltd. Edinburgh, 1965
7. Worboys M: The emergence of tropical medicine: a study in the establishment of a scientific specialty. p. 75. In Lemaine G, Macleod R, Mulkay M, Weingert P (eds): Perspectives on the Emergence of Scientific Disciplines. Mouton, The Hague, 1976
8. Worboys M: The emergence and early development of parasitology. p. 1. In Warren KS, Bowers JZ (eds): Parasitology: A Global Perspective. Springer Verlag, New York, 1983
9. Manson P: On the development of the *Filaria sanguinis-hominis* and the mosquito considered as a nurse. Trans Linnean Soc Zool 14:304, 1878
10. Warren KS: The present status of the parasitology literature. p. 142. In Warren KS,

Purcell EF (eds): The Current Status and Future of Parasitology. Josiah Macy Jr Foundation, New York, 1981
11. Warren KS: The guerrilla worm. N Engl J Med 282:810, 1970
12. McKeown T: The Modern Rise of Population. Academic Press, Orlando, FL, 1976
13. Rifkin, SB, Walt G: Why health improves: defining the issues concerning ''comprehensive primary health care' and 'selective primary health care.'' Soc Sci Med, 23:559, 1987
14. Weinstein PP: Teaching parasitology. p. 51. In Warren, KS, Purcell EF (eds): The Current Status and Future of Parasitology. Josiah Macy Jr Foundation, New York, 1981
15. Warren KS, Goffman G, Chernin E: The status of the parasitology literature: linkages to modern biology. In Warren KS, Bowers JZ (eds): Parasitology: A Global Perspective. Springer Verlag, New York, 1983
16. Walsh JA, Warren KS: Selective primary health care: an interim strategy for disease control in developing countries. N Engl J Med 301:967, 1979
17. Lederberg J: The future of parasitology: an overview. p. 157. In Warren KS, Purcell EF (eds): The Current Status and Future of Parasitology. Josiah Macy Jr Foundation, New York, 1981
18. Warren KS: Foreword. p. X. In Warren, KS, Purcell EF (eds): The Current Status and Future of Parasitology. Josiah Macy Jr Foundation, New York, 1981

2 The Worldwide Burden of Parasitic Disease

Donald Heyneman

THE NUMBERS—UNRELIABLE YET MIND-BOGGLING TOTALS

An appreciation of the burden of parasitic diseases initially requires that a clear epidemiologic distinction be made between infection, illness and disability, and mortality. Estimates for each category for the underdeveloped regions[1,2] are overwhelmingly high in comparison with anything known in the western (northern) world, however unreliable the data may be. This presentation will focus on levels of parasitism in the developing world to provide an introductory overview of the impact of the protozoans and the helminths that infect humans in such numbers. Information about the principal viral and bacterial infections of the developing countries will also be presented to provide perspective. Only a fraction of persons infected actually suffer from debilitating illness from these infections, and, of course, a far smaller but still significant number of them die. Within each category the total number is nonetheless enormous, cumulatively representing an overwhelming human burden.

Parasitic Disease Total: Mortality Estimates

The diarrheal diseases constitute by far the most common cause of death in the developing world, causing approximately one-third of the 15 to 20 million deaths estimated for 1980–81 (Table 2-1).[1–3] Respiratory disease killed an additional 4 to 5 million[4] and malnutrition (in terms of frank starvation) killed over 2

Table 2-1. Killers in the Developing World, (Africa, Asia, Central America, South America) 1983

Rank	Cause	Deaths per Year (millions)
1	Diarrheal diseases	5.0–7.0
2	Respiratory diseases	4.0–5.0
3	Malnutrition (i.e., starvation)	2.0
4	Malaria	1.5
5	Measles	0.9
6	Schistosomiasis	0.5–1.0
7	Whooping cough	0.3–0.9
8	Tetanus	0.6
9	Tuberculosis	0.5
	Hepatitis B	0.5
10	Amebiasis	0.4–1.1
	Total	16.2–21.0
	All Causes	42.0±15

(Data from World Health Organization,[1] Walsh,[2] and Snyder.[3])

million.[1,2] This last tragedy is only the lethal tip of the iceberg of severe malnutrition, which exacerbates the impact of *all* infectious agents causing morbidity and mortality in the tropical world.[5–12] Malaria is the prime killer involving a single agent, *Plasmodium falciparum,* which continues to play a role it has doubtlessly held for many hundreds of years.[13]

A major concern of the high death levels by the infectious agents listed in Table 2-1 is that 80 percent of these deaths in the developing world are of infants and children under the age of 5. The striking contrast between these deaths and those due predominantly to chronic, noninfectious ailments of older individuals in temperate America and Europe is dramatically evident (Table 2-2). Deaths from infectious agents in the developed world are chiefly terminal infections of the chronically ill. Figure 2-1 illustrates the proportions of total deaths in various geographic regions that are accounted for by children. The astonishing levels of child deaths in developing countries is tragically evident. China, however, demonstrated by 1981 a remarkable drop in child deaths, from over 50 percent of total deaths to approximately 30 percent.[2] In the other major developing areas infants and children account for more than half of all deaths[14] (imagine the repercussions were this true in the United States!). In tropical and northern Africa the totals range from 60 to 70 percent—an unconscionable loss. The estimated number of deaths from all causes among all ages in 1980–81 is 42 million for the developing world and approximately 50 million for the entire world.

Temperate-Tropical, Developed-Undeveloped World Comparisons: Chronic versus Infectious Patterns

United Nations demographic estimates for 1984 (Table 2-2) give us the birth versus death totals for the year,[1] which show that birth totals in the

Table 2-2. World Demographic Estimates, 1984

	Population $\times 10^6$	Rates per 1,000		Population Increase			Total $\times 10^6$			Infant and Child Deaths	
		Birth	Death	per 1000	%	Doubling Time (yr)	Births	Deaths	Increase	% of total	$\times 10^6$
Northern group											
North America	261	16	9	7	0.7	100	4.18	2.34	1.84	4	0.09
Europe	490	14	11	3	0.3	233	6.86	5.39	1.47	6	0.32
USSR	276	19	9	10	1.0	70	5.24	2.48	2.76	35	0.87
East Asia (China, Japan, Korea)	1,239	18	7	11	1.1	64	22.30	8.67	13.63	28	2.43
Southern group											
Latin America	397	32	8	24	2.4	29	12.70	3.18	9.52	50	1.59
Africa	537	46	17	29	2.9	24	24.70	9.13	15.57	55	5.02
South Asia (India; west, southeast Asia)	1,539	35	13	22	2.2	32	53.87	20.01	33.86	50	10.01
Oceania (Australia, NZ, Pacific Isl.)	24.5	21	8	13	1.3	54	0.51	0.196	0.31	35	0.07
World	4,763	27	11	17	1.7	41	130.36	51.40	78.96	40	20.40

(From United Nations,[41] with permission.)

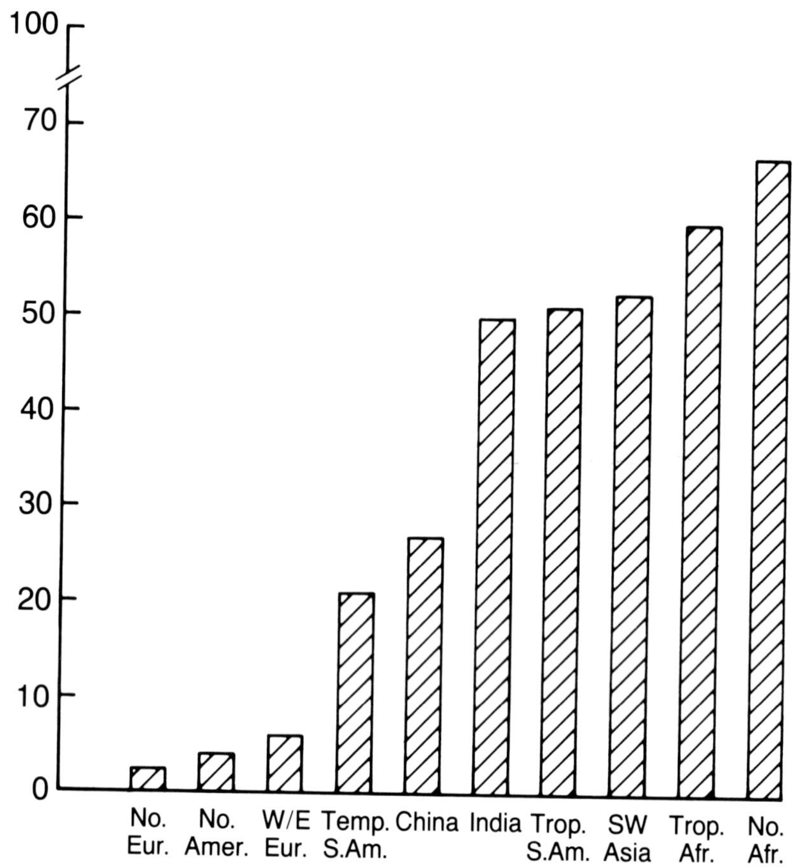

Fig. 2-1. Deaths from infectious agents in the developed world are chiefly terminal infections of the chronically ill. This graph shows the percentage of total deaths of children under the age of 5 in each geographic area. (Data from Walsh.[2])

developing regions swamp the death totals despite the tragic toll of infants and young children: the worldwide population increment is approximately 80 million, equal to more than one Mexico added each year, and going up! High sustained birth rates throughout the developing world are now accompanied by dramatic declines in death rates to levels quite comparable with those of the developed world. The differential is a net increase of 24 persons per 1,000 for the developing nations (see Table 2-2, southern group). One can also view these changing population patterns in terms of the years required for the population to double (Table 2-2), conveniently derived by dividing 70 by the percentage of population increase). The total doubling time for the developing world is about 29 years, less than *half* the period projected for the Soviet Union, which itself has *one-third* the population doubling time of the Scandinavian nations.

The enormity of these birth versus death discrepancies is emphasized by noting that *80 percent* of the world's total of 130 million births estimated for 1984 occurred in the underdeveloped, chiefly tropical, world. A more sobering fact is that along with the high proportion of births contributed by the developing world, a still higher proportion (95 percent) of all deaths among infants and children were from the same developing areas. In striking contrast, the primary causes of death in the United States for 1977 are ranked in Table 2-3. Chronic diseases (circulatory diseases, neoplasms, respiratory, and digestive diseases) affecting our aging population are the chief causes of death. Their chronic rather than infectious nature is suggested by the relatively low average number of years estimated to have been cut off from life expectancy. Most of these losses are under 20 years per death, in contrast with the far longer losses caused by deaths among children in the tropics, or by violent and accidental deaths in the United States, which rank third in Table 2-3. The other obvious causes of death in the United States preventing a full life span are pregnancy losses and congenital anomalies. Of the various killers in the developing world listed in Table 2-1, only one item, respiratory disease, is even represented among the 16 top causes of death in the United States for 1977, and in that instance it generally is the pneumonia that ends the lives of the chronically ill or aged ("the old person's friend") rather than the acute respiratory diseases of infants that are so characteristic of the tropics.

Table 2-3. Deaths in the United States, 1977

Rank	Cause	Number $\times 10^3$	Years Lost per Death
1	Circulatory diseases	978	12
2	Neoplasms	392	16
3	Accidents, poisonings, violence	156	36
4	Respiratory system diseases	110	14
5	Digestive system diseases	69	19
6	Unclassified	55	6
7	Endocrine, nutritional, and metabolic diseases	41	16
8	Genitourinary diseases	26	13
9	CNS/sense organ diseases	17.5	27
10	Infective, parasitic diseases	17	26
11	Congenital anomalies	13	64
12	Mental disorders	10	21
13	Blood, hematopoietic diseases	5	20
14	Musculoskeletal diseases	5	19
15	Diseases of skin and subcutaneous tissues	2.5	15
16	Diseases of pregnancy, childbirth, and puerperium	0.4	51
	Total	1,900.0	17

(Data from National Center for Health Statistics, Division for Vital Statistics and Division of Analysis.)

Parasitic Disease Totals: Morbidity Estimates

In reviewing the lifelong burden of disease in the developing world, one must distinguish the extraordinarily high levels of *infection* from (Table 2-4) the levels of *disease*. Many infectious agents are so abundant in developing countries as to be considered part of the way of life; such infections are an integral part of the environment in which most people live. This is well expressed in the latest statement reviewing major parasitic infections published in the World Health Statistics Quarterly[1]:

> Despite the emphasis laid in the last 30 years on the quantitative epidemiology of parasitic diseases, global prevalence estimates of either infected people or those at risk are of such staggering magnitude that the mind has difficulty in conceiving the descriptive statistics. The total number of protozoan and helminthic infections currently existing far outnumbers the total world population since multiple infections are the rule, and not the exception, in most tropical areas. Statistical estimates of infection rates merely represent the rates of diagnosis, which depend on the sensitivity of the techniques used. Hence the true prevalence of the parasitic diseases may be much higher than the official estimates, and this fact, combined with the known inadequacy of health statistics over much of the world, makes it highly probable that the parasitic diseases have, in numerical terms, been grossly underestimated in the past.

Table 2-4. Infections in the Developing World (Africa, Asia, Central America, South America) 1984

Rank	Cause	Infections per Year (millions)
1	Tuberculosis	2,000
2	Ascariasis	800–1,300
3	Hookworm	900
4	Malaria	800
5	Trichuris	500–700
6	Trachoma	500
	Amebiasis	500
7	Giardiasis	250
8	Poliomyelitis	240
9	Schistosomiasis	200
10	Hepatitis B virus	170
11	Filariasis[a]	100
Opportunists—widespread in all populations:		
	Toxoplasmosis	1,300
	Cryptosporidiosis	?
	Pneumocystosis	?

[a] Based on estimates from microfilaremic individuals. Other estimates run far higher (250 million).

(Data from World Health Organization, Parasitic Diseases Program[2] and other sources.)

Tuberculosis is present in approximately 40 to 50 percent of the 3.7 billion persons living in the developing world as of 1981.[15] Malaria parasites are harbored by 800 million, chiefly at low levels in individuals partially immune or relatively unaffected except for an occasional fever. Hookworms infect 700 to 900 million persons; again for the most part the numbers of worms per infected individual are small and cause little damage, perhaps 1 to 2 ml of blood loss per day. However a daily loss of even that small amount of blood may be a significant cause of anemia in a child marginally nourished or in an undernourished nursing mother. The total combined daily blood loss can be unbelievable. As a conservative estimate, if 800 million people harbor an average of 10 hookworms, each worm sucking 0.1 ml blood per day, a total of 800,000 L of blood would be lost daily. This is equivalent to the *daily* loss of the entire blood volume of a city of 150,000 population.

Trichuris and *Ascaris* are the nematodes that are enormously successful as parasites of mankind throughout the tropical and developing world. *Ascaris* is the more adaptable, as it is distributed deeply into the temperate zone as well, probably infecting well over 1 billion persons worldwide. Current estimates run as high as 1.3 billion.[16] Pawlowski lists 17 nations, representing about half the world's population, in which over 50 percent of the people during the 1973–83 period harbored *Ascaris* worms, at an average of about six worms per person.[16] These countries are Afghanistan, Bangladesh, Brazil, Burma, China, Colombia, India, Indonesia, Iran, Kenya, Malaysia, Mexico, Peru, Philippines, Tanzania, Turkey, and Viet Nam. At about 2g per worm, six worms per person, and 1.2 billion persons infected, one comes up with about 15,000 metric tons of worms! Similarly, *Trichuris* is the ever-present nematode of the tropics, where 60 to 80 percent of children characteristically harbor the worm; in the Cameroons, the Caribbean region, and Malaysia over 90 percent of the population is thought to be infected! These infection levels essentially mean that *everyone* has or has had one or both of these nematode infections.

Entamoeba histolytica and *Giardia lamblia* appear and reappear in the intestine of most if not all children of these regions, causing infections capable of producing severe disease in malnourished individuals or in those otherwise stressed into reduced immunologic competence. The *Mycobacterium* of tuberculosis, the virus of hepitatis B or of poliomyelitis, the *Entamoeba* of amebic colitis, and the blood fluke of schistosomiasis all are potent pathogens. However, each is more often a widespread chronic agent of low-level mild or asymptomatic infections, a small proportion of which induce the full clinical syndrome characteristic of each disease. Yet, the pathologic capacity of these agents can be devastating.

This is being abundantly, tragically, and increasingly demonstrated among the immunosuppressed victims of the acquired immunodeficiency syndrome (AIDS), who suffer fatal host-parasite imbalance, which permits opportunistic agents heretofore seldom considered important to overwhelm the patient.[17] Four protozoans have emerged as important opportunistic infections in patients with AIDS. *Cryptosporidium,* formerly thought to be confined to calves and other domestic animals, has now been recognized as a significant parasite of mankind and a cause of severe diarrhea in AIDS patients. Worldwide *Cryptosporidium* has a prevalence we can only speculate upon. *Pneumocystis carinii,* formerly considered responsible only for a rare interstitial plasma cell pneumonitis of the aged and of premature infants, is now recognized as the primary killer of more than half of AIDS victims. It is thought to be present throughout the human environment, infecting one-third to perhaps one-half of the entire human population. Similarly, *Toxoplasma,* which may infect 1 of 3 persons worldwide, has been for many years a threat to the children of women infected for the first time during pregnancy. It is now a cause of severe cerebritis in immunosuppressed individuals, especially those with AIDS. Species of the genus *Isospora* have also been associated with severe diarrhea in patients with AIDS. Whether other parasitic microorganisms will emerge as important pathogens in AIDS will only become clear as the AIDS epidemic spreads out of urban areas of the tropics into regions where the parasites are more prevalent.

Many of the widespread, perhaps universal, agents of human infection appear to be present in *all* populations but are clinically visible only when the normally protective cell-mediated immunity and other modes of host protection are undeveloped, lost, or compromised. In other words, we survive, live, and thrive in a world of multiple infections as a result of prolonged exposure and evolutionary adaptation. We must withstand the continuing presence of a surrounding aura of parasitic agents, largely rendered harmless except among those who have lost this evolutionary armament. It is not man, but man *and* his full complement of environmental worms, protozoa, bacteria, viruses, and other pathogens that must be taken into account in order to measure and evaluate human health and survival in this inordinately complex amalgam.[18–21]

Table 2-5 deals with the numbers of individuals who do suffer illness, and thus represent the pathologic by-product of this lost adaptation to parasitic infection. One again notes in the table the enormity of diarrheal disease, the most important cause of pathology as well as death among any group of agents afflicting mankind.[3,22] This is a preventable but continuing tragedy, as oral rehydration therapy (ORT) is an answer that is both economically available and easily administered by all peoples in all areas of the world.[23,24] It unquestionably can reduce this huge loss to a small proportion of the present level. Nonetheless, agents of dysentery in 1981 killed one-third all children who died before the age of 5 (which means one-fourth of *all* deaths for the year in the Third World) and they continue to afflict humanity, causing severe illness, again chiefly among children, in astronomic numbers (3 to 5 *billion* cases per year). Even if we use the overly high estimate that 50 percent of the population of the developing world consists of children under 15, 3 to 5 billion cases means 1.5 to 2.5 severe cases of diarrheic illness per child per year. In fact, in many of the malnourished areas of the tropics, *monthly* episodes of severe diarrhea and dehydration are not unusual. At present ORT reaches perhaps one-fifth of these patients. Until such time as it can be extended throughout the developing world as an immediately available life-saving therapeutic regimen, these enormous totals and unnecessary losses will continue.

Malaria infects over 800 million, causes serious disease in 150 million, and

Table 2-5. Illness in the Developing World (Africa, Asia, Central America, South America) 1980–81

Rank	Cause	Cases per Year × 10^6 (millions)
1	Diarrheal diseases	3,000.0–5,000.0
2	Malaria	150.0
3	Measles	80.0
4	Amebiasis	35.0–50.0
5	Whooping cough	30.0
6	Schistosomiasis	20.0
7	Tuberculosis	20.0
8	Malnutrition	5.0–8.0
9	Poliomyelitis	3.0
10	Onchocerciasis[a]	
	Skin	2.0–5.0
	Blindness	0.2–0.5
11	Filariasis	2.0–3.0
12	Hookworm	1.5
13	Dengue	1.0–2.0
14	Chagas' disease	1.2
	Leishmaniasis	1.2
	Leprosy	1.2
15	Ascariasis	1.0
	Tetanus	1.0
	Giardiasis	1 ?
	Cysticercosis	?

[a] Transmission of onchocerciasis in the seven West African states of Burkina, Faso, Benin, Côte d'Ivoire, Ghana, Mali, Niger, and Togo apparently has been blocked as a result of *Simulium* larviciding activities of the World Health Organization Onchocerciasis Control Programme in the Volta River basin area over the past 10 years (WHO Tropical Diseases Research program, funded by the World Bank, U.S. Agency for International Development, and the U.N. Development Program).

(Data from Walsh.[2])

kills 1 to 2 million a year. It is the most destructive and dangerous single infectious agent of mankind in the developing world.[13,25,26] Among children and mothers in this population, malaria remains the major cause of anemia. It is responsible for more energy loss, more debilitation, more loss of work capacity, and more total economic damage than any other human ailment.

Measles too often is dismissed, owing to our restricted view, as being of minor importance, a mild childhood disease that rarely exhibits more serious toxicity. Yet, it is the cause of nearly 1 million deaths annually in the developing world and the third major cause of illness (80 million cases). Its toxic side effects include blindness, serious neurologic disease, and a variety of other pathologies far more widespread and serious than we appreciate from our protected vantage point.

Of the 200 million persons who harbor schistosome worms in their mesenteric veins or hepatic portals, approximately 10 percent suffer the more debilitating forms of this chronic granulomatous disease. Of these 20 million, 2 to 5 percent will die each year. Many other killers listed in Table 2-1 are, as would be expected, also represented in Table 2-5, which lists the major causes of illness in the same population. Massive infection levels (480 million) and disease levels (36 million) are attributed to human amebiasis.[27] Its lethality (40,000 annually) ranks only after that of malaria and schistosomiasis among parasites but is considerably below the level of the more lethal microbial scourges of Table 2-1. Yet its impact, as with most parasitic infections, is as a significant cause of disease rather than death. Its total impact as an agent of suffering and impoverishment is probably greater than that of more lethal agents, owing to its vast presence in the tropics and its severity.

Malnutrition, a special case, is not thought of as a primary cause of death, despite the terrible loss in 1981 of 2 million persons, who, as usual, were mostly children and who died of frank starvation. This number, as we know, subsequently rose still higher during the tragedy of Sahelian starvation. Malnutrition, however, acts chiefly as a predisposing factor accentuating *all* debilitating infections, in which strength of the host response is needed to neutralize or control infection.[5–12] Malnutrition underwrites disease pathology throughout the developing world, affecting at least 10 to 15 million persons annually. Essentially all deaths from infectious agents in the developing countries include undernutrition as a component.

Onchocerciasis (river blindness) is so poignantly apparent that it has become an object of focused concern by the World Health Organization (WHO) in a so far remarkably successful 20-year program in West Africa. The form of filariasis that involves the gross elephantine limbs or genitalia of elephantiasis, although accounting for only about 10 percent of the total number of person with filarial disease, nonetheless is so dramatic as to bring the disease to immediate attention or to generate fear as well as social isolation. Hookworm, which infects children at critical points in their development, can cause iron deficiency anemia, leading to suppression of growth and modified development of the central nervous system. In the southeastern United States early in this century, hookworm anemia was a major impediment preventing children from reaching their full genetic potential and manifested itself in large numbers of depressed, small, slow-learning children. The worms are still with us in the southeastern United States, although in lesser numbers. They are abundant, however, in many immigrant farm workers in the southern and southwestern United States. Chagas' disease is the principal cause of premature death from heart disease in Latin America. Cutaneous leishmaniasis, leprosy, and tetanus are other afflictions whose agents take individual and collective tolls that significantly reduce human potential in the developing world. An affliction of serious proportions, but for which no reasonable estimate of total numbers is available, is cysticercosis.[28] In Mexico and other regions of Latin America increasing numbers are recognized as having central nervous system damage from the presence of these tapeworm larvae, which compress and destroy brain tissue space or block ventricular conduits.

A fragmentary sense of the impact of these infections and their disease-causing agents can be obtained from Table 2-6, which lists the top 11 or so causes of major disability, causing each individual affected to lose 3 months or more of work capacity. For some diseases, lifetime affliction is involved, as with paralytic poliomyelitis, onchocerciasis, leprosy, or elephantiasis.

SOCIAL IMPACT—THE BURDEN OF PARASITISM

However unreliable, these figures make it evident that the preponderant cause of infection, illness, disability, and death throughout the tropical developing world is parasitic infection, and the major impact is on children under the age of 5. Other approaches, however, may be more persuasive and more illustrative of the impact than is the impersonal listing of agents, diseases, and numbers affected. Numbers beyond a few dozen quickly lose human relevance and meaning. One can, however, suggest some of the burdens imposed by human parasites in terms of their social impact.

Blindness—the Ultimate Curse

Perhaps the most tragic and imprisoning burden that can be imposed on an individual and a community is blindness, such as is seen throughout west and central Africa from chronic infection with *Onchocerca volvulus*. This infection, the cause of river blindness, is associated with the presence of masses of river-breeding, blood-sucking black flies (*Simulium*, well named *S. damnosum*) infected with the filaria. Wherever the vector occurs in sufficient concentration near human habitats, life becomes a travail we can hardly envision. The period between infection and blindness usually takes 5 to 15 years. The infection is

Table 2-6. Disability in the Developing World (Africa, Asia, Central America, South America: 1980–81)

Rank	Cause	Average Days of Disability per Case
1	Poliomyelitis	3,000+
2	Onchocerciasis	
	Skin	3,000
	Blindness	3,000
3	Leprosy	500–3,000
4	Filariasis	1,000
5	Schistosomiasis	600–1,000
6	Chagas' disease	600
7	Tuberculosis	200–400
8	Hepatitis B virus	300
9	African trypanosomiasis	150
10	Leishmaniasis	100–200
11	Hookworm	100

(Data from Walsh.[2])

accompanied by intractable, sometimes intolerable levels of pruritis induced by the microfilariae of *Onchocerca,* which leave the dermal nodule containing the adult worms and migrate through the skin, destroying elastic and other fiber elements. Children, especially boys, grow up in these hyperendemic areas with the knowledge that they, too, will probably become blind, as have their fathers, usually before the age of 40.

Social Disruption—Village Abandonment and Cultural Dissolution

In riverine valleys plagued by onchocercal blindness, whole regions have been subjected to village abandonment to seek surcease in less agriculturally productive but safer areas away from the river bottoms, where the best farming conditions—and the black flies—abound. So the social cycle continues: sustained, repeated exposure in the rich agricultural river valleys, followed by skin disease and blindness, then village abandonment, struggle and malnutrition, and eventual return to the river bottoms after some years, followed by another cycle of disease and social disruption.

Similarly, African sleeping sickness, trypanosomiasis, denies vast tracts of central and southeast Africa to human occupation—for fear of sleeping sickness among the inhabitants, or, equally tragic economically, in their cattle. The history of Africa over the past two centuries is inextricably linked both to malaria and sleeping sickness.

Population Impact: Children Lost to Parasites—the Population Paradox

Perhaps of greatest concern, as was already noted, is the burgeoning population in all portions of the tropics, particularly in Africa but other areas as well (Table 2-2). Whether one calls it a population bomb, a population level beyond the carrying capacity of the land, or a population level at which quality existence is no longer possible and is rapidly declining, the message is clear.[29–32] The role of parasitic infection and the disease and death it causes constitute a paradox of immense importance in this matter of population control. *Reduction* of these infant and child deaths may prove to be the answer to overpopulation. Wherever parents lack the confidence that their children can survive the malnutrition, the diarrheas, the malaria and other parasitic diseases that plague them, they will continue to produce more children. This necessity becomes associated with a sociocultural acceptance and demand for large families to follow the basic need. The average family size in Kenya is over nine children per family. The rate of population increase in Kenya is approximately 3.5 percent, a doubling time of 20 years. I first visited to Egypt in 1950, when its population was under 20 million, or about 40 percent of what it is today. What would the Egyptian economy and the social well-being of its people be like with a present-day population *half* its present level? In spite of all the family planning efforts by private or government effort, by education, or by financial incentives, large families will remain a social necessity so long as half the babies are going to die. Short of a China-style total effort (limited to a highly homogeneous and cooperative population), the surest way for parents to reduce their family size voluntarily is through their confidence that enough boys will live to work the farm or care for cattle, sheep, and goats, that girls will grow up to receive dowries, and that both will be present to care for aging parents—their only social security. The need to provide money for the children's education later becomes important as living standards improve. With increasing urbanization comes rapid recognition that education is essential for a job, as is money for a better life and, inevitably, for payment of taxes. Nonetheless, as long as more than 100 infants per 1,000 live births do not survive their first year and malnutrition takes another significant share, along with the huge losses from dehydration through diarrheic illness, the need and the striving for large families will continue despite all efforts to condemn the practice or to provide financial incentives to parents of small families. The population increase in the southern group of nations listed in Table 2-2 is attributable almost entirely to the maintenance of high birth rates, more that twice the average levels of the northern group. Death rates in the two regions (except for Africa) are remarkably comparable if not identical. Latin America, for example, has a death rate *lower* than that of North America, while its birth rate continues at a rate twice as high, giving a net population increase in Latin America three times that of North America. *Some* sort of resolution of the continuing population explosion is inevitable. Either the parasite-induced burden of excessive child deaths in the tropics will be reduced by our combined efforts or there will be a rapid rise in total deaths from starvation, more disease, and other factors reestablishing the ancient pattern of high birth rate/high death rate. The inevitability of either a controlled or an uncontrolled resolution of the present dangerous imbalance is increasingly evident.

Parasitism as an Occupational Hazard—Role of the Land, Place, Habits

Other expressions of the social impact of parasitism in the developing world may be less clearly evident but are nonetheless present. The occupational hazard of parasitism is the presence of parasitic disease associated with inescapable exposure and infection: frequent exposure of agriculturalists to numerous bites of black flies carrying onchocerciasis while they work their riverine farms; swarming of vast numbers of *Leishmania*-bearing sand flies around lumbermen who cut the trees harboring the flies; cattle and herders alike fearfully crossing a tsetse belt in Tanzania, hastening to escape sleeping sickness; malaria- and/or filaria-infected mosquitoes breeding near or within villages and feeding almost continuously upon villagers during evening and nocturnal hours. Guinea worm larvae, cause of dracunculiasis, are carried within intermediate host copepods and drunk in contaminated rainpool water in Africa and from step-in wells in the Near and Middle East. The soilborne nematodes *Ascaris, Trichuris, Strongyloides* as well as hookworms all are associated with agricultural pursuits in soil contaminated with human feces. This is especially evident where human excrement (night soil) is a necessity for the fertilization of crops, as it is in much of east Asia.

Energy Parasitism—Losses at Work and at School, in Outlook and in Hope

All these parasitic agents drain energy as well as blood and nutrients. The so-called lazy tropical dweller is more likely a person handicapped by significant anemia over a sustained period and thereby denied a normal growth and development history and the ability to learn at levels considered normal in temperate zones or to work the long periods required for survival. Discouragement, depression, and lack of interest and ambition are as much a part of hookworm anemia as is a low hematocrit and low energy level and are also related to the maintenance of a satisfactory state of immunity.

Poverty and Parasitism—the Endless Cycle

The age-old cycle of poverty and parasitism is continuously repeated but is now recurring at an accelerating rate and a higher level than ever before: poverty, crowding, poor housing with inadequate sanitation, contaminated water, exposure to pathogens, a diet low in protective protein, increased susceptibility, infection, and disease leading to a further decrease in energy and initiative—again resulting in more poverty and a new cycle of exposure, susceptibility, and disease. This is the way of life for multiple millions in tropical and other underdeveloped regions of the world. The loss of infant and other young lives to this sequence and to the parasites that come with it adds immeasurably to the dilemma; frequent childhood death is the most discouraging, cruel, and destructive social insult of all.

PARASITISM AND IMMUNOSUPPRESSION—A NEW AWARENESS

Immunosuppression is a component of the parasitic syndrome that only recently has been recognized as accompanying malaria, filariasis, schistosomiasis, leishmaniasis, and trypanosomiasis. Most if not all the parasitic diseases have some immunosuppressive action. The fear and furor raised by the acquired immunodeficiency syndrome (AIDS) has opened a whole new dimension of concern, with greatly increased general awareness of the vital role played by immunity in controlling all infectious agents. Today AIDS is a problem of rapidly increasing dimension and threat in Africa, where it is far more severe than in the more publicized San Francisco, Los Angeles, and New York-New Jersey sectors of the United States.

"New" Disease and the Ever-Present Opportunists

The protozoan diseases cryptosporidiosis, toxoplasmosis, and pneumocystosis, along with fungi causing thrush and other mycotic infections and a variety of microbial agents, are now recognized as widely, perhaps universally, present potential pathogens but usually at immunologically controlled low levels and hence unnoticed. Until recently they have not been part of our medical concern, not part of the "prepared mind" of the good diagnostician. They remained out of sight, out of mind—until AIDS appeared. Now we appreciate that these agents are part of a spectrum of opportunistic infections always present, ready, and waiting to surge into clinical recognition as soon as the host's immune barriers to parasite multiplication are down.

Strongyloides is the only common helminth capable of continuous recycling in the human body. Therefore, it must be included with protozoan and microbial opportunists able to take advantage of a breakdown of host defense against pathogen multiplication. Immunologically controlled, *Strongyloides* can recycle and remain in small numbers for a person's lifetime, as World War II survivors of the bridge of the River Kwai can attest; uncontrolled, the parasite can destroy a human in a brief fulminating, migratory assault—like those that have killed a number of AIDS patients.

Malnutrition, Migration, Refugees, Crowding, Multiple Infection

We now can reevaluate the interlocking network of insults or traumas (i.e., stress, immunosuppression, and disease) that have such a deleterious impact, especially on children in the tropics. The common pathway is an immunosuppression, which exposes these hidden or emergent diseases or the normally well-controlled parasitic infections. Malnutrition, war, migration, refugee encampment, sudden or overwhelming exposure to pathogens after breakdown of sanitary controls, infection with parasites not previously encountered, multiparasitism, even fear and social upheaval—all can impose stress. Whether physical, psychic, social, or parasite-induced, these stresses affect an individual's capacity to maintain immunologic surveillance and a controlling cell-mediated and/or humoral response.

The Host-Parasite Balance, a Continuing Struggle through Evolution and Readjustment

Parasitologists long have been concerned with host-parasite relationship, the continuous process by which invasive mechanisms and other infection modes are countered by host-defense measures and these in turn are nullified by ingenious parasitologic reactions that avoid, neutralize, or escape the host's immune responses. The result is a continuing seesaw of changing balance in time, ultimately tending towards an evolutionary equilibrium. First one, then the other may be favored, but ultimately a host-parasite balance evolves that permits survival of both the host species and its assortment of parasites. Humans are subject to 100 or more parasitic agents of various descriptions. Very few are invariably lethal, as they presumably would not survive the resulting evolutionary imbalance for more than a few generations. AIDS, however, is returning us to that pre-equilibrium state of host helplessness to lethal parasitic takeover.

Effect of Parasitism on AIDS?

The recognition of immunosuppressive effects of parasitic infections has caused some parasitologists to wonder if AIDS may, in fact, *follow* rather than cause the reduced human immune capacity. High concentrations of intestinal parasites, associated with male homosexual activities, have been suggested as predisposing these individuals to subsequent infection by the AIDS lymphocyte-associated virus. In the Tropical Diseases Laboratory at the University of California, San Francisco we noted that enormous concentrations of *Entamoeba histolytica, Endolimax nana,* and *Dientamoeba fragilis* were frequently found in male homosexual patients several years before AIDS was recognized. However, considering the 2- to 8-year incubation period of the AIDS virus, the massive overgrowth of intestinal protozoans that we first observed a few years ago could still have followed the virus. It does, however, reflect the extraordinarily high levels of exposure associated with the homosexual life style. AIDS found in hemophiliacs and other nonhomosexual risk groups, however, argues against such a causative association.

One unresolved paradox is the apparent absence of invasive strains of *Entamoeba histolytica* (by zymodeme analysis) in the male homosexual population. Even among pre-AIDS homosexuals, who are so highly susceptible to *Pneumocystis, Cryptosporidium,* mycotic infection, *Strongyloides,* and other systemic pathogens, there appears to be a remarkable absence of clinical amebic dysentery and hepatic amebiasis. Clearly, a great deal remains to be learned about that complex host-parasite interaction.

Meanwhile, as AIDS moves beyond the homosexual population, its tragic impact, both real and by hysteria, rises exponentially. The current AIDS epidemic in central Africa, which also affects a highly parasitized population as well as a significant proportion of nonimmune newborns in the populations studied (estimates of 10 percent are current), poses a frightening threat to millions in that beleagured continent.

MAN AND HIS PARASITES—THE COMBINATION: A MORE BALANCED WORLDWIDE PICTURE

The state of host-parasite modulation of infection provides a useful approach to studying human illness from the public health standpoint, where the focus is on populations rather than on individual patients. It leads us to recognize, for example, that the germ theory as the primary explanation of disease is incomplete, although obviously essential. As we have seen, disease does not necessarily follow exposure or even infection. The human elements—behavior, age, prior infection, state of general health, and immunologic competence—all are relevant and any or all may be keys to disease development.

Treatment may, in fact, be contraindicated, even apart from concerns with drug toxicity. Treatment of cutaneous leishmaniasis induced by *Leishmania major* shortcuts the immunologic process and renders the patient susceptible to reexposure and to new, perhaps more severe, disease. Treatment of loiasis in patients from West Africa while they reside in the United States not only may subject them to neuropathy from the interaction between diethylcarbamazine and wandering adult worms in the brain, but should they return to endemic areas and be reexposed, they may suffer from serious anaphylactoid reactions. Low-level infection with falciparum malaria in Africa may actually protect against a severe challenge infection. Curing the infection could be a distinct disservice, exposing the patient to extreme manifestations of a new infection once the original infection has been exorcised through chemotherapy.

Vaccination? Eradication or Control?

Vaccinations as well as treatment must be evaluated with the greatest care in terms of their possible epidemiologic impact. A population may be rendered vulnerable to serious disease should a short-lived vaccine-induced immunity not be sustained or should the level of serum proteins be so affected by malnutrition that antibody production is severely reduced. The frequency of vaccination required to maintain the immune state and the age at which it must first be given to protect infants will be primary research considerations with the new malaria vaccines currently being tested.

Similarly, the simplistic view that eradication is a feasible answer to most tropical diseases has long since been replaced.[33] No single recipe for eradication is possible owing to the biologically varied requirements of different vectors and reservoirs, the range of human behavior that may be involved, and the differing mix of other epidemiologic variables. The successful eradication of smallpox is an extraordinary exception but one unlikely to be duplicated. Dracunculiasis has been targeted as a possible subject of eradication, owing to its simple epidemiology, which involves copepods infected with worm larvae shed from a skin ulcer of an infected human who waded into the pool and contaminated the drinking water 2 weeks before. The apparent lack of an animal reservoir of human infection would permit an eradication campaign to focus on water filtration devices. Poliomyelitis and measles are other candidates for possible eradication since excellent vaccines are available. However, the failure to make significant inroads in the frequency and intensity of these infections in Africa despite the availability of vaccines—just as we see yaws returning in Africa despite penicillin[14]—illustrates the complexity of eradication, even when the tools and the technology are available to achieve it. Consequently, emphasis now is toward regional disease *control,* not eradication, based on epidemiologic understanding, integration with human behavior patterns, and the exigencies of economic necessity. We have learned to evaluate the host-parasite interaction as part of a total biologic complex with specific parameters that vary greatly from one area to another.[34–37] The quest for a single-cure magic bullet regimen ranges from unrealistic to impossible.

Epidemic versus Endemic; Acute versus Chronic

Part of an understanding of the epidemiology of human parasitic infection is the distinction between epidemic and endemic disease. The former occurs in populations lacking immunity, the latter under the continuing immunizing presence of the parasitic agent, which elicits various human protective responses. Epidemic disease usually strikes unpredictably against all ages, often acutely, with high levels of morbidity and mortality. In contrast, endemic disease occurs continuously, rendering the population, in effect, accustomed to the presence of the parasite. Morbidity levels are usually relatively low, and mortality is restricted to the very young, the very old, and others rendered equally immunoincompetent. Ultimately, these endemic infections become limited to diseases of childhood since infection is well tolerated above the age of infancy and is infrequently observed as clinical disease in adolescents or adults. The contrast between endemic and epidemic is well exemplified by the mild action of measles virus in the developed world and its lethal impact in epidemic form in Africa.

The other side of the coin turns up in the case of falciparum malaria, which was lethal to the majority of early European colonial settlers in West Africa. According to some estimates, as many as 80 percent were lost. The acute manifestations of cerebral malaria, with extremely high mortality to newcomers, is comparable with the local impact of falciparum malaria on infants in the same hyperendemic regions. Similarly, malaria can strike swiftly and lethally in a population at a low stage of immunity, as in the Natal area of Brazil in the early 1930s, when the superefficient vector *Anopheles gambiae* was carried across the south Atlantic from West Africa. The resulting explosive epidemic struck over 100,000 persons and killed 14,000. In contrast, the infection is mild, widespread, chronic, and maintained at easily tolerated low levels among indigenes exposed from childhood. For these individuals malaria usually is limited to an occasional fever outbreak, typically after loss of one infection and during the onset of another. This state of infection-immunity is termed *premunition* or *concomitant immunity,* in which a living infection somehow prevents establishment of a rival challenge infection and permits a host-parasite balance to be maintained at a low, generally asymptomatic, level.

Such a moderated or "tame" infection resembles our infections with the common cold virus, occasionally suffered by nearly all residents of the temperate zone. If one's immunity is at a low ebb, the cold persists, but otherwise it is only a nuisance of varying severity. Influenza epidemics, on the other hand, tend to be severe and rapidly spreading, as they usually are introduced variants against which the endemic population has no prior experience and therefore no immunity. The 20 million victims of the 1919 influenza pandemic attest to its life-taking potential, which, however, is quickly reduced in potency when even partial immunity is achieved.

Quality of Life in a 10-Billion Person World?

A final speculation in this rather broad-ranging review of the impact of parasitic infection and disease would be to guess the effect of a continued massive increase of human population on the host-parasite balance. There is already painfully clear evidence that human crowding induces social stress, poverty, malnutrition, poor housing, and loss of minimal standards of sanitation. All these, as has been emphasized, will affect human capacity to resist disease by reducing the state of immune responsiveness.

United Nations projections of the world population at the forthcoming turn of the millenium range from 5.9 to 6.5 billion, with a combined urbanization level of approximately 50 percent, ranging from 45 percent in less developed to 80 percent in more developed regions. Estimates beyond that date obviously are of greatly diminished reliability, but they tend to merge towards the worldwide figure of 10 billion toward the end of the twenty-first century.[38–41] Other projections suggest a level of 8 to 8.5 billion late in the twenty-first century, depending on the rapidity of fall of the birth rate; this may in turn depend, as has been suggested, on the speed and effectiveness of reduction and control of parasite-induced mortality of infants and pre-5-year-olds. Intimately tied to these population projections are estimates of per capita food production. These have lagged somewhat behind the rate of population increase in the last decade, showing, in fact, a *decreased* production per capita in Africa and Latin America during this period. Whatever the eventual population level at which our children and grandchildren will be living, it is going to be a far more crowded world than we now generally encounter. Unless there are vast improvements in agricultural productivity and, in particular, in pest-free storage and more equitable distribution during the next 50 years, this increased crowding will be accompanied by further impoverishment and malnutrition, continued violence, and growing conflict between haves and have-nots. Since the problems of parasitic disease and immunosuppression are far from solved, they may well compound the problems causing additional population pressures during the next half century.

Reduction of infant and child mortality in the developing world is a critical start towards reducing the rate of population increase. This can best begin with control of diarrheal disease through widespread adoption of oral rehydration therapy. Focused attacks on specific tropical diseases, such as the WHO Onchocerciasis Control Programme in West Africa, clearly constitute an essential aspect of parasitic disease prevention. Equally important is the well organized, selective treatment of the severely ill or most heavily infected rather than *all* infected patients. This is a feasible, effective, and efficient approach to an otherwise insoluble problem.[36,42] Long-term efforts to provide clean water remain the top public health priority, which is still far from accomplished; improved housing and culturally acceptable sanitary measures are also essential and must be simultaneously pursued. Clearly needed is a dedicated cadre of internationally funded public health professionals, available for program leadership, staff training, and continuity of effort—an effort needed at a scale that has never been approached, although the example of the former International Health Division of the Rockefeller Foundation is the best model we have.[21] Field research to determine the local epidemiology, local transmission patterns, and local behavioral and cultural factors are essential. Intersectoral, multiphasic approaches, reaching down to the level of the village dweller in terms of behavior modification and participation, are required if there is to be any relief from the terrible scourge of human suffering and death caused by avoidable parasitic disease.[43] The alternative is increasing physical and emotional exhaustion with loss of cultural and individual humanity in the desperate struggle to survive in a more and more crowded, violent, and angry world.

The complexity of all these physical, social, and epidemiologic interactions is readily apparent. It is clear, however, that parasitic disease is a critical part of the problem. Reduction of clinical morbidity and of mortality to socially and economically tolerable levels, maintained by immunologic competence, will go a long way toward the improvement of human well-being in general and the interacting problems of overpopulation, poverty, malnutrition, and parasitic disease in particular. Any disease-controlling measures that ensure greater survival of children will permit parents to aim toward improved standards of living for fewer offspring in a more stable environment and society. This would be the greatest possible gift we could give to our children.

REFERENCES

1. World Health Organization, Parasitic Diseases Programme: Major parasitic infections: a global review. World Health Stat Q 39:145, 1986
2. Walsh JA: Estimating the burden of illness in the tropics. p. 1073. In Warren KS, Mahmoud AAF (eds): Tropical and Geographical Medicine. McGraw-Hill, New York, 1984

3. Snyder JD, Merson MH: The magnitude of the global problem of acute diarrhoeal disease: a review of active surveillance data. Bull WHO 60:605, 1982
4. Leowski J: Mortality from acute respiratory infections in children under 5 years of age: global estimates. World Health Stat Q 39:138, 1986
5. Scrimshaw NS, Taylor CE, Gordon JE: Interactions of nutrition and infection. Am J Med Sci 237:368, 1959
6. Brasitus TA: Parasites and malabsorption. Am J Med 67:1058, 1979
7. Chandra RK: Nutritional deficiency and susceptibility to infection. Bull WHO 57:167, 1979
8. Beisel WR: Single nutrients and immunity. Am J Clin Nutr, suppl., 35:417, 1982
9. Latham MC, Stephenson LS, Hall A, et al: Parasitic infections, anaemia and nutritional status: a study of their interrelationships and the effect of prophylaxis and treatment on workers in Kwale District, Kenya. Trans R Soc Trop Med Hyg 77:41, 1983
10. Harris AD, Danis VA, Heatley RV: Influence of nutritional status on immune functions in patients with Crohn's disease. Gut 25:465, 1984
11. Pawlowski ZS: Implications of parasite-nutrition interactions from a world perspective. Fed Proc 43:256, 1980
12. Crompton DWT: Influence of parasitic infection on food intake. Fed Proc 43:239, 1984
13. Wernsdorfer WH: The importance of malaria in the world. p. 1. In Kreier JP (ed): Malaria. Epidemiology, Chemotherapy and Metabolism. Vol 1. Academic Press, Orlando, FL, 1980
14. Gwatkin DR: How many die? A set of demographic estimates of the annual number of infant and child deaths in the world. Am J Public Health 70:1286, 1980
15. Hershfield ES: Tuberculosis in the world. Chest, suppl., 76:805, 1979
16. Pawlowski ZS: Strategies for the control of ascariasis. Ann Soc Belge Med Trop 64:125, 1984
17. Owen RL: Enteric disease in acquired immunodeficiency syndrome (AIDS). Proc Southeast Asian Parasitology Symposium, Dec. 9–12, 1983
18. Bradley DJ: Prevention of disease in the tropics: questions in health economics. Epidemiol Community Health 33:66, 1979
19. Ghana Health Protective Team: A quantitative method of assessing the health impact of different diseases in less developed countries. Int J Epidemiol 10:73, 1981
20. Taylor C: Health for all-most. Harvard Med Alumni Bull 55:36, 1981
21. Weller TH: Too few and too little: barricades to the pursuit of health. Rev Infect Dis 5:994, 1983
22. Mata L: How harmful is diarrhoea? World Health:5, Apr 1986
23. Santosham M, Reid R: Diarrhoea management. World Health:8, Apr 1986
24. Goodall RM: UNICEF: 11 years in the field. World Health:12, Apr 1986
25. Brown PJ: Socioeconomic and demographic effects of malaria eradication: a comparison of Sri Lanka and Sardinia. Soc Sci Med 22:847, 1986
26. World Health Organization, Expert Committee on Malaria: Eighteenth Report. WHO Tech Rep Ser 735, 1986
27. Walsh JA: Problems in recognition and diagnosis of amebiasis: estimation of the global magnitude of morbidity and mortality. Rev Infect Dis 8:228, 1986
28. Schenone H, Villarroel F, Rojas A, et al: Epidemiology of human cysticercosis in Latin America. In Flisser A, Willms K, Laclette JP, et al (eds:) Cysticercosis: Present State of Knowledge and Perspectives. Academic Press, New York, 1982
29. Ehrlich PR, Ehrlich AH, Holdren JP: The history and future of the human popula-

tion. p. 181. In Ecoscience. Population, Resources, Environment. WH Freeman, San Francisco, 1977
30. McNamara RS: The world's population problem. Possible interventions to reduce fertility. Public Health Rep 93:124, 1978
31. Walton S: Stop the world; we'd better get off: Global 2000 projects grim future. BioScience 30:629, 1980
32. Brown LR, Wolf E, Starke L, et al: State of the World 1984. WW Norton, New York, 1984
33. Warren KS: The present impossibility of eradicating the omnipresent worm. Rev Infect Dis 4:955, 1982
34. Francis D: Selective primary health care: strategies for control of disease in the developing world. III. Hepatitis B virus and its related diseases. Rev Infect Dis 5:322, 1983
35. Arfaa F: Selective primary health care: strategies for control of disease in the developing world. XII. Ascariasis and trichuriasis. Rev Infect Dis 6:364, 1984
36. Mott KE: Schistosomiasis: a primary health care approach. World Health Forum 5:221, 1984
37. World Health Organization: The Control of Schistosomiasis: Report of a WHO Expert Committee. WHO Tech Rep Ser 728. Geneva, 1985
38. Mauldin WP: Population trends and prospects. Science 209:148, 1980
39. Murphy EM: World Population: Toward the Next Century. p 18. Population Reference Bureau, Washington, 1981
40. Office of Technology Assessment: World population and fertility planning technologies. The next 20 years. Congress of the United States, Washington, 1982
41. United Nations: World Summary. p. 143. In Demographic Yearbook 1984. Issue 36. Department of International Economic and Social Affairs, Statistical Office, United Nations, New York, 1986
42. Warren KS, Mahmoud AAF: Targeted mass treatment: a new approach for the control of schistosomiasis. Trans Assoc Am Physicians 89:195, 1976
43. Mahler H: Partnership for health for all. Address to the WHO Regional Committee for South-East Asia. WHO Chron 35:203, 1981

3 Variation of Parasitic Antigens: Purpose, Strategy, and Underlying Molecular Mechanisms

Nina Agabian
George R. Newport
Richard S. Stephens

Parasites have evolved various strategies for evading the vertebrate immune system. These are thought to include: (1) intracellular localization of one or more life cycle stages; (2) peripheral adsorption of host antigens; (3) presentation of hostlike antigens; (4) sequestration within protected anatomic sites; (5) suppression or subversion of host protective effector mechanisms (some parasites either hydrolyze bound immunoglobulins or secrete factors that suppress antiparasitic immune responses); (6) sequential presentation of stage-specific antigens; and (7) antigenic variation among parasites of a particular life cycle stage. Detailed molecular evaluation of how parasites avoid immunologic destruction should provide valuable insights into the biologic basis of parasitism and may thus provide a basis for development of vaccines or therapeutic compounds.

Antigenic diversification and variation have long been recognized as strategies used by many organisms to overcome hostile environmental surroundings. Particularly in the case of parasitic organisms dependent on vertebrate hosts for sustenance, the evolutionary pressure to develop mechanisms for evading recognition by the immune system has proved unrelenting. Understanding of this trend, coupled with understanding of the immunogenic and genetic characteristics of structurally related but immunologically distinct molecules, can provide insight about how parasites have become so biologically successful and how mechanisms for generating antigenic diversity operate.

We define antigenic variation, in its strictest sense, as a process involving the purposeful diversification of functionally equivalent molecules or of molecules that originate from genetic homologues. While related at the level of structure and function, these molecules are nevertheless antigenically distinct and are recognized as foreign by the host as a result of their innate immunogenicity. The criterion that imposes preservation of structure-function relationships among these molecules might ordinarily suggest that variability is likely to occur in regions of a molecule that can vary considerably without affecting biologic function, unless, however, generation of antigenic diversity itself is the primary role of the antigen.

ANTIGENIC VARIATION IN AFRICAN TRYPANOSOMIASIS

The most striking and best studied example of antigenic variation is that displayed by subspecies of *Trypanosoma brucei,* the parasitic protozoa that cause African sleeping sickness.[1,2] Trypanosomes proliferate in the bloodstream of the mammalian host and are usually diagnosed by direct examination of blood smears. The blood stage parasites have no characterized tissue or cell surface interactions with the host. While in the bloodstream the parasite is covered with a surface coat composed of a single glycoprotein, which is thought to be required for its viability in the mammalian host.[3] As infection persists, blood samplings of infected patients or animals reveal repeated waves of parasitemia that extend for days or weeks, depending on the host-parasite pair. Figure 3-1 illustrates the pattern of parasitemia exhibited by a patient with *Trypanosoma brucei gambiense* infection. This subspecies of the parasite is primarily a human pathogen and commonly results in chronic rather than acute trypanosomiasis. Successive samplings of blood reveal parasites whose surfaces are antigenically distinct.[4] This phenomenon also occurs in experimental animals even when infections are initiated with a single clonally derived organism. Thus, the ability to change antigenic character is an inherent genetic characteristic of these protozoa.

Studies by Vickerman in the early 1970s demonstrated that the surface glycoprotein coat of the bloodstream parasite is itself the variable antigen, whence it is named the variable surface glycoprotein (VSG).[5] Infections initiated with a single trypanosome can manifest as many as 100 different antigenic types, and experiments at the genetic level indicate that each parasite genome may encode in excess of 1,000 different VSG gene sequences.[6,7] The VSGs

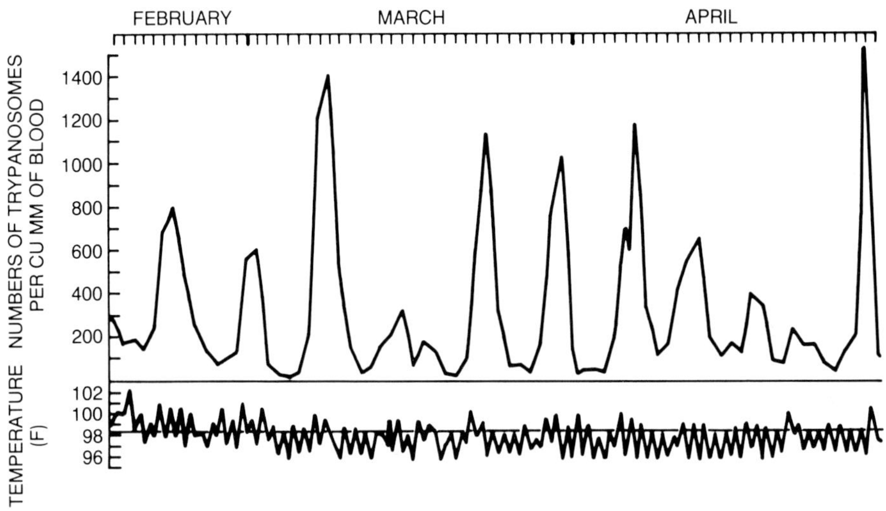

Fig. 3-1. Relapsing nature of parasitemia and fever in a patient infected with *Trypanosoma brucei gambiense*. In the upper portion of the graph parasitemia number of trypanosomes per milliliter of blood is plotted, and in the lower portion the patient's temperature in degrees Fahrenheit is plotted. Samplings took place over a 3-month period.

range in molecular weight from 55,000 to 65,000 and differ in primary amino acid sequence throughout most of the polypeptide chain.[8] Figure 3-2 shows a schematic diagram of the VSG gene and its product.

Except for a region of homology at the carboxy terminus of the polypeptide, VSG amino acid sequences are distinct. Nevertheless, expression of each VSG gene results in the synthesis of structurally related proteins (as inferred from x-ray crystallographic data), which perform a common function and are transcribed, translated, processed, and assembled via a common pathway. In addition to the VSG genes encoded in a single trypanosome genotype, there are many different subspecies, geographic isolates of the parasite, which have their own antigenic repertoire.[9] The magnitude of permissible variation in this class of proteins is thus staggering.

With the application of molecular genetic technology, antigenic variation in trypanosomes has become a paradigm of a process that seems to have mechanistic equivalents in *Borrelia*-induced relapsing fever and in the serologic diversity of gonococcal and *Moraxella* pilus antigens.[10,11] Interestingly, *Paramecium* also undergoes antigenic variation,[12] although the biologic significance of the process in this free-living protozoan is not at all clear.

After the molecular reagents for studying VSG gene expression were developed by now well established techniques,[13] the mechanism of antigen switching became accessible to analysis. Quickly it was learned that the variability in VSGs expressed at the cell surface resulted from the expression of one of a vast number of possible VSG genes in the parasite genetic repertoire.[14]

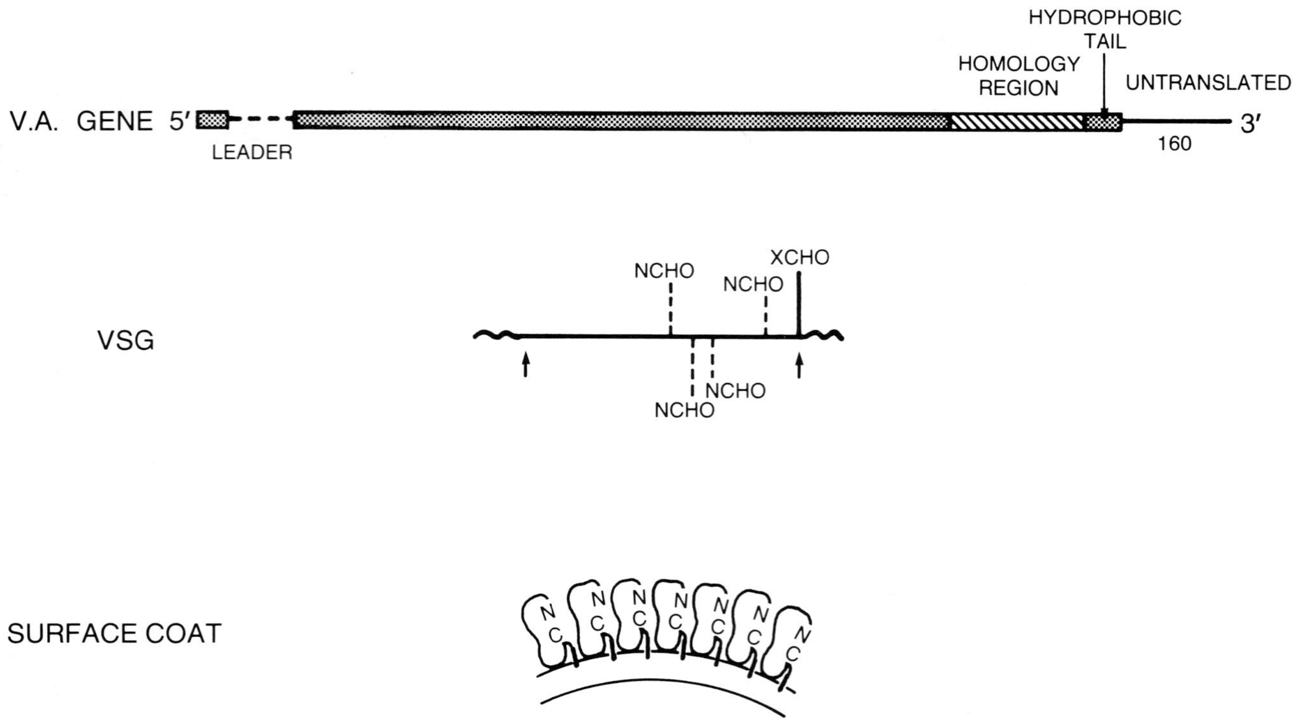

Fig. 3-2. Organization of a typical variant antigen. The gene encoding the variant antigen protein (top line) has the following features: it contains no introns, most of the gene encodes the variable portion of the protein (dark, thick line); the variable region is followed by a shorter stretch encoding a region of VSG homology; and the gene does not encode a 5′ spliced leader sequence that is found on all trypanosome RNAs. The protein itself (VSG, middle line) is glycosylated (NCHO) and is assembled on the surface (bottom line) in such a way that the amino terminus faces the aqueous environment. The carboxyl terminus, which contains the region of homology, is highly glycosylated and is anchored to the membrane by covalent linkage with a myristic acid unit.

VSG genes were found to be organized in a supergene family, which represented the repertoire of each isolate.[7] Expression of a single VSG from this repertoire is regulated at the level of transcription; mRNA is only transcribed from a single VSG gene in the repertoire at any given time.[15] Molecular analysis of the organization of VSG genes, both during expression and in subsequent relapses when a different VSG antigen was elaborated at the cell surface, revealed major genomic rearrangements associated with antigen switching; VSG genes changed in number and in chromosomal position during successive relapses.[13,14]

Figure 3-3 outlines the major types of genetic rearrangements associated with antigen switching and the genomic organization of VSG genes. The trypanosome genome is composed of a large number of chromosomes (estimates range from 100 to 500), which occur in three size classes—a large proportion of the genome is found in chromosomes in excess of 10,000 kilobase (kb), in a medium-size class of about 2,000 kb and a minichromosome class of about 50 kb.[14] The number of chromosomes in each class and thus the karyotype vary among isolates and species, but it seems clear that every size class of chromosome is capable of accommodating a VSG gene. Minichromosomes are characteristic of African trypanosomes that are capable of antigenic variation and are

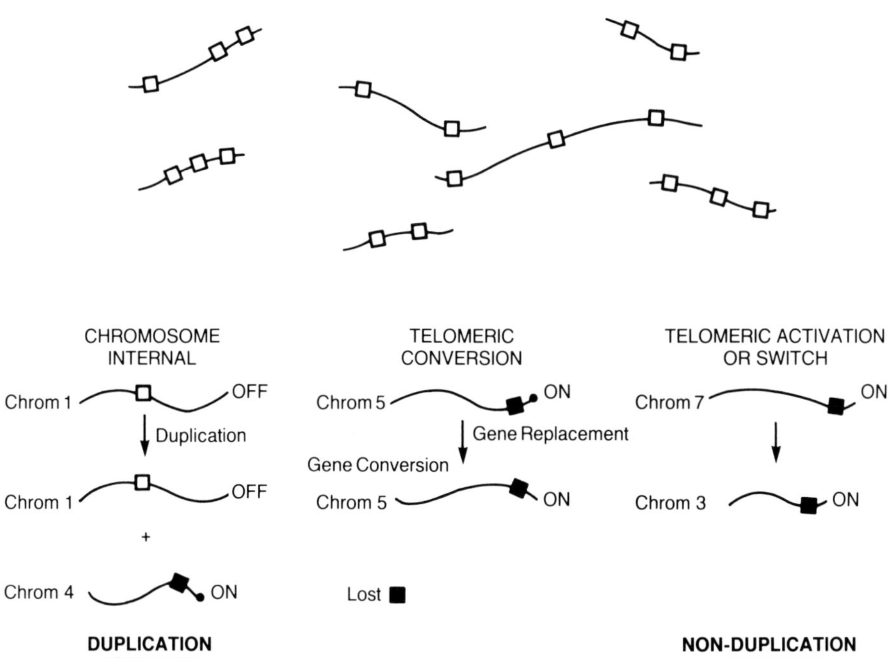

Fig. 3-3. Schematic diagram showing multiplicity of trypanosome chromosomes that vary in size (top). Each chromosome contains one or more variant antigen genes (□). In the bottom half of the figure, three different mechanisms for VSG gene switching are shown. See text for details.

not found in *Trypanosoma cruzi, Leishmania,* and other trypanosomatids that are not. Some believe that the complexity of this chromosome class is related to the diversity of the VSG gene repertoire in each species. The special relationship of the minichromosome class of VSG genes to the rearrangement and expression of the VSG repertoire remains unresolved.

VSG genes are organized into subfamilies encoding closely related sequences. Some antigenic types contain gene families with as many as 10 to 20 members while others contain only a single copy of a particular VSG type.[7] We still do not know if all the members of these multigene families can be expressed or if their role in antigenic variation is related to the generation of new VSG genes or to some other aspect of VSG gene expression.

In general, VSG genes occupy two positions in the genome: they may be found internally within a chromosome and/or at the ends of chromosomes (telomeric copies). Occupation of a telomeric location appears to be a necessary condition for the expression of a given VSG gene since transcription of a VSG gene from a chromosome-internal position has never been documented. However, telomeric location in and of itself is not sufficient for expression since there are many telomeres occupied by VSG genes, but only one telomeric copy is transcriptionally active in any one variant antigen type trypanosome.[13,14]

The gene rearrangements and the duplications of VSG genes all seem to have as a primary objective the placement of a VSG gene at a telomeric site so that it has the potential for expression. These events can proceed by several alternate routes; Figure 3-3 (bottom, left) illustrates the duplicative transposition events first recognized by Borst[15] and colleagues. Here an internal copy in chromosome 1 is duplicated, and the extra copy is transposed to a telomeric expression site on chromosome 4 by a mechanism involving recombination. Examination of VSG gene arrangement in DNA isolated from trypanosomes during expression of a given VSG gene and in a subsequent relapse revealed an extra copy of the VSG gene in the expressor population. In most cases this extra copy of the VSG gene disappears in relapse populations. Duplicative transposition, however, is only one of the rearrangements that can lead to VSG gene expression. As shown in Figure 3-3 (bottom, middle), a VSG gene can be replaced with another variant type in situ by gene conversion (i.e., at the same telomere); in this case the expressing copy of the VSG gene is lost from the genome. A third mechanism also exists for switching VSG gene expression, as shown in Figure 3-3 (bottom, right). In this case two telomeric VSG genes from antigenically different VSG gene families are shown on two different chromosomes. By a mechanism we do not understand transcription ceases from one telomeric expression site and is initiated at another telomere. Any of the quiescent telomeric VSG genes may potentially be activated by this telomeric switch.

Analysis of a number of VSG genes during expression and relapse has shown that any single VSG gene can be expressed by any or all of these mechanisms. Although antibodies against specific VSGs are sufficient to kill parasites in the mammalian host, the parasite's ability to switch between VSG genes and telomeric expression sites is random enough and rapid enough to preclude the use of VSG genes in the development of recombinant antigens for vaccination purposes. Therefore, repertoire size and antigenic diversity of VSG genes, as well as frequency of antigen switching, become crucial factors in immune evasion and chronicity in this disease.

ALLELIC VARIATION OF THE MAJOR OUTER MEMBRANE PROTEIN IN *CHLAMYDIA TRACHOMATIS*

A second form of antigenic variation, which we call here *allelic variation,* was suggested by molecular and immunochemical examination of *Chlamydia trachomatis* isolates. In *C. trachomatis* more than 15 serologically distinct groups (serovars) characteristic of lymphogranuloma venereum and trachoma pathology have been identified. By using polyvalent[16] and monoclonal antibodies[17] to the major outer membrane protein (MOMP) of *Chlamydia,* it was discovered that each of the MOMPs appears to be a genetic mosaic of epitopes: The MOMPs possess major immunodominant epitopes[17] that are unique (serovar-specific) as well as epitopes that are shared within the species and among multiple serovars. The origin of these immunodominant regions of three of the MOMPs has been studied at the molecular genetic level by Stephens and coworkers.

The gene-encoding MOMP from serovar L2 was isolated after cloning of L2-specific genomic DNA fragments into an expression vector, in this case λgt11.[18] Recombinant DNA clones expressing the L2 antigen were identified by screening of the L2 library with polyvalent antisera raised against L2 MOMP. Positive clones were characterized with both monoclonal and polyclonal antibodies. One clone, encoding a 20,000 molecular weight portion of the carboxyl-terminal peptide fragment of the L2 MOMP (designated L2 33) was chosen for further molecular studies.

If *Chlamydia* alter their type-specific antigens in a manner analogous to that described above for trypanosomes, one might expect that an appropriate gene probe would detect several genomic fragments corresponding to a repertoire of serotypes. The complexity of nucleotide sequences associated with the MOMP antigenic phenotype was evaluated by use of the MOMP gene probe L2 33, which encodes both species- and subspecies-specific antigenic determinants. The hybridization pattern of the L2 33 probe with restriction digests of genomic DNA from serovars L2, C, and B is shown in Figure 3-4. In all three cases the L2 33 probe hybridized with a unique DNA fragment at both high and low stringency.[19] The most likely interpretation of these results is that the common species-specific determinants of the MOMP retain sufficient homology to recognize alternative MOMP genes in different *Chlamydia* serovars. This was confirmed directly by DNA sequence analysis.[19]

In order to study the relationship between serovar sequences in more detail, the MOMP genes from serovars C, B, and L2 were cloned and se-

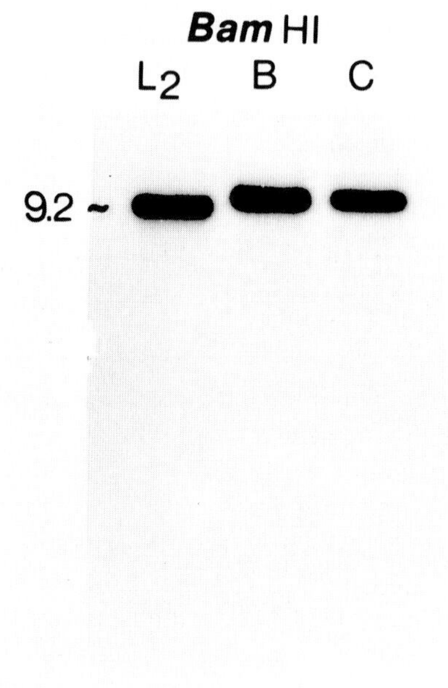

Fig. 3-4. Southern hybridization of *Bam* H1-digested DNA obtained from *C. trachomatis* serovars L_2, B, and C probed with phosphorus 32–labeled λgt11/L2/33 insert DNA. (From Stephens,[19] with permission.)

quenced.[20] Figure 3-5 summarizes these studies. The entire amino acid sequence of L2, deduced from the DNA sequence, is compared with the sequence determined for the C and B serovar MOMP genes. The MOMPs are homologous for most of their sequence except as indicated. Four domains of the MOMP were identified in which the translated amino acid sequences varied. Truncated fusion products of the L2 gene expressed in λgt11 provided polypeptides for mapping of epitopes for species, subspecies, and type-specific determinants using the monoclonal antibodies developed for typing these strains. Species- and subspecies-specific epitopes are found in the carboxyl-terminal variable region of the molecule whereas type-specific epitopes are found in the amino-terminal region. Variability in the amino-terminal variable regions accounts for the antigenic diversity of the serovars.

Molecular genetic analysis of the sequence and genomic context of MOMP genes suggests that antigenic differences are related to that MOMP allele which is present in each *C. trachomatis* isolate rather than to an alternative expression of one of several genes present within the genome of a single isolate. DNA hybridization analysis provides no evidence for multiple MOMP genes within a single genome, and restriction endonuclease patterns of L2, B, and C further indicate that each of these MOMP genes is found in similar genomic context, as expected for genetic alleles.

Because of the highly circumscribed domains of variation within MOMP it will be interesting to determine the extent of variation possible within this class of molecules. MOMP is multifunctional and appears to participate in attachment, endocytosis, toxicity, porin activity, and the structural integrity of the

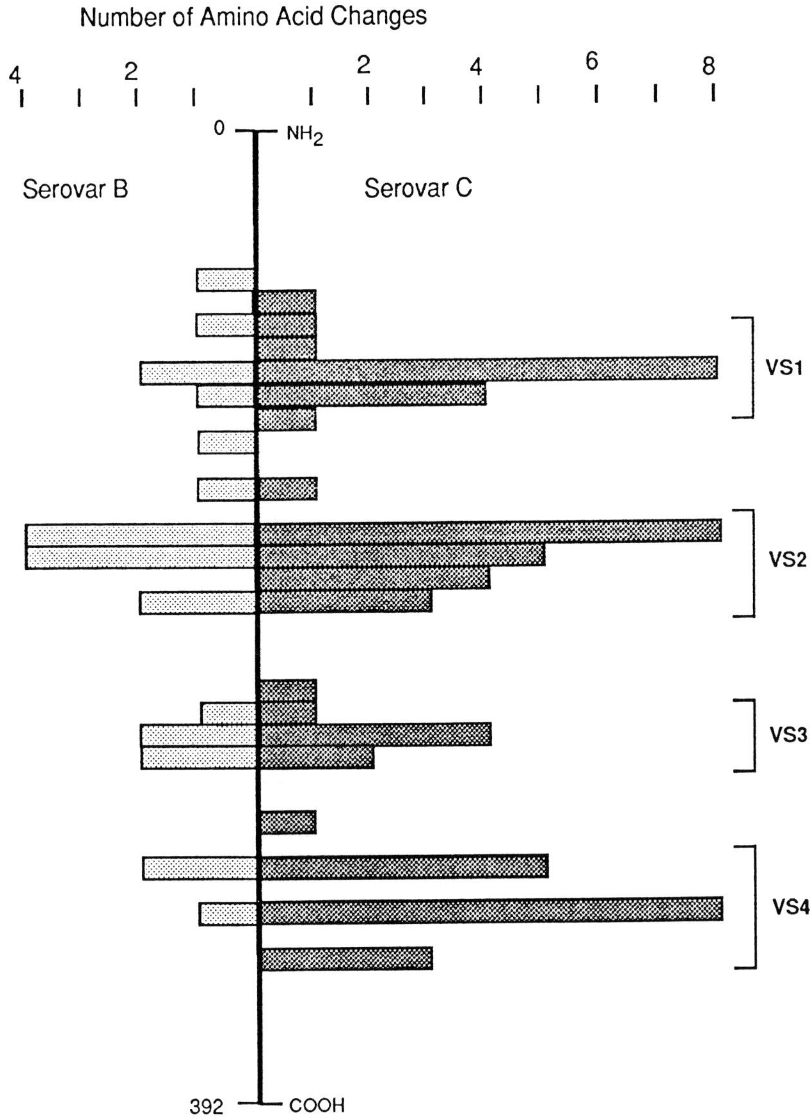

Fig. 3-5. Frequency and distribution of amino acid differences for the major outer membrane proteins for serovar B and serovar C from the serovar L_2 sequence. Brackets delineate four variable sequence (VS) domains. (From Stephens,[20] with permission.)

Chlamydia outer membrane.[21] In order to preserve these functions, the number of permissible mutations within the restricted protein domains may in fact result in a limited number of variations in sequence and hence in a limited amount of antigenic variation.

In diseases such as those caused by *Chlamydia,* where there is constant reinfection of a single host, the ability of *Chlamydia* populations to exhibit alternative serotypes might ensure the continuation of long-term infections within the host population. The frequency of appearance of alternative serovars might then be expected to be a function of the frequency of reinfection, the incidence of different serovars in the population, and the longevity and intensity of the specific host immune response. These factors in sum would contribute to the chronicity and persistence of disease both in the individual and in the population.

INTERSPECIFIC DIVERSITY AMONG GENETIC HOMOLOGUES IN SCHISTOSOMIASIS

Many genera of parasites exhibit strict specificity for a particular host species; this characteristic is manifest in the host-parasite range, the pathology associated with infection, and the specificity of acquired immunity of the host as indicated by cross-protection or lack thereof. For example, while each species of *Plasmodium* initiates infection with a sporozoite, the species of *Plasmodium* and the species of the host determine the severity of the disease and whether, in fact, infection actually occurs. Thus *P. lophurae,* a parasite of birds, cannot establish itself in humans, although the natural history of the parasite is similar to that of *P. falciparum*. The sporozoite of each *Plasmodium* species produced (i.e., during development in the mosquito) is sheathed in an antigenic coat called the *circumsporozoite* (CSP) antigen.[22] While functioning similarly in each parasite species, each CSP antigen is nevertheless antigenically distinct.[23] Thus, *P. falciparum, P. vivax,* and *P. malariae,* all of which infect humans, possess CSP antigens that are functionally equivalent but immunologically distinct. Clearly, then, no cross-species immunity is provided by these antigens, although within the host-parasite pair protection may be afforded against homologous challenge.

The CSP antigen of *Plasmodium* illustrates a third type of antigenic variation (i.e., species-specific antigenic differences among functionally homologous proteins). Recently, we have had occasion to discover another case of such variation in helminth infections caused by *Schistosoma* species. In the schistosomiasis disease complex, infections with *S. mansoni, S. japonicum,* and *S. haematobium* are pathologically distinct; this distinction is dictated by the site of worm maturation within the mammalian host. In those cases in which protective immunity can be demonstrated, it is largely species-specific.

A λgt11 expression library containing cDNA sequences from *S. mansoni* adult worms was screened with a variety of antisera from infected humans, mice, and rats and with serum from mice vaccinated with irradiated cercariae. Recombinant DNA clones, which expressed an epitope encoded by a native antigen of 70,000 molecular weight, were detected at a frequency of about 1 : 1,000. An unusual property of this antigen was the uniformity of its recognition by individual immune sera, including sera from donors with either chronic (high and low worm burden) or acute infections. This property of uniform antigenicity was especially notable since the spectrum of antigens recognized by individual serum samples was highly variable.[24]

Sera from patients infected with another schistosome, *S. japonicum,* similarly detected an antigen of 70,000 molecular weight among the in vitro translation products of the adult worm mRNA. Moreover, while the sera from *S. japonicum*–infected individuals was highly variable in the spectrum of antigens recognized, a 70,000-molecular-weight antigen was again detected by the sera of all patients examined, as established in the case of *S. mansoni.*[25] The similarity in molecular weight between the *S. japonicum* and *S. mansoni* immundominant antigens suggested that these might be antigens shared by *Schistosoma* species. To test this possibility, adult worm mRNA from *S. mansoni* and *S. japonicum* was translated in vitro, and the proteins produced were immunoprecipitated with both homologous and heterologous sera. The results are shown in Figure 3-6. Antisera from both *S. mansoni*- and *S. japonicum*–infected individuals detected an immunodominant antigen of 70,000 molecular weight; however each antigen was detected only by homologous and not by heterologous infection serum.

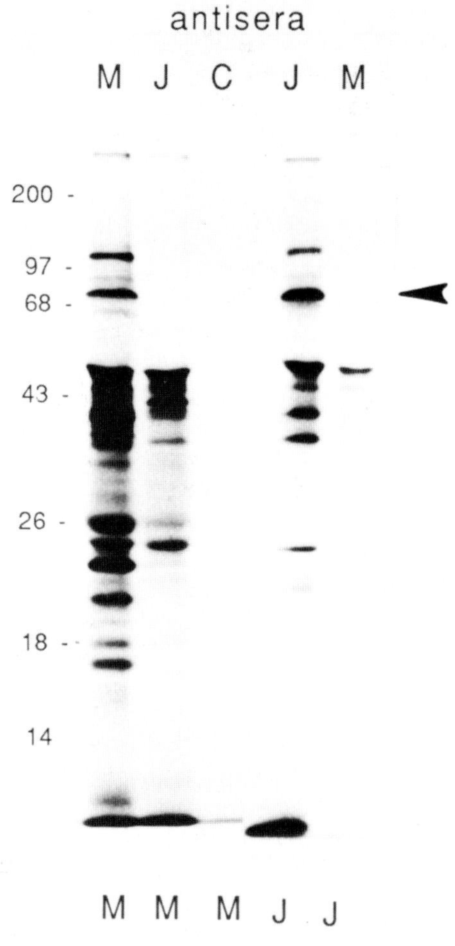

Fig. 3-6. Immunoprecipitation of adult schistosome mRNA translation products with human antisera M (*S. mansoni*), (*S. japonicum*), and C (normal control) The arrow points to the 70 kd peptide.

Remembering that there is species-specific immunity to schistosomes, which does not provide for cross-protective immunity, it seemed likely that these molecules might represent immunologically different but functionally homologous proteins. The cDNA clone from *S. japonicum,* which contains an epitope corresponding to the immunodominant epitope of the 70,000-molecular-weight antigen, was hybridized to its *S. mansoni* analogue and to itself (Fig. 3-7) under stringent conditions. Furthermore, Southern analysis of both *S. mansoni* and *S. japonicum* genomic DNA using either clone resulted in hybridization with identical restriction fragments. Thus, while these sequences are completely non-cross-reactive at the immunologic level, they are homologous at the DNA sequence level.

Figure 3-8 shows a comparison of the amino acid sequences of both the *S. mansoni* and *S. japonicum* clones as deduced from their respective DNA sequences. Also shown is the sequence of the *Drosophila,* human,[26] and malarial heat-shock protein HSP70.[27] The *S. mansoni* peptide is 71 percent homologous with the *Drosophila* and 80 percent homologous with human HSP-70 homologues. The identification of the schistosome immunogen encoding clones as HSP70 was revealed by a computer search of amino acid sequence libraries.[28]

Identification of the schistosome immunodominant antigens as heat shock protein homologues was unexpected. The HSP70 proteins are among the most highly conserved protein families known in nature.[29] They are synthesized as a stereotyped response to stress, the most commonly characterized of which is

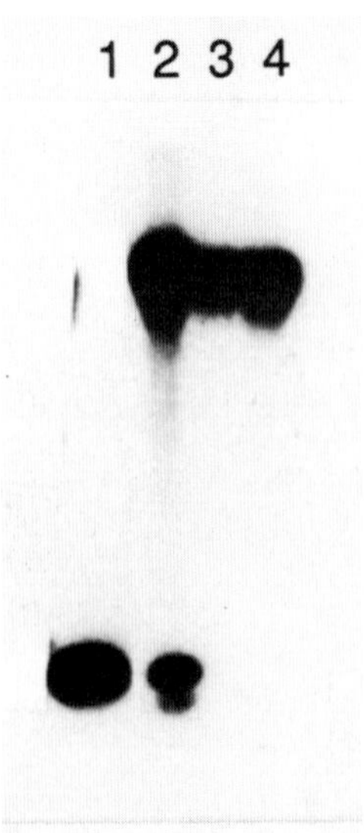

Fig. 3-7. Cross-hybridization of 70 kd cDNA clones from *S. mansoni* and *S. japonicum*. A positive control (*S. mansoni*) and *S. japonicum* cDNAs were hybridized with the *S. mansoni* cDNA under conditions of high stringency. 1 = Positive control (purified insert from λcSmA-F1). 2 = Eco R1 digestion of λcSj-J4. 3,4 = Eco R1 digestion of unrelated λcSjA clones.

```
Sm          ERALTKDNNLLGKFELSGIPPAPRGTPQIEVTFDIDANGILNVSAVDKGTGK
Sj          **TM**************C*******V*********************A***
Hs          ***M*********R************V****************T*TKDS***
Dm          ***M******A**T*D**********V********L*********KEMS***
Pf          ***************H*D*******KV****************T**E*S***

Sm    QNKITITNDKGRLSKEEIERMVADADKYKAEDEKQRDRVASKNSLESYVYTMKQQVEG
Sj    E*****************D**INE*****S*****KN*IC**********S***S***
Hs    A****************QE*E*******V**E******A****AFN**AFN***SA**
Dm    AKN***K*******QA**D***NE****AD****H*Q*IT*R*A******NV**S**Q
Pf    **H***********QD**D***N**E*******EN*K*IEAR****N*C*GV*SSL*D

Sm    E-LKEKIPESDH-QVIISKCEDTISWLDVHQSAEKHETESKREELEKVCAPIITKVYQ
SJ    DEM*D**S***RKNRIL****E**R*M*NN*L***E*F*E*KS******M****AMNR
Hs    EG**G**S*A*KKK*-LD**QEV*****ANTL***D*F*H**K***Q**N***SGL**
Dm    APA-G*LD*A*K-NSVLD**NE**R***SNTT***E*FDH*H***TRH*S**M**MH*
Pf    QKI***LQPAEIETC--MTITTILE**EKN*L*G*D***A*QK*A*S*****MS*I**

Sm    -AGG--------MPGGMHEAS--GAGGSG--------------KGPTIEEVD
Sj    -***---GVPSG*****---P--****G*--------------*********
Hs    -***-----G-G-***-FG*Q-GPK****--------------S********
Dm    Q--*AA--------**-PG*NCGQAGGF*GY------------S********
Pf    D*A*AAGGMPGG*****PGGMPG*MNFA*GMPGAGMPGNAPAGS***V***A
```

Fig 3-8. Nucleotide sequence of cDNAs encoding the carboxy terminus of the HSP70 of various species. Sm = *Schistosoma mansoni*, Sj = *S. japonicum*, HS = human, Dm = *Drosophilia melanogaster*, and Pf = *Plasmodium falciparum*. The human and *Drosophila* sequences are from Hunt and Morimoto[26] and the malarial one is from Bianco et al.[27] Asterisks denote regions of identity with the *S. mansoni* sequence. The dashes indicate that there are no intervening amino acids in the HSP70 of that species.

heat shock, and are thought to mediate the removal of structurally abnormal (e.g., denatured) proteins. Additionally, heat shock proteins are generally found in the cell nucleus after induction, where they are believed to regulate gene activity in such a way as to compensate for the extremes experienced by biosynthetic mechanisms taxed by elevated temperature. Recently, it has been discovered that the heat shock proteins themselves are encoded by complex gene families containing homologues that are expressed constitutively, as well as in response to stress. Constitutively expressed cognates of HSP70 appear to be involved in the disassembly and assembly of protein aggregates.

While the existence of considerable homology between schistosome and human HSP70s is consistent with the observed conservation of sequences among this class of proteins, the ability of the helminth protein to invariably elicit a strong and specific immune response is not. The immunodominant epitope of the schistosome HSP70 has been localized to the carboxyl terminus of the molecule. Surprisingly, the *S. mansoni* and *S. japonicum* heat shock proteins are antigenically unique even though they differ from one another in this region at only 14 positions over a stretch of 113 amino acids. These sites generally correspond to points of divergence between the human and fruit-fly homologues as well. Although the function of the schistosome protein is currently unknown, we have noted that its synthesis is highly induced during the transformation of cercaria to schistosomulum, which thus implies a developmental role for HSP70. In addition, HSP70 is an early schistosome antigen, stimulating an immune response within 30 days in experimental animals, and it may thus prove useful for diagnosis.

The strict specificity of host responses to schistosome HSP70s offers a model system for studying the phenomenon of antigen presentation by parasites. The kinetics of the immune response to HSP70 indicates an association with adult and juvenile worms; the antigen is not a surface component. Immunization of animals with chicken HSP70 results in a broad cross-reactive response directed against the entire polypeptide. The question of how the schistosome ensures that only the antigenically unique carboxyl terminal domain is presented to the host is an intriguing problem for future study.

CONCLUSION

The application of molecular genetics to the study of parasites has already revealed phenomena of antigenic variation that fall in three major categories.

First, as outlined in the case of the African trypanosomes, clonally derived populations can express phenotypically variable antigens as a result of the intrinsic ability of a parasite genome to alternately regulate the transcription of genes from a particular gene family (i.e., antigenic variation is manifest as a phenotypic variation caused by the expression of alternate genes from a given genomic repertoire). In addition to trypanosomes, *Borrelia recurrentis*, a tick-borne parasite that causes relapsing fever, and perhaps *Plasmodium falciparum,* with its strain-specific surface antigens, provide examples of such classes of molecules.[10,30]

A second form of antigenic variation, allelic variation, was exemplified by studies of the *C. trachomatis* MOMP. In this case, isolates within a species possess alternative alleles for immunodominant antigens, which themselves are serologically distinct. While a single genotype does not have the capacity to switch between antigenic types, the population as a whole possesses several alleles for a particular antigen class, thus expanding the parasite's antigenic repertoire.

A third form of antigenic variation, recognized in studies of malaria and schistosomiasis, is interspecific variation, which occurs among protein antigens that are functionally homologous. Different species and subspecies of related parasites personalize some of these polypeptides antigenically. The CSP antigens of *Plasmodium* species and the heat shock protein HSP70 of *Schistosoma* species are examples of this class.

At least two major variables emerge from considering these alternative mechanisms of antigenic variation: the period of interaction-exposure of the parasite with the host immune system and the function of the protein encoding the variable epitopes.

The evolutionary pressure of cohabitation is great—the greater the parasite's exposure to the host's immune system, the more extensive its armory of defenses must be for the organism to persist. If the parasite's main arsenal in evading the immune system is antigenic variation, its success is dependent upon the size of its antigenic repertoire and the efficiency and frequency with which it can call this repertoire into play. The parasites must also have a means for preventing the simulataneous presentation of all possible antigenic forms by a given population. To complicate matters, if the variable antigens are functionally important to the parasite's biology, then variability must occur within constraints that ensure the functional integrity of the polypeptide; deficiencies in either area doom the organism either as the immune system catches up with the parasite or as diversity obscures function and the parasite can no longer exist within the host.

It is relatively easy to see why African trypanosomes would evolve complex mechanisms for varying their antigenic repertoire and rapidly switching between antigenic types. In as much as they are constantly and directly exposed to the immune system as blood stage parasites, it is their ability to switch VSGs that allows survival in the mammalian host. Parenthetically, African trypanosomes must also persist long enough in the mammalian stages to ensure their transmission to the tsetse fly vector—a rather inefficient and intricate process in itself.

Some parasites minimize the period of their exposure to the immune system by intracellularization, emerging only to reinitiate another proliferative cycle. *Chlamydia, Leishmania, Toxoplasma, Plasmodium,* and many other parasites thus limit their interactions with the host immune system. The ability of the host to mount an effective immune response is then related to the immunogenicity of the parasite components and the time between rounds of parasite dissemination and penetration of susceptible host cell types. Depending upon the efficiency of each of these processes, it may be distinctly advantageous for the parasite to have a repertoire of alternative antigens or, if reinfection is frequent, to maintain several different antigenic populations to perpetuate the species.

The chlamydial MOMP, as well as other parasite macromolecules that are antigenically plastic despite structural and functional constraints, poses another interesting parameter to consider when one seeks to understand how much variability is permissible. Stated another way: How much can a protein change in sequence and antigenicity without affecting function? Is there a limit to the number of different forms a functionally restricted structure can take? If one were to look at VSGs the answer appears to be no—there is a seemingly endless number of protein sequences that are capable of functioning as VSGs, although preliminary crystallographic data suggest that all VSGs share a common shape and interaction with neighboring VSG molecules. In this extreme case, however, the function of these antigens may be to vary, and therefore their synthesis and assembly may be relatively permissible as compared with MOMP or the CSP antigens of *Plasmodium*. In these latter cases the antigen must vary within the constraints of the receptor-ligand relationship; otherwise the parasite will not be able to infect its host. Extending this concept to the last example of antigenic variation—interspecific variation—the functional role of the variable molecules in parasite pathogenesis becomes intriguing. Do these molecules represent a chronicle of the evolution between host and parasite, the end results of which are highly stereotyped and interwoven biologic programs? A specific example of such a cat-and-mouse game has been recently suggested to have occurred between a schistosome elastase-mediating breach of the skin barrier[31] and a family of vertebrate protease inhibitors.[32] The latter have evolved at an unprecedentedly rapid rate, presumably to keep up with an equally rapid rate of parasite protease evolution.[32]

Antigenic variation by infectious organisms is a dynamic process, completely understood only within the context of the host-parasite interplay. While new technologies promise to illuminate the genetic mechanisms called on by both parasites and hosts, antigenic variation by the parasite challenges our own strategies for vaccine development.

ACKNOWLEDGMENTS

The research underlying the scientific results presented herein was supported in part by funds provided by the John D. and Catherine T. MacArthur, Edna McConnell Clark, and Rockefeller foundations. Nina Agabian is a Burroughs Wellcome Scholar of Molecular Parasitology.

REFERENCES

1. Moulder JW: Comparative biology of intracellular parasitism. Microbiol Rev 49:298, 1985
2. Ross R, Thomson D: A case of sleeping sickness studied by precise enumerative methods: further observations. Ann Trop Med Parasitol 4:395, 1911

3. Vickerman K, Luckins AG: Localization of variable antigens in the surface coat on *Trypanosoma brucei* using ferritin conjugated antibody. Nature 244:1125, 1969
4. Levaditi C, McIntosh J: Mechanisme de la création de races de trypanosomes resistantes aux anticorps. Bull Soc Pathol Exot 3:368, 1910
5. Vickerman K: On the surface coat and flagella adhesions in trypanosomes. J Cell Sci 5:163, 1969
6. Turner MJ: Biochemistry of the variant surface glycoprotein of salivarian trypanosomes. Adv Parasitol 21:69, 1982
7. Frasch ACC, Borst P, Van den Burg J: Rapid evolution of genes coding for variant surface glycoproteins in trypanosomes. Gene 17:197, 1982
8. Olafson RW, Clarke MW, Kielland SL, et al: Amino terminal sequence homology among variant surface glycoproteins of African trypanosomes. Mol Biochem Parasitol 12:287, 1984
9. Gray AR: Antigenic variation in a strain of *Trypanosoma brucei* transmitted by *Glossina morsitans* and *G. palpalis*. J Gen Microbiol 41:195, 1965
10. Meyer TF, Billyard E., Haas R, et al: Pilus expression in *Neisseria gonorrhoeae* involves chromosomal rearrangement. Cell 30:45, 1982
11. Meier JT, Simon MI, Barbour AG: Antigenic variation is associated with DNA rearrangements in a relapsing fever *Borrelia*. Cell 41:403, 1985
12. Beale GH: Adaptation in *Paramecium*. p. 294. In Davis R, Gale E (eds): Adaptation in Microorganisms. Symp. Soc. Gen. Microbiol. Vol. 3, 1953
13. Englund PT, Hajduk SL, Marini JC: The molecular biology of trypanosomses. Ann Rev Biochem 51:1982
14. Borst P: Discontinuous transcription and antigenic variation in trypanosomes. Ann Rev Biochem 55:701, 1986
15. Borst P, Cross GAM: Molecular basis for trypanosome antigenic variation. Cell 29:291, 1982
16. Caldwell HD, Schachter RJ: Antigenic analysis of the major outer membrane proteins. Infect Immun 38:960, 1982
17. Stephens RS, Tam MR, Kuo CC, et al: Monoclonal antibodies to *Chlamydia trachomatis*: antibody specificities and antigen characterization. J Immunol 128:1083, 1984
18. Stephens RS, Kuo CC, Newport G, et al: Molecular cloning and expression of *Chlamydia trachomatis* major outer membrane protein antigens in *Escherichia coli*. Infect Immun 47:733, 1985
19. Stephens RS, Mullenbach G, Sanchez-Pescador R, et al: Sequence analysis of the major outer membrane protein gene from *Chlamydia trachomatis*. J Bacteriol 168:1277, 1986
20. Stephens RS, Sanchez-Pescador R, Wager EA, et al: Diversity of *Chlamydia trachomatis* major outer protein genes. J Bacteriol 169:3879, 1987
21. Schachter J, Caldwell HD: Chlamydiae. Ann Rev Microbiol 34:285, 1980
22. Nussenzweig V, Nussenzweig RS: Circumsporozoite proteins of malarial parasites. Cell 42:401, 1985
23. Galinski MR, Arnot DE, Cochrane AH, et al: The circumsporozoite gene of the *Plasmodium cynomolgi* complex. Cell 48:311, 1987
24. Newport G, McKerrow J, Barr P, et al: Stage-specific expression of schistosome proteases. p.121. In Agabian N, Nogueira N, Goodman H (eds): Molecular Strategies of Parasitic Invasion. Alan R Liss, New York, 1987
25. Hedstrom R, Culpepper J, Schinski V, et al: Schistosome heat-shock proteins are immunologically distinct host-like antigens. Mol Biochem Parasit (In Press)

26. Hunt C, Morimoto RI: Conserved features of eucaryotic HSP70 genes revealed by comparison with the nucleotide sequence of human HSP70. Proc Natl Acad Sci USA 82:6455, 1985
27. Bianco AE, Favaloro JM, Burkot TR, et al: A repetitive antigen of *Plasmodium falciparum* that is homologous to heat shock protein 70 of *Drosophila melanogaster*. Proc Natl Acad Sci USA 83:8713, 1986
28. Hedstrom R, Culpepper J, Harrison RA, et al: A major immunogen in *Schistosoma mansoni* infections is homologous to the heat-shock protein HSP-70. J Exp Med 165:1430, 1987
29. Lindquist S: The heat shock response. Ann Rev Biochem 55:1151, 1986
30. Leech JH, Barnwell JH, Miller LH et al: Identification of a strain-specific malarial antigen exposed on the surface of *Plasmodium falciparum* infected erythrocytes. J Exp Med 159:1567, 1984
31. Newport G, McKerrow J, Hedstrom R, et al: Schistosome elastases: biological function, structure, and stage-specific expression. Symp Biochem Soc 53: (in press)
32. Hill RE, Hastie ND: Accelerated evolution in the reactive center regions of serine protease inhibitors. Nature 326:96, 1987

4 The Role of Proteinases in the Pathogenesis of Parasitic Diseases

James H. McKerrow

Proteinases are enzymes that cleave the peptide backbone of proteins at an internal site. As such, they may be called *endoproteases* or *endopeptidases,* which distinguishes them from those enzymes that are capable of cleaving an amino acid only from the amino terminus or carboxy terminus of a protein (such as leucine *amino*peptidase or *carboxy*peptidases). Proteinases may play a variety of roles in the pathogenesis of infectious diseases, as listed below for parasitic infections:

1. Invasion of host
2. Metabolism within host
3. Evasion of immune response
4. Interaction with host protease systems (plasmin, kallikrein, complement)
5. Targets of immune response

TISSUE INVASION

Invasion of Skin by Helminth Larvae

Many parasites have a larval form that invades or migrates through host tissue. One of the best characterized examples of this invasion is that of intact skin by schistosome cercariae. The aquatic cercaria finds the human host by following a thermal gradient; when it contacts host skin, penetration is stimulated by medium-chain free fatty acids present in the lipid that covers the surface of this skin.[1] The barrier that cercariae must transgress is complex; regardless of whether they penetrate directly through the surface of the skin or migrate down a hair shaft, they ultimately must cross the epidermis, the dermal-epidermal basement membrane, the extracellular matrix of the dermis, and a second basement membrane before entering a small blood vessel or lymphatic in the superficial dermis. It has been known for some time that when cercariae are stimulated to penetrate, they release the contents of a set of glands known as the *acetabular glands*. Some of the material from these glands[1] has proteolytic activity. Recently the principal (and probably sole) proteinase of these secretions has been purified and characterized[2] as a proteinase of the serine class* with an ability to degrade elastin, a quality shared by only a few proteinases.

The elastin molecule is relatively resistant to degradation and is found in abundance in two organs that are common sites of parasitic invasion, the skin and the lung. If one were to choose an enzyme to facilitate tissue invasion, an elastase would be a wise choice because they characteristically have a broad substrate specificity and therefore, can cleave a number of connective tissue or basement membrane macromolecules in addition to elastin.[3] The cercarial enzyme is no exception; in addition to its ability to degrade elastin, it can degrade fibronectin, laminin, keratin, the peptide backbone of proteoglycans, and type IV collagen.[4–6]

Keratin, of course, is found in the cornified layer at the surface of the epidermis. Laminin and type IV collagen are two of the most important molecules in maintaining the structure of basement membrane. Fibronectin performs a similar function in connective tissue and has a number of domains that allow interaction of connective tissue macromolecules, such as collagen and proteoglycans, with each other and with nearby cells. Therefore, in addition to being able to degrade the extensive elastin network found in the superficial dermis, the cercarial enzyme is uniquely suited to disrupt the interactive framework of both basement membrane and connective tissue extracellular matrix.

While the cercarial elastase was the first helminthic proteinase to be studied extensively, more recently a number of other parasites with similar pathways of invasion have come under scrutiny. Of particular interest has been the fact that whenever the characteristics of the proteolytic enzymes released by these parasites have been studied in detail, enzymes with broad substrate specificities capable of degrading elastin have been elaborated. For example, L3 larvae of the hookworm parasite *Ancylostoma caninum* release a metalloelastase, which probably functions in much the same way as the cercarial elastase to facilitate larval invasion of skin.[7] Interestingly, in the adult worm this same enzyme acts as an anticoagulant, primarily by degrading fibrinogen.[8] Thus, the parasite takes advantage of the broad substrate specificity of elastase to perform two critical functions with a single enzyme.

---

* Other members of the serine class of proteinases are pancreatic elastases I and II, trypsin, chymotrypsin, complement factors, and blood coagulation proteases.

There is at least preliminary evidence suggesting that enzymes similar to either the hookworm elastase or the cercarial elastase are present in a number of nematode parasites (Table 4-1). These findings have led us to propose that a family of functionally and probably structurally related enzymes are produced by all nematode and trematode parasites for which there is a skin or lung invasive stage. While support for this hypothesis must await purification and characterization of several of these enzymes, it is clear at least that two distinct subgroups of enzymes exist. The first group, represented by the cercarial enzyme consists of serine proteinases; the second group, represented by the hookworm elastase, consists of metalloproteases. Since both the hookworm and cercarial enzymes have been purified and cDNA clones isolated from them, it will be possible to use cDNA probes or antibodies to the purified enzymes to check for structural homology by DNA or RNA hybridization and by immunologic assay. For example, Table 4-2 shows that there is immunologic cross-reactivity among the hookworm and schistosome proteinases and putative enzymes in *Onchocera volvulus,* the causative agent of African river blindness.

What are the clinical implications of these findings? From a diagnostic standpoint, these enzymes may be used as serodiagnostic reagents. Both the hookworm and cercarial enzymes have proved to be excellent markers of their respective diseases (P. Hotez, personal communication; Toy, McKerrow JH, et al., unpublished data).[9] However, in the case of the cercarial elastase there is cross-reactivity with other schistosome species (unpublished data) as well as with filarial nematodes (Table 4-2). Nevertheless, since these enzymes are often the first proteins released in the host, they may have utility as markers of exposure to larvae for epidemiologic studies and as indicators of infection early in the course of the disease.

Table 4-1. Trematode and Nematode Parasites that Appear to Express Proteinases for Tissue Invasion

Organism	Type of Proteinase	Reference
Ancylostoma caninum (hookworm)	Metalloproteinase	7
Dirofilaria immitis		
L3	Metalloproteinase	UD[a]
microfilariae	Serine proteinase	29,30
Brugia pahangi L3	ND[b]	UD[a]
Brugia malayi microfilariae	ND[b]	UD[c]
Toxocara canis L3	Metalloproteinase, probably an elastase	UD[d]
Onchocerca volvulus microfilariae adults	ND[b]	29
Schistosoma mansoni cercariae	Serine elastase	2
Strongyloides ransomi filariform larvae	Metalloproteinase	31
Haemonchus contortus juveniles	Metalloproteinase	32
Necator americanus	ND[b]	33

[a] McKerrow JH, Wong M, unpublished data
[b] Not as yet determined
[c] Bianco AE, McKerrow JH, unpublished data
[d] Robertson B, Bianco AE, McKerrow JH, unpublished data

Table 4-2. Reactivity to Purified Proteinases of Sera from Patients with Onchocerciasis or Schistosomiasis and Rabbit Antisera to Hookworm Elastase

	Sera			
Antigens	Human Anti-schisto	Human[a] Anti-oncho	Rabbit[b] Anti-hookworm	Control
Adult schisto hemoglobinase	1.05	0.62	0.22	0.20
Cercarial elastase	1.09	0.48	0.82	0.22
Hookworm elastase[b] (fusion peptide)	0.67	0.20	0.98	0.38
Hookworm elastase[b] (native protein)	0.51	0.94	0.95	0.43

Values are A_{414} from ELISA using 1 μg antigen and sera at 1 : 100 dilution
Mean of four determinations, SD = 0.09
Control = healthy American students
Schisto = pool of sera from Egyptian patients with schistosomiasis and no other parasitic infections
Oncho = Canadian tourist with onchocerciasis and no other parasitic infections
[a] Provided by Dr. Bruce Greene, Case Western Reserve University.
[b] Provided by Dr. Peter Hotez, The Rockefeller University.

Another area of interest in these enzymes is their possible use as vaccine components. For example, the hookworm elastase has two important functions in the hookworm life cycle: it probably facilitates initial larval invasion of the human host, and later it facilitates adult feeding in the intestinal wall by preventing blood coagulation. Preliminary studies suggest that vaccination with this proteinase may ameliorate the anemia that results from heavy intestinal infestation and parasite feeding (P. Hotez, personal communication).

The elastase of schistosome cercariae and similar enzymes of the invasive larvae of nematode parasites are also attractive targets for an induced immune response since they may be some of the first proteins released into the host. An immune response to such components might arrest disease before parasites reach body sites at which an immune response might contribute to pathology rather than to its prevention.

Proteases That Mediate Intestinal Wall Invasion by a Protozoan Parasite—*Entamoeba histolytica*

In contrast to the elastase-like proteases produced by helminthic larvae that invade skin or lung, the intestinal parasite *Entamoeba histolytica* produces proteases with significant collagenase activity but no elastase activity. Two major enzymes have been implicated. The first, studied by Rojkind and colleagues, is a metallocollagenase, which is apparently associated with the surface membrane of *E. histolytica* trophozoites.[10] It may be packaged in small vesicles, which ultimately are released from the surface and become associated with collagen fibers of the extracellular matrix of the lamina propria after the surface epithelium of the bowel is denuded. The second enzyme is a cysteine (thiol) proteinase secreted by trophozoites, which also degrades collagen but not with the classic 3/4–1/4 cleavage of vertebrate collagenases.[11] The cleavage pattern is more like that of cathepsin B and results in numerous fragments of various molecular weights. Also, like cathepsin B, this enzyme cleaves peptide substrates such as Z-Arg-Arg-AMC.[11] In addition to degrading collagen, this enzyme acts as a plasminogen activator by cleaving proteins on the carboxy-terminal side of positively charged amino acids. It also degrades laminin and fibronectin and can therefore cause disruption of the epithelial basement membrane of colonic mucosa and the underlying extracellular matrix of the lamina propria. The expression of both the collagenase and cysteine proteinase increases relative to the virulence of the strain of *E. histolytica* (as defined by its ability to produce hepatic abscesses in experimental animals or by cytopathic effects on cells in culture).

Like some helminthic proteinases, the cysteine proteinase of *E. histolytica* has proved to be an excellent marker of disease. Patients with amebic colitis or hepatic abscesses have high antibody titers against this enzyme, but patients with mild or asymptomatic infections do not (Keene, Wu, McKerrow, manuscript in preparation). This finding, coupled with the fact that the enzyme is present in increased quantities as the virulence of the strain increases, suggests that it is a critical virulence factor in amebic invasion of the intestinal wall. Both the cysteine proteinase and the collagenase are being studied as possible targets for amebic vaccine development.

Unfortunately, little is known about the types of proteolytic enzymes in other protozoan parasites. Thiol-dependent cysteine proteinases have been reported in African trypanosomes[12] and *Plasmodium falciparum*.[13] The catalytic properties and inhibition profile of these cysteine (thiol) proteinases suggest that they are similar to lysosomal cathepsin B, as is the ameba enzyme. The trypanosome enzyme has a much narrower pH optimum than the ameba enzyme, but the *Plasmodium* proteinase is active from pH 4.5 to 6. The function of these enzymes is unclear. Their more acidic pH optimum as compared with the thiol proteinase of *E. histolytica* suggests that they function more like lysosomal cathepsin B in terms of intracellular protein degradation. In the case of the *Plasmodium* enzyme, it has been suggested that hemoglobin degradation may be one particularly important function.[13]

Recently, it was shown that the major surface protein of *Leishmania* promastigotes (called p63) is a protease.[14] This protein is evolutionarily conserved in all *Leishmania* species studied, and the protease domain appears to be anchored to the surface membrane by a glycophospholipid. Its substrate specificity and function remain unknown at present.

PROTEINASES AS DIGESTIVE ENZYMES IN PARASITES

Cathepsin B–like thiol proteinases are also found in helminths. The best characterized of these enzymes is the so-called hemoglobinase of *Schistosoma mansoni*. Monoclonal antibodies and enzyme histochemistry have localized this proteinase in the gut of schistosomula and adult schistosomes.[15,16] It has an acid pH optimum and readily degrades hemoglobin; it is therefore thought to be the enzyme primarily responsible for the initial degradation of the hemoglobin released from lysed red blood cells. This is a major source of nutrition for the adult worms, which can survive in the human bloodstream for over 10 years.

Like cathepsin B lysosomal enzymes, the schistosome hemoglobinase cleaves specific peptide substrates with sequences such as Phe-Arg or Arg-Arg. It appears to occur in two molecular forms with nearly identical catalytic properties. These forms differ in their molecular weights (27,000 versus 30,000 to 32,000) and have sufficient tertiary structural differences to give non-cross-reacting epitopes when monoclonal antibodies are produced.[17] Two groups have purified the 30,000 to 32,000 molecular weight hemoglobinase to homogeneity.[17,18] Davis and co-workers,[19] using rabbit antisera to a hemoglobinase preparation, isolated clones from an adult schistosome cDNA library that hybridized to a 1.4-kilobase (kb) message on Northern blot analysis of adult RNA.

The adult hemoglobinase, particularly the 32,000 molecular weight species, has proved to be an excellent marker of *S. mansoni* infection. Both Dresden and co-workers (Chappell and Dresden, personal communication), and McKerrow and co-workers (Toy, et al., unpublished data) have shown that purified hemoglobinase can be used in enzyme-linked immunosorbent assay (ELISA) to distinguish infected human or animal sera from control sera. Even in human infections in which only a few worm pairs are present there is a marked antibody response to the regurgitated hemoglobinase. Furthermore, Toy, Maddison, and McKerrow (unpublished data) showed that in infected monkeys the serum antibody reactivity to hemoglobinase does not appear until 3 weeks postinfection. It is at this stage in the parasite's life cycle, when the gut is developed sufficiently, that ingestion and lysis of red cells and subsequent degradation of hemoglobin become a significant metabolic event. Since the gut of the schistosome is blind-ended, digestive products, including digestive enzymes, are regurgitated into the host's bloodstream.

The abrupt antibody response to the hemoglobinase at 3 weeks postinfection corresponds very well with the results of Dresden and Basch's assays[20] of the production of hemoglobinase activity in cultured schistosomula. Also, Northern blot analysis by Davis's group has shown that transcripts for the hemoglobinases are barely detectable in sporocyst or cercarial mRNA but increase dramatically in adult mRNA, which suggests control at the level of transcription.

Enzymes similar to the schistosome hemoglobinase in proteinase class and pH optimum have been tentatively identified in *Paragonimus ohirai*[21] and *Fasciola hepatica* (AW Senft, personal communication). There is also significant cross-reactivity in the antibody response to the hemoglobinase among all three major species of schistosome (McKerrow, et al., unpublished data). McKerrow and co-workers have shown that there is no significant cross-reactivity to the purified schistosome hemoglobinase in sera from patients with hydatid cyst, tapeworm, or protozoan infections, including *E. histolytica* (unpublished data).

THE POTENTIAL ROLE FOR PARASITE PROTEINASES IN EVASION OF THE HOST IMMUNE RESPONSE

Pathogenic bacteria have been reported to express proteinases capable of degrading immunoglobulins. *Neisseria* secretes an IgA proteinase,[22] and *Pseudomonas aeruginosa* expresses an elastase that can degrade complement factors and is thought to interfere with chemotaxis of inflammatory cells to sites of infection and possibly also to block direct killing of the organism.[23] Capron and co-workers[24] have suggested that a surface-associated proteinase of *S. mansoni* performs a similar function. They found that proteolytic enzyme activity in membrane fractions of adult schistosomes could degrade immunoglobulin G and proposed that this was one mechanism by which the organism eludes the host immune response during its long residence in the human bloodstream. Samuelson and Caulfield[25] have offered an alternative explanation for this phenomenon, namely, shedding of bound immunoglobulin via small membranous vesicles from the parasite surface. Nevertheless, there do appear to be several surface-associated peptidases or proteinases on the complex tegument of schistosomes.[26,27] The schistosome surface is folded to produce a topographically complex and large surface area much like an inside-out intestine. Surface peptidases or proteinases may, in fact, be intimately involved in parasite metabolism and possibly also may perform some type of protective function, either against the immune response or by preventing fibrin deposition.

INTERACTION OF PARASITE PROTEINASES WITH HOST PROTEASE SYSTEMS

The elaboration of proteolytic enzymes with similar substrate specificity to some host proteinases suggests possible activation of host proteinase systems and therefore amplification of proteinase-related phenomena. While as yet no example of activation of coagulation by parasite proteases has been observed, the adult hookworm produces a proteinase that appears to interfere with coagulation and increases clotting time, allowing the organism to feed.[8]

Serratia marcescens, isolated from a human corneal lesion, elaborates a proteinase that activates the Hageman factor–prekallikrein cascade, thus increasing vascular permeability.[28] The thiol (cysteine) proteinase, produced by trophozoites of *E. histolytica,* has a substrate specificity quite similar to that found in a number of host protease systems, including the Hageman factor–prekallikrein cascade. It has already been shown to act as a plasminogen activator[11] and therefore may activate plasmin at sites of tissue invasion, amplifying the tissue-destructive effect of parasite-derived enzymes. This would entail a mechanism similar to that proposed for invasion of tissue by certain malignant tumors that elaborate plasminogen-activating proteinases.

ACKNOWLEDGMENT

Supported by Grant DCB-8603689 from the National Science Foundation, Grant AI20452-04A1 from National Institute of Allergy and Infectious Diseases, and the University-wide Task Force on AIDS of the University of California.

REFERENCES

1. Stirewalt MA: *Schistosoma mansoni:* cercaria to schistosomule. Adv Parasitol 1:115, 1974
2. McKerrow JH, Pino-Heiss S, Lindquist RL, Werb Z: Purification and characterization of an elastinolytic proteinase secreted by cercariae of *Schistosoma mansoni.* J Biol Chem 260:3703, 1985
3. Banda MJ, Werb Z, McKerrow JH: Elastin degradation. In Colowick SP, Kaplan NO (eds): Methods in Enzymology (Structural and Contractile Proteins, Part C). Academic Press, Orlando, FL, in press
4. McKerrow JH, Jones P, Sage H, Pino-Heiss S: Proteinases from invasive larvae of the trematode parasite *Schistosoma mansoni* degrade connective tissue and basement membrane macromolecules. Biochem J 231:47, 1985
5. Tzeng S, McKerrow JH, Fukuyama K, et al: Degradation of purified skin keratin by a proteinase secreted from *Schistosoma mansoni* cercariae. J Parasitol 69:992, 1983
6. Landsperger WJ, Stirewalt MA, Dresden MH: Purification and properties of a proteolytic enzyme from the cercariae of the human trematode parasite *Schistosoma mansoni.* Biochem J 201:137, 1982
7. Hotez P, Trang N, McKerrow JH, Cerami A: Isolation and characterization of a proteolytic enzyme from the adult hookworm *Ancylostoma caninum.* J Biol Chem 260:7343, 1985
8. Hotez P, Cerami A: Secretion of a proteolytic anticoagulant by *Ancylostoma* hookworms. J Exp Med 157:1594, 1983
9. Pino-Heiss S, Petitt M, Beckstead JH, McKerrow JH: Preparation of mouse monoclonal antibodies directed against the preacetabular gland proteinase of *Schistosoma mansoni* cercariae. Am J Trop Med Hyg 35:536, 1986
10. Munoz MA, Calderon J, Rojkind M: The collagenase of *Entamoeba histolytica.* J Protozool 31:468, 1984
11. Keene WE, Petitt MG, Allen S, McKerrow JH: The major neutral proteinase of *E. histolytica.* J Exp Med 163:536, 1986
12. Lonsdale-Eccles JD, Mpimbaza GWN: Thiol-dependent proteases of African trypanosomes. Analysis by electrophoresis in sodium dodecyl sulphate/polyacrylamide gels co-polymerized with fibrinogen. Eur J Biochem 155:469, 1986
13. Vander Jagt DL, Hunsaker LA, Campos NM: Characterization of a hemoglobin-degrading, low molecular weight protease from *Plasmodium falciparum.* Mol Biochem Parasitol 18:389, 1986
14. Etges R, Bouvier J, Bordier C: The major surface protein of *Leishmania* promastigotes is a protease. J Biol Chem 261:9098, 1986
15. Bogitsch BJ, Dresden MH: Fluorescent histochemistry of acid proteases in adult *Schistosoma mansoni* and *Schistosoma japonicum.* J Parasitol 69:106, 1983
16. Chappell CL, Dresden MH: *Schistosoma mansoni:* Proteinase activity of "hemoglobinase" from the digestive tract of adult worms. Exp Parasitol 61:160, 1986

17. Chappell CL, Dresden MH: A monoclonal antibody and polyclonal sera from infected animals recognizes a purified proteinase secreted by *Schistosoma mansoni* adults. p. 149. In Proceedings of the Joint Meeting of the Royal and American Society of Tropical Medicine and Hygiene. Allen Press, Lawrence, KS, 1983
18. Lindquist RL, Senft AW, Petitt M, McKerrow JH: *Schistosoma mansoni:* purification and characterization of the major acidic proteinase of adult worms. Exp Parasitol 61:398, 1986
19. Davis AH, Nanduri J, Blanton R, Mahmoud AAF: J Cell Biochem, suppl., 10A:160, 1986
20. Dresden MH, Payne DC, Basch PF: Acidic thiol proteinase activity of *Schistosoma mansoni* cultured in vitro. Mol Biochem Parasitol 6:203, 1982
21. Yamakami K: Purification and properties of a thiol protease from lung fluke adult *Paragonimus ohirai.* Comp Biochem Physiol 83B:501, 1986
22. Halter R, Pohlner J, Meyer TF: IgA protease of *N. gonorrhoeae.* EMBO J 3:1595, 1984
23. Schultz DR, Miller KD: Inactivation of complement components and complement-derived chemotactic and phagocytic factors. Infect Immun 10:128, 1974
24. Auriault C, Ouiassi MA, Torpier G, et al: Proteolytic cleavage of IgG bound to the Fc receptor of *Schistosoma mansoni* schistosomule. Parasite Immunol 3:33, 1981
25. Samuelson JC, Caulfield JP, David JR: Schistosomula of *Schistosoma mansoni* clear concanavalin A from their surface by sloughing. J Cell Biol 94:355, 1982
26. Keene WE, Jeong K, McKerrow JH, Werb Z: Degradation of connective tissue matrix by larvae of *Schistosoma mansoni.* II. Degradation by newly transformed and developing schistosomula in vitro. Lab Invest 49:201, 1983
27. Auriault C, Pierce R, Cesari IM, Capron A: Neutral protease activities at different developmental stages of *Schistosoma mansoni* in mammalian hosts. Comp Biochem Physiol 72B:337, 1982
28. Matsumoto K, Yamamoto T, Kamata R, Maeda H: Pathogenesis of serratial infection: activation of Hageman factor–prekallikrein cascades and serratial protease. J Biochem 96:739, 1984
29. Petralanda I, Yarzabol L, Piessons WK: Studies on filarial antigens with proteolytic activity of collagen and elastin. (Abstract). Am Soc Trop Med Meeting, 1986
30. Scott AL, Tamashiro WK, Rao M: J Cell Biochem, suppl., 10A:174, 1986
31. Dresden MH, Rege AA, Murrell FD: *Strongyloides ransomi:* proteolytic enzymes from larvae. Exp Parasitol 59:257, 1985
32. Rogers WP: Enzymes in the exsheathing fluid of nematodes and their biologic significance. Int J Pharmacol 12:495, 1982
33. Matthews BE: Skin penetration by *Necator americanus* larvae. Parasitenkunde 68:81, 1982

5 Immunopathology and Resistance in Helminthic Infections

G. Richard Olds

Helminths are large, multicellular organisms, which reside in the bodies of over half the world's human inhabitants.[1] Worms have several characteristics that separate them from other agents that cause infectious diseases of humans. They have very complex life cycles, often with different stages present at the same time within the infected host and separate stages in intermediate hosts. Each stage may be dramatically different both morphologically and biochemically. Unlike viral, bacterial, or protozoan pathogens, helminths do not, in general, multiply within the human host. Thus, increasing parasite numbers can only occur through reinfection.[2,3]

Most clinically important helminthic infections are characterized by their chronicity. Adult worms appear to be almost totally resistant to immune attack from the parasitized host. Resistance to reinfection is at best partial and is directed toward more immature invasive larval stages of the parasite.[4] Disease or clinical illness occurs in a relative minority of infected individuals[5] and appears either to be related to intensity of infection or to be caused by the host's overexuberant immune responses directed toward one or more stages of the parasite.

The immunology of parasitic infections has mainly focused on two aspects of the host-parasite interaction. The first aspect is the host's ability to destroy new invading parasites, or resistance to reinfection;[4] this area has as its ultimate goal vaccine development. The second aspect is a better understanding of the immunopathogenesis of disease associated with infection.[5] Such insights might ultimately lead to a vaccine to prevent illness rather than to prevent infection. In the present chapter an overview will be presented of these two major areas of immunoparasitology. In a third section the interaction of these two immunologic processes will be discussed, along with their potential interference with vaccine development.

ACQUIRED RESISTANCE

Resistance to reinfection can either be innate,[6] as when schistosomes penetrate into an abnormal host,[7] or acquired.[4] Resistance in animals to various helminthic infections can be enhanced through the use of immunoadjuvants such as BCG or *Cryptosporidium parvum*.[8] This type of acquired resistance is often nonspecific in that it enhances the host's resistance to a wide variety of infectious agents and tumors.[8] Unfortunately, this form of acquired resistance tends to be of short duration and difficult to apply to humans. Most researchers have focused on the enhanced resistance acquired through past or present exposure to the parasite.[4,9] This type of acquired resistance is quite specific and often will not induce resistance even to other species, and on some occasions not even to other strains[10] of the same helminth.[11]

Teleologically, inducing partial resistance to reinfection in the parasitized host is of survival advantage to the adult worms, since it allows maintenance of a chronic infection without overpopulating the host.[12] Experimentally, animals develop enhanced resistance to a new challenge with infective larvae if they actively harbor adult worms.[9] The best evidence for this type of acquired resistance in humans comes from field epidemiology studies in which a population is constantly exposed to a given parasite.[13] In such studies the highest prevalence and the heaviest infections are usually found among the young.[13] With chronic exposure, most older individuals either are uninfected or harbor relatively few adult worms. In some field studies a subset of individuals appears to be highly susceptible to reinfection despite past or present exposure.[14,15] Such individuals do not follow the usual trend and rapidly reacquire heavy worm infections following curative chemotherapy.[16] The immunologic basis for the apparently high susceptibility of these people is unknown but may be related to their genetic background.[17,18] This is a particularly important group for the development of protective vaccines. If immune response genes present in the genome of these highly susceptible individuals prevent them from developing an appropriate protective immune response following natural infection, will they do so following artificial vaccination?

The targets of almost all forms of acquired resistance to helminthic infections are the stages of the parasite that make initial contact with the host.[4] Prior to completing their life cycle in human hosts parasites have often been adapted to life in another host (snails for schistosomiasis, biting flies for onchocerciasis, mosquitoes for some forms of filariae) or have been free-living in the environment. Although worms are adept at rapidly adapting to new environments and evading the host immune response,[19] they are often most vulnerable soon after penetration into the host.[4] Schistosomes, for example, lose their ability to be killed by many host effector mechanisms within 24 hours of penetration through mammalian skin.[20–21]

Unlike viral infections, in which neutralizing antibody mediates solid protection from reinfection, or mycobacterial infections, in which acquired resistance is entirely dependent on cell-mediated immunity, resistance to helminthic infections appears to be mediated by both T- and B-cell–dependent effector mechanisms.[4] Worm-specific, antibody-dependent parasite killing has received the greatest attention since it is the easiest to induce through vaccination, and resistance can be transferred passively by serum from one animal to another.[9] It is important, however, to point out that such a passive transfer of B cell products (worm-specific antibody) has never achieved as high a level of acquired resistance in naive animals as that found following a natural infection. Therefore vaccines that stimulate only B-cell responses may only mimic one component of naturally acquired resistance to helminths.

Vaccine development

Most vaccines against living organisms and even transplantable tumors have been developed along the same basic principles[22] (Fig. 5-1). The targets of the vaccine (parasites, cancer cells, bacteria, viral-infected cells, etc.) have antigens on their surface, which can be detected by the host immune system as foreign. These key surface antigens stimulate B- and/or T-cell immune responses, which mediate the destruction of the organism or tumor on subsequent challenge. These key antigens are depicted in Figure 5-1 and on all subsequent figures as hatched triangles. Many older vaccines (e.g., pertussis, typhoid, or cholera vaccines) have used homogenized organisms that presum-

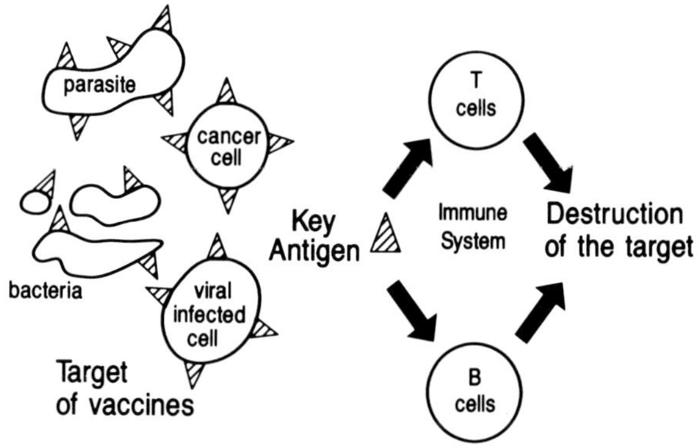

Fig. 5-1. Principles of vaccine development. The targets of potential protective vaccines are antigens (◬) found on the surface of parasites, bacteria, tumors, or virally infected cells. These key antigens are capable of stimulating the immune system to destroy the target on subsequent challenge. This stimulation could involve T or B cells or both, depending on the target's susceptibility to antibody- versus cell-mediated immunity.

ably contain these key antigens. In order to obtain a more potent vaccine with fewer side effects recent vaccines (e.g., hepatitis B vaccine or tetanus toxoid) have used purified antigens. The ideal vaccine would contain only the antigen molecules or the key structural segment (epitope) of that molecule responsible for inducing resistance to reinfection.

An understanding of the mechanisms of acquired resistance has been useful in developing effective vaccines but is not a prerequisite. Cowpox (vaccinia) was used as an effective vaccine against smallpox several hundred years before the infectious agent was even identified. As early as 1939 it was recognized that immunization of dogs with small subcutaneous injections of hookworm larvae would induce resistance.[23] Recently, this has led to a successful vaccine[24] without a clear understanding of all the mechanisms of resistance. Vaccines have been developed against a wide variety of helminths.[25–27] In addition, vaccines have also been produced that partially protect laboratory animals[28,29] cows,[30] sheep,[31] and even primates[32–34] against a challenge with infective cercariae of several schistosome species. These vaccines have all used infective larval forms of the parasite that have been attenuated by sublethal irradiation. The parasites penetrate into the host but are unable to mature and are destroyed. Recently, similar protection has been induced against schistosomes and *Brugi malayi* by using worm extracts.[35,36] All these preparations presumably have on their surface the key antigens capable of inducing immunity. Although crude in their preparation, these vaccines have established that animals and potentially humans can be protected against helminthic infections through active immunization with larval forms.

Vaccination with intact living attenuated organisms is impractical when one considers both the difficulty in producing large numbers of larvae and the logistics that would be required to deliver such a highly perishable vaccine to the third world. The best vaccine would be based on one or more key protective antigens that are capable of inducing protective immune responses. Most antihelminth vaccines presently planned for human use have therefore taken advantage of recently developed technologies in molecular and cellular biology[37] to produce highly purified antigen or subunit vaccines.

The development of new vaccines for various helminthic infections has generally taken the same scientific approaches. Since living invasive larvae both actively immunize the host and are the targets of protective immune responses, it has been assumed that the key antigen(s) are present on the larval surface. These antigens are recognized by the host immune system and ultimately mediate their destruction on subsequent challenge (as depicted in Fig. 5-1). These protective antigens can be identified and characterized by polyclonal[9] or monoclonal antibodies,[38–44] which bind to the surface of living infective larvae and mediate acquired resistance upon passive transfer into naive laboratory animals. In some experiments antigens purified by using one of these protective monoclonal antibodies induced resistance to schistosomes in mice.[45] From this point vaccine development has branched out in two different directions.

Recombinant DNA Technology

Recombinant DNA technology now allows us to mass-produce many protein molecules encoded in the DNA of living organisms[46] (Fig. 5-2). Messenger RNA is extracted from the organism and DNA copies made. These pieces of genetic information are then inserted into bacteria by use of a phage or other vector. The bacteria, containing a small piece of the worm's genetic information, are now capable of producing a foreign (worm) protein encoded by the inserted DNA. A large selection (10^6 to 10^9) of growing clones of such bacteria, each encoding a unique foreign protein, is called a *cDNA library*.[46] In Figure 5-2 these various parasite-derived molecules, each being expressed by a colony of growing bacteria, are depicted as different geometric symbols. Hopefully one of these proteins is the desired one. These protective key antigens are sought from among the millions of recombinant proteins by using the protective polyclonal or monoclonal antisera as a probe. Once identified, the genetic material that encodes for this protein can be used to produce large quantities of highly purified antigen. This molecule can be extracted from other contaminating bacterial antigens and used as a vaccine to actively induce resistance. Such an approach has already been used to express schistosome antigens of *Schistosoma mansoni*.[47] Alternatively, the DNA encoding this protein can be removed, purified, and inserted into a carrier virus such as vaccinia.[48] Immunization with this genetically altered virus not only protects the host from smallpox (the original use of vaccinia) but also induces resistance to a given helminthic infection through the presentation of protective (key) antigens on virally infected cells within the host. This approach is already being used experimentally

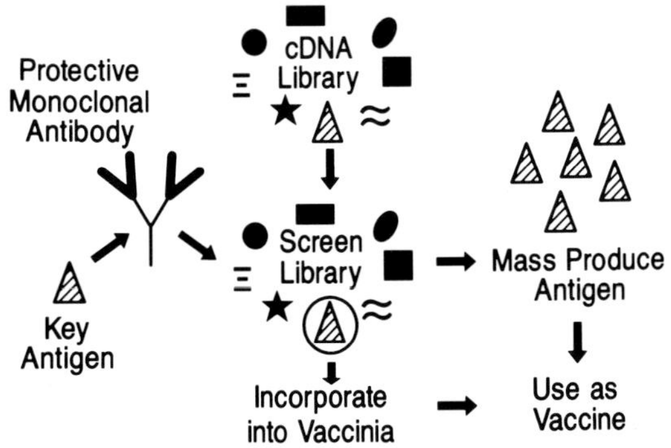

Fig. 5-2. The molecular biology approach to vaccine development. The key antigen responsible for inducing protection is identified by a monoclonal antibody. This antibody is screened for binding to the parasite and for protection of naive animals following passive transfer in vivo. The key antigen is sought from within a cDNA expression library constructed from the messenger RNA of the worm, by using the monoclonal antibody to screen the library. Once identified, the key antigen can be mass produced in bacteria or the genetic information encoding for the antigen can be inserted into a carrier virus such as vaccinia.

in vaccine strategies against some viruses and malaria.[48] Finally, the knowledge of the DNA sequence that encodes for these molecules could allow synthetic production of short protein sequences capable of inducing protection on their own.[22] Such an approach has been used successfully to protect cattle from foot-and-mouth disease.[49]

Although numerous methodologic obstacles exist for any given parasitic infection, recombinant DNA technology now exists to produce such vaccines.[46] There are, however, some problems intrinsic to this strategy. It has been easiest to construct cDNA libraries from RNA extracted from adult worms,[47] since they represent the largest stage in the life cycle and contain the most messenger RNA. Protective antigens, however, are usually contained in the invasive larval stages. Larvae are generally smaller by orders of magnitude than adult worms and are both technically difficult and expensive to obtain in large numbers. It is hoped that the RNA message that encodes for protective antigen molecules is present in both the infective larvae and adults.

A potentially greater obstacle could arise if the immunogenic part of the protective antigen is a carbohydrate or lipid rather than a protein. There is significant precedent for this with viral capsid antigens.[50] This is also a very real possibility in helminths since many potential protective antigens in schistosomiasis are glycoproteins.[51] As yet, molecular biologic technology has only been successful in producing glycoprotein molecules in large quantities. Although new technologies are being developed for translation of glycosylate recombinant molecules,[46] this could be a major technical obstacle if the protective epitope (that portion of the molecule that induces resistance) is a carbohydrate.

Finally, immunogenetics may produce another obstacle to successful vaccination. If the basis for unusual susceptibility to infection is a genetic failure to respond to the protective antigen(s), then a vaccine based on these molecules might not work in the very subset of individuals who most need vaccination. In human schistosomiasis japonica, for example, low responsiveness to worm antigens appears to be genetically controlled.[52,53]

Anti-idiotopic Vaccines

An alternative strategy for vaccine development has arisen from the theories of N. K. Jerne,[54] who has postulated that a complex interaction of complementary structures controls immune responses to antigens (Fig. 5-3). When the immune system is presented with a new antigen, the body produces an antibody (Ab_1), which binds to unique epitopes (small structural components) on the antigen molecule. This Ab_1 molecule is itself a protein and contains many structural components that it shares with other immunoglobulin molecules of the same class and isotype. It also contains structural areas that are unique to that clone of immunoglobulin molecules. One such area is its antigen binding site found in the hypervariable region, portrayed by the two dark V's on the Ab_1 molecule in Figure 5-3. Other unique structural areas on the Ab_1 molecule

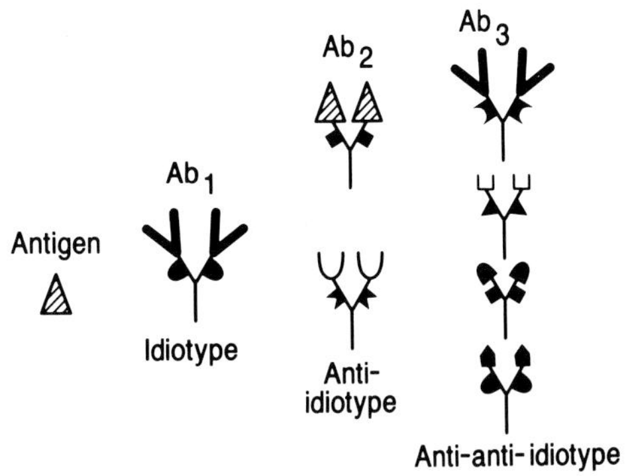

Fig. 5-3. Network interactions. Antigen (▲) stimulates the immune system to produce anti-antigen antibodies (Ab_1). These molecules contain unique structural areas, called *idiotypes,* which differentiate them from all other antibody molecules. The Ab_1 molecules stimulate a second antibody response; the Ab_2 antibodies thereby formed bind to these unique areas and are called *anti-idiotypic* antibodies. These molecules in turn can stimulate another cascade of immunoglobulin molecules, called *anti-anti-idiotypic* antibodies (Ab_3).

may be outside the antigen combining site; these are portrayed in Figure 5-3 as half circles.

Jerne postulated that the immune system could recognize these unique structural areas on the Ab_1 molecule (termed *idiotopes*) and produce a second cascade of antibody molecules (Ab_2) directed toward these structures on the first (Ab_1) antibody. These Ab_2 antibodies are termed *anti-idiotypic* antibodies and are portrayed in Figure 5-3 as belonging to two types: one binding to the antigen combining site of the Ab_1 molecule (upper Ab_2 molecule) and others binding epitopes that are not antigen combining sites (lower Ab_2 molecule). In turn, other Ab_3 and even Ab_4 molecules could be generated in the same way, forming a complex network of complementary binding proteins. This naturally occurring network has been demonstrated experimentally in many purified antigen systems[55,56] and has provided many new insights into the control of an immune response.[57]

A careful structural analysis of the original antigen and the Ab_1, Ab_2, and Ab_3 molecules demonstrates that some Ab_2 molecules are the mirror image of the original antigen (*antigen mimics*). This subset of Ab_2 molecules can be used to induce an Ab_3 response very similar to the Ab_1 response induced by the original antigen (compare the top Ab_3 molecule in Figure 5-3 with the original Ab_1 molecule). This structural interrelationship allows the artificial manipulation of the system by immunizing with Ab_2 molecules (antigen mimics) rather than with the original antigen.[58,59] This approach is particularly appealing since monoclonal antibody molecules can be produced with very restricted specificities and in unlimited quantities through hybridoma technology.[60] In this strategy, presented in Figure 5-4, the key antigen (△) is again identified by a protective monoclonal antibody, and the steps followed are the same as those used in

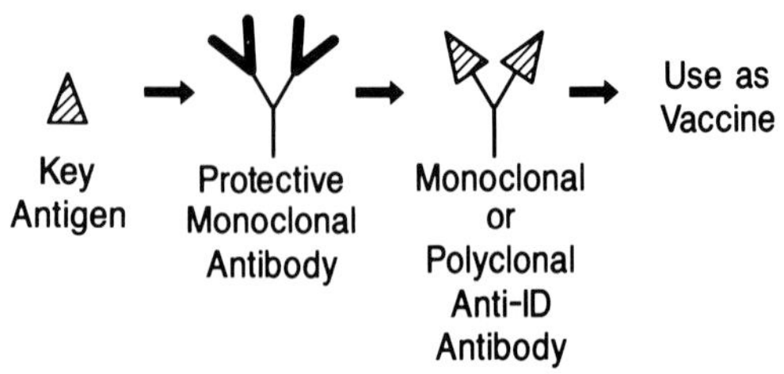

Fig. 5-4. The anti-idiotypic approach to vaccine development. The key antigen responsible for inducing protection is identified by a protective monoclonal antibody. This antibody molecule (Ab_1) is then used to produce a monoclonal or polyclonal anti-idiotypic antibody (Ab_2), which is an antigen mimic. This molecule is then used as a vaccine.

the molecular biology approach to a vaccine (Fig. 5-2). This protective monoclonal antibody is used to produce monoclonal or polyclonal anti-idiotypic antibodies that are antigen mimics; these rather than the original antigen are then used to actively immunize the host.

Anti-id vaccines have already been produced against a variety of infectious organisms[58] and recently have been used to protect primates from challenge with hepatitis B virus.[61] The use of an immunoglobulin molecule to actively immunize the host is a concept foreign to most physicians, who normally envision the use of immunoglobulin as passively protecting the host from an infectious organism and use this approach clinically with such viruses as hepatitis A and B and rabies. In general, passive protection is short-lived and lasts only as long as the foreign antibody is present in the circulation. An anti-idiotypic (anti-id) vaccine, however, stimulates the immune system (just as does the antigen itself) and induces long-term protection through production of protective Ab_3 molecules and Ab_3-bearing memory B cells. In schistosomiasis mansoni a polyclonal anti-id vaccine has already been developed by using a protective anti-schistosomula monoclonal antibody[62] and has been shown to protect rats from a challenge with *S. mansoni* cercariae.

Such an approach has several advantages over other types of vaccines. It is not necessary to isolate and purify the protective antigen and the antigen need not be a protein. For example, anti-id vaccines have been used to induce neutralizing antibody against the glycoprotein capsular antigens of the rabies virus[63] and against carbohydrate epitopes of streptococci.[64] This is a particular advantage over vaccines generated by recombinant DNA techniques. Anti-id vaccines are effective even when immunogenetics have blocked an effective Ab_1 response.[65] For example, inbred mice genetically unable to produce a particular Ab_1 antibody can be induced to produce an Ab_3 with similar specificities through use of an anti-id vaccine.[65] Anti-id vaccines against infectious organisms (e.g., Sendai virus) induce immunity that is less genetically restricted than that resulting from immunization with live virus.[66] Finally, anti-id vaccines are effective in inducing both B- and T-cell responses,[67] since idiotypic and anti-idiotypic receptors are present on both B and T cells. Anti-id vaccines have been used, for example, to stimulate T-cell responses in vitro against the Sendai virus.[66]

Anti-id vaccines do, however, have some drawbacks.[58,65] They tend to be very dose-dependent; an immune response can be depressed rather than stimulated with sub- or supraoptimal doses of anti-idiotype, and multiple immunizations are often required. Furthermore human hybridoma technology has not at present advanced to the stage at which human monoclonal anti-idiotypes can be produced in large quantities. Murine monoclonals are quite stable and can be produced in unlimited quantities, but they require the repeated injection of a foreign antigen (mouse immunoglobulin), with potential adverse allergic reactions.

Both these major approaches to antihelminth vaccines (recombinant DNA technology and anti-id vaccine) are being actively pursued against the trematode *Schistosoma mansoni* and the nematode *Brugia malayi* in experimental animals. It seems likely that within the next decade these technologies will be applied to a wide variety of other helminths and used to protect humans from schistosome and filaria infections.

IMMUNOPATHOLOGY

Fortunately for humans, only a relatively small percentage of individuals infected with helminths develop clinical disease; the vast majority tolerate parasitism without apparent symptoms.[5] For most intestinal worms symptoms develop only with heavy infection. For helminths that live within host tissues, however, disease is often related to the immune response directed toward specific stages of the parasite. In strongyloidiasis severe disease develops from rhabdoid larvae, which penetrate into host tissues.[68] In filariasis dead or dying worms evoke severe lymphangitis.[69] In onchocerciasis blindness is presumed to be initiated by the host's immune attack directed against microfilariae present in the eye,[70] while in schistosomiasis most disease is related to the granulomatous reaction directed toward parasite eggs trapped in host tissues.[71]

Most infected hosts are unable to eradicate adult helminths despite their presence within host tissues for many years.[2,3] Only when they die do they evoke a significant reaction. Adult worms produce microfilariae or eggs, which complete their life cycle. Those that are unsuccessful in getting out of the body often evoke an exuberant inflammatory immune response within the host, which forms the basis for the immunopathology and the subsequent development of clinical disease.[5] Since the host is unable to eradicate the source (adult worms), its only defense is to dampen or modulate its immune response directed at these latter stages of the parasite.

Modulation is the term used to describe this beneficial immunologic adjustment, which is commonly found in experimental animals and has been documented in humans with chronic helminth infections.[5] The ideal modulatory response would be efficient destruction of the foreign material (eggs, microfilariae, etc.) but at the minimum cost of inflammatory mediators and subsequent pathologic sequelae. Decreased immune responses to parasite antigens are common findings in chronic parasitic infections,[72–74] which often resolve with heightened responsiveness following parasitologic cure.[75] Various mechanisms for immune modulation have been described in animals and man[5,76,77]; they include antigen-specific and nonspecific suppressor T cells, suppressor adherent phagocytic cells, and inducible suppressor T cells,[78] as well as suppressive serum factors[79] such as anti-idiotypic antibodies,[80] immune complexes,[81] and circulating T-suppressor factors.[82]

As with infection, the development of clinical disease in several helminthic infections may be related to the immunogenetics of the host.[17] In schistosomiasis mansoni the development of clinical disease is found to cluster within families and to be related to the genetic background of the infected individual.[83]

Our understanding of the immunologic basis for immunopathology and its regulation has been greatly aided by new insights into the complex interactions that control the immune response to parasite antigens.[5] These include an understanding of network interactions, presented earlier, and our ability to clone the specific cells involved in the immune response.

Idiotypic (ID) and anti-idiotypic (anti-id) antibody molecules contain unique complementary structures[54] (whose interrelationship in regulation of immunoglobulin synthesis has been previously discussed). Similar structures are present on T cells.[84] These surface molecules, also referred to as *clonotypic*,[85] are unique to a specific clone of T cells and are critical to antigen-specific regulation of the immune response and are structurally related to the original antigen [i.e., they bind antigen (ID) or bind anti-antigen (anti-id)].

Our understanding of T cell interactions in health and disease has been greatly aided by recent advances in cell biology. It is now possible to produce large quantities of a single clone of T cells or to produce T-cell hybrids that secrete regulatory molecules "captured" from lymphocytes involved in the immune responses to a specific antigen.[86] In the same way that B-cell hybrids produce monoclonal antibodies, T-cell hybrids can produce and secrete lymphokine molecules.[87] These technologies have allowed characterization and production of such essential cell hormones as interleukin II and III and macrophage-activating factors.[87] Lymphokines involved in specific immune responses can be characterized in the same way.

By using this technology regulatory T-cell circuits have been well characterized in highly purified antigen systems.[88,89] A general illustration of such T-cell interactions is given in Figure 5-5. The cells responsible for eliciting and maintaining an immune response to an antigen are T-helper cells (T_H), which rapidly develop after immunization with a given antigen. These cells can be identified in mice by the surface marker L_3T_4 and in humans with the monoclonal antibody OKT_4. In addition, T-helper cells have unique surface receptors (ID-positive) present only on a specific clone of cells. They respond to presentation with antigen by secreting various lymphokines, which recruit other cells and mediate inflammation.

This exuberant immune response is damped or modified by a suppressor cell cascade,[88,89] which is initiated by a T suppressor-inducer cell (Ts_1), which also binds antigen (ID-positive). The Ts_1 cells secrete antigen-specific (also ID-positive) soluble factors (TsF), which recruit a second population of T cells (Ts_2) out of the spleen or thymus.[90] Ts_2 cells have surface structures complementary to those of Ts_1 cells, which bind ID rather than antigen. These anti-idiotypic bearing suppressor lymphocytes suppress T-helper cells either directly through secretion of anti-id T-suppressor factor(s)[90] or indirectly through recruitment of another cascade of suppressor cells (Ts_3).

In response to helminthic infection T-cell circuits appear similar. Inflammation is maintained by antigen-specific helper-T cells, which have been well characterized in schistosomiasis[76] and filariasis[91,92] and recently cloned in both diseases.[91–96] In schistosomiasis japonica T-helper cells appear to be idiotype-positive[97] and can be regulated by anti-idiotypic antisera.[80] In addition some T cells involved in the suppressor cell cascade have been defined,[76,78] as well as some of the T-suppressor factors (TsF) secreted by these cells.[98,99] The specific antigens responsible for eliciting the immune response have not been well characterized in most worm infections but in schistosomiasis appear to be glycoproteins.[100] Although our knowledge of the mechanism involved in the immune response to infection with helminths is in its infancy, it appears similar to that outlined in purified antigen systems.[88]

The long-term goal of such studies is to understand the basis for the observation that clinical disease is a relatively uncommon event in most helminthic infections. It is presumed that most infected individuals modulate exuberant and potentially pathologic immune responses as a defense against the development of severe clinical disease. Insights into these processes may allow us to identify high-risk groups in which to concentrate curative chemotherapy. Alternatively, it may be possible to develop a vaccine to prevent disease rather than

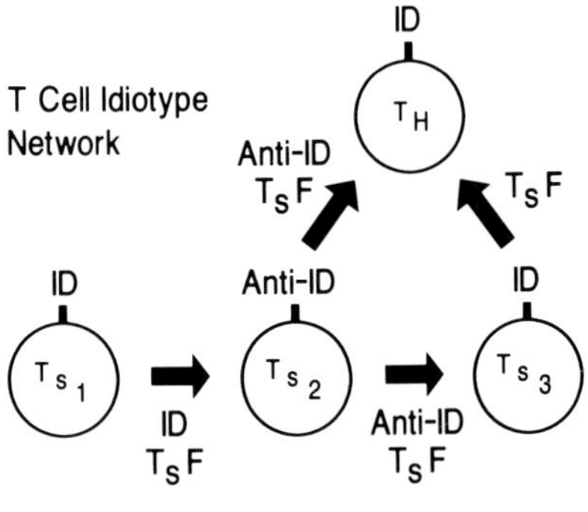

Fig. 5-5. T-cell idiotype network. T-helper cells (T_H) maintain the immune response induced by antigens. T_H cells have unique structural molecules (idiotopes or ID) on their surface, which bind antigen and differentiate them from other T_H cells. These cells are regulated by a suppressor cell cascade (Ts_1, Ts_2, and Ts_3) involving several clones of cells with complementary idiotypic and anti-idiotypic surface markers. These cells regulate each other through the local release of T-cell suppressor factors, which also carry ID and anti-id determinants.

pursuing the usual goal of infection prevention. In helminthic infections if the small subset of infected persons who develop clinical illness could be adjusted immunologically to behavior like that of the vast majority of infected but asymptomatic individuals, most helminthic infections would no longer be clinically important.

INTERACTION BETWEEN IMMUNOPATHOLOGY AND RESISTANCE

In general the two major areas of immunologic interest to the host-parasite interaction have been explored independently. Ideally we would like to induce solid protection from reinfection through vaccination; realistically, however, acquired resistance will be at best partial. Thus, even if vaccination were combined with curative chemotherapy, a significant percentage of vaccinated individuals would be reinfected. If the immunization process leads to enhanced immunopathology, then the result might be to lower the prevalence and intensity of infection but increase the number of individuals who develop clinical disease.

Immunologic manipulation could be a two-edged sword, beneficial to one aspect of the host-parasite interaction but detrimental to the other. Human studies with filariasis and schistosomiasis would suggest that those with the most suppression of immune responsiveness to worm antigens are the most heavily infected individuals.[101–104] Conflicting immune responses have been observed in animal models.[105–108] In murine schistosomiasis mansoni, acquired resistance to reinfection wanes as animals modulate their immunopathology.[105] The Lyt 2+ cyclophosphamide-sensitive T-suppressor cells responsible for smaller hepatic granulomas and lower portal pressures also suppress T-cell-mediated macrophage activation, one of the known mechanisms for acquired resistance.[4] In animal models of *Trichinella spiralis* infection, selective suppression of IgE antibody titers, presumably involved in the immunopathogenesis of disease, resulted in decreased resistance to infection.[106]

The effect on immunopathology of attenuated larval vaccines has only been examined once. Damian et al.[107] examined the effect on granuloma size around parasite eggs following vaccination of baboons with irradiated cryopreserved schistosomula. Interestingly, the vaccine did not protect against reinfection but it did induce a modulatory effect on the immunopathology. This study strongly suggests that these two immunologic processes (resistance and immunopathology) are interrelated in schistosomiasis. In *Brugia pahangi* Klei et al. have shown that immunization with *Brugia* microfilariae leads to increased resistance to infection but also increases immunopathology (lymphatic lesions).[108]

In human schistosomiasis japonica Japanese investigators have characterized a genetic D-locus phenotype associated with low responsiveness to worm antigens.[52] This low responsiveness was mediated by the development of a worm antigen–specific T-suppressor cell in these individuals.[109] This human genetic phenotype was also associated with more severe hepatic disease induced by *Schistosoma japonicum*.[110] The interrelationship between genetics, resistance, and disease in this group of individuals has yet to be determined, but low responsiveness to worm antigens and more severe disease would seem to be the worst of both ends of the immunoparasitologic spectrum.

This problem is made more complicated by the fact that there is a significant amount of antigenic cross-reactivity between various helminths and even between different stages of the same parasite. Thus it is not surprising that messenger RNA from adult schistosome worms has significant cross-reactivity with invasive larvae.[47] This may benefit the search for protective larval antigens in cDNA libraries constructed from adult worms but increases the likelihood that such antigens might be involved in the immunopathogenesis of disease.

The best evidence for potential cross-reactivity between resistance and immunopathology comes from the study of protective monoclonal antibodies. Monoclonal antibodies bind to small structural components of an individual antigen molecule (epitopes), but in schistosomiasis mansoni they have significant cross-reactivity between different stages of the parasite.[38–44] Several protective monoclonal antibodies, used to identify putative protective antigen molecules on the surface of cercariae or schistosomula, cross-react with egg antigens of the same species[41,43,44,111] (Table 5-1). It is also worth noting that not all protective monoclonal antibodies react with adult worms, which raises some questions about screening cDNA libraries constructed from this stage of the parasite. Hopefully the epitopes involved in acquired resistance will turn out to be different from those involved in the immunopathology. However, this problem remains as a potential major obstacle to vaccine development against helminths.

CONCLUSION

Our understanding of the immunology of worms has developed rapidly over the last two decades. Recent advances in biotechnology should allow us to have protective vaccines against several of the clinically most important helminthic infections of man within the next decade. In addition, our understanding of the immunopathogenesis of helminthic infection and its regulation has progressed to the point that it may soon be defined at the subcellular and molecular levels. How these two spectra of the immune response to parasitism interrelate, however, will be critical to their overall impact on disease. Such insight may allow us both to decrease disease transmission and to reduce clinical disease in the billions of individuals presently infected with helminths. On the other hand, this interrelationship may prove to be the Achilles' heel of vaccine development.

Table 5-1. Cross Reactivity of Protective Monoclonal Antibodies in Schistosomiasis Mansoni

Study	Reference	Isotype of Monoclonal	Antigen Size Detected	Reactive with		
				Schistosomula	Adult Worms	Eggs
Zodda	41	IgG_1	130,160	Yes	No	Yes
Smith	40	IgM	53,155	Yes	Yes	Yes[a]
Grzych	43	IgG_{2a}	38	Yes	Yes	N.R.[b]
Harn	44	IgG_{2b}	130,160	Yes	No	Yes
Hazdai	38	IgG_1	200	Yes	Yes	N.R.[b]
Harn	39	IgG_1	22	Yes	Yes	N.R.[b]
King	111	IgM	68	Yes	Yes	Yes

[a] Reactive with miracidia from freshly hatched eggs.
[b] Not reported

REFERENCES

1. Warren KS: Diseases due to helminths. p. 1562. In Mandell GL, Douglas RG, Bennett JE (eds): Principles and Practice of Infectious Diseases. John Wiley, New York, 1985
2. Warren, KS: The guerrilla worm. N Engl J Med 282:810, 1970
3. Warren, KS: The control of helminths: nonreplicating infectious agents of man. Annu Rev Public Health 2:101, 1981
4. Ellner JJ, Mahmoud AAF: Phagocytes and worms: David and Goliath revisited. Rev Infect Dis 4:698, 1982
5. Mahmoud AAF: Regulation of immunopathology in parasitic infections. p. 267. In Proc 8th Int Convocation on Immunology. Ogra PO, Jacobs DM (eds): S Karger, Basle, Switzerland 1983
6. Peck CA, Carpenter MD, Mahmoud AAF: Species-related innate resistance to schistosomiasis mansoni. Role of mononuclear phagocytes in schistosoma killing in vitro. J Clin Invest 71:66, 1983
7. von Lichtenberg F, Sadun EH, Bruce JI: Tissue responses and mechanisms of resistance in schistosomiasis mansoni in abnormal hosts. Am J Trop Med Hyg 11:347, 1962
8. Mahmoud AAF: Nonspecific resistance to parasitic infection. p. 99. In Cohen S, Warren KS (eds): Immunology of Parasitic Infections. Blackwell Scientific Publications, Boston, 1982
9. Dean DA: A review: *Schistosoma* and related genera: acquired resistance in mice. Exp Parasitol 55:1, 1983
10. Moloney NA, Garcia EG, Webbe G: The strain specificity of vaccination with ultraviolet attenuated cercariae of the Chinese strain of *Schistosoma japonicum*. Trans R Soc Trop Med Hyg 79:245, 1985
11. Cheever AW, Hieny S, Duvall RH, Sher A: Lack of resistance to *Schistosoma japonicum* in mice immunized with irradiated. *S. mansoni* cercariae. Trans R Soc Trop Med Hyg 77:812, 1983
12. Bradley DJ, May RM: Consequences of helminth aggregation for the dynamics of schistosomiasis. Trans R Soc Trop Med Hyg 72:262, 1978
13. Mahmoud AAF: Schistosmiasis. p. 179. In Gilles HM (ed): Recent Advances in Tropical Medicine. Churchill Livingstone, New York, 1984
14. Butterworth AE, Capron M, Cordingley JS et al: Immunity after treatment of human schistosomiasis mansoni. II. Identification of resistant individuals and analysis of their immune response. Trans R Soc Trop Med Hyg 79:393, 1985
15. Schad GA, Anderson RM: Predisposition to hookworm infection in humans. Science 228:1537, 1985
16. Dineen JK, Donald AD Wayland BM, Turner JH: Predisposition to heavy infection has been demonstrated for helminth parasites (*Nematodirus spathiger*) in sheep. Parasitology 55:103, 1965
17. Mahmoud AAF: Genetics in schistosomiasis. p. 303. In Michel F (ed): Tropical Diseases Research Series 4. A.B. Basel, Schwabe & Co., 1981
18. Abdel-Salam E, Kalik A, Meguid A, et al: Association of HLA class I antigens (A1, B5, and CW2) with disease manifestations and infection in human schistosomiasis mansoni in Egypt. Tissue Antigens 27:142, 1986
19. Cohen S: Host-parasite interface: evasion. In Warren KS, Mahmoud AAF (eds): Tropical and Geographic Medicine. McGraw-Hill, New York, 1984
20. Tavares CAP, Cordeiro MN, Mota Santos TA, Gazzinelli G: Artificially trans-

formed schistosomula of *Schistosoma mansoni*: mechanisms of acquisition of protection against antibody-mediated killing. Parasitology 80:95, 1980

21. McLaren DJ, Clegg JA, Smithers SR: Acquisition of host antigens by young *Schistosoma mansoni* in mice: correlation with failure to bind antibody in vitro. Parasitology 70:67, 1975
22. Liew FY: Review: new aspects of vaccine development. Clin Exp Immunol 62:225, 1985
23. Otto GF, Kerr KB: The immunization of dog against hookworm *Ancylostoma caninum* by subcutaneous injection of graded doses of living larvae. Am J Hyg 29D:25, 1939
24. Miller TA: Hookworm infection in man. Adv Parasitol 17:315, 1979
25. Yates JA, Higashi GI: *Brugia malayi:* vaccination of jirds with ^{60}cobalt-attenuated infective stage larvae protects against homologous challenge. Am J Trop Med Hyg 34:1132, 1985
26. Gould SE, Gomberg HJ, Bethell FH, et al: Studies on *Trichinella spiralis*. IV. Effect of feeding irradiated *Trichinella* larvae on production of immunity to reinfection. Am J Pathol 32:949, 1955
27. Tayler AER, Muller R (eds): Symposium of the British Society for Parasitology. Vaccines against Parasites. Blackwell Scientific Publications, London, 1980
28. Bickle QD, Andrews BJ, Doenhoff MJ, et al: Resistance against *Schistosoma mansoni* induced by highly irradiated infections: studies on species specificity of immunization and attempts to transfer resistance. Parasitology 90:301, 1985
29. Lewis FA, Stirewalt MA, Leef SL: *Schistosoma mansoni:* vaccination of mice with 10 Krad-irradiated, cryopreserved schistosomulas. Exp Parasitol 57:261, 1984
30. Hsu SYL, Hsu HF, Xu, ST, et al: Vaccination against bovine schistosomiasis japonica with highly x-irradiated schistosomula. Am J Trop Med Hyg 32:367, 1983
31. Bickle QD, Tayler MG, James ER, et al: Further observations on immunization of sheep against *Schistosoma mattheei* and *S. bovis* using irradiation-attenuated schistosomula of homologous and heterologous species. Parasitology 78:185, 1979
32. Hsu HF, Hsu SYL, Osborne JW: Further studies on rhesus monkeys immunized against *Schistosoma japonicum* by administration of x-irradiated cercariae. Z Tropen Med Parasitol 14:401, 1963
33. Stek M, Minard P, Dean DA, Hall JE: Immunization of baboons with *Schistosoma mansoni* cercariae attenuated by gamma irradiation. Science 212:1518, 1981
34. James ER, Otieno M, Harrison R, et al: Partial protection of baboons against *Schistosoma mansoni* using radiation-attenuated cryopreserved schistosomula. Trans R Soc Trop Med Hyg 80:378 1986
35. James SL, Pearce EJ, Sher A: Induction of protective immunity against *Schistosoma mansoni* by a nonliving vaccine. I. Partial characterization of antigens recognized by antibodies from mice immunized with soluble schistosome extracts. J Immunol 134:3432, 1985
36. Kazura JW, Cicirello HG, McCall JW: Induction of protection against *Brugia malayi* infection in jirds by microfilarial antigens. J Immunol 136:1422, 1986
37. Knopf PM, Srisastaua BS, Baker RH Jr: Application of cloning techniques to development of a synthetic vaccine against schistosomiasis. Vet Parasitol 10:255, 1982
38. Hazdai RT, Levi-Schaffer F, Brenner V, et al: Protective monoclonal antibody against *Schistosoma mansoni* antigen isolation, characterization and suitability for active immunization. J Immunol 135:2722, 1985

39. Harn DA, Mitsuyama M, Huguenel ED, Davis JR: *Schistosoma mansoni* detection by monoclonal antibody of a 22,000 dalton surface membrane antigen which may be blocked by host molecules on lung stage parasites. J Immunol 135:2115, 1985
40. Smith MA, Clegg JA, Snary D, Trejidosiewicz AJ: Passive immunization of mice against *S. mansoni* with an IgM monoclonal antibody. Parasitology 84:83, 1982
41. Zodda D, Phillips SM: Monoclonal antibody-mediated protection against *Schistosoma mansoni* infection in mice. J Immunol 129:2326, 1983
42. Taylor DW, Butterworth AE: Monoclonal antibodies against surface antigens of schistosomula of *Schistosoma mansoni*. Parasitology 84:65, 1982
43. Grzych JM, Capron M, Bazin H, Capron A: In vitro and in vivo effector function of rat IgG2a monoclonal anti-*S. mansoni* antibodies. J Immunol 129:2739, 1982
44. Harn DA, Mitsuyama M, David JR: *Schistosoma mansoni:* anti-egg monoclonal antibodies protect against cercarial challenge in vivo. J Exp Med 159:1371, 1984
45. Smith MA, Clegg JA: Vaccination against *Schistosoma mansoni* with purified surface antigens. Science 227:535, 1984
46. Davies JE: Genetic engineering and vaccines. Ann Inst Pasteur/Immunol 136D:143, 1985
47. Davis AH, Blanton RE, Rottman F, et al: Isolation of cDNA clones for differentially expressed genes of the human parasite *Schistosoma mansoni*. Proc Natl Acad Sci 83:5534, 1986
48. Perkus ME, Piccini A, Lipinskas BR, Paoletti E: Recombinant vaccinia virus: immunization against multiple pathogens. Science 229:981, 1985
49. DiMarchi, Brooke RG, Gale C, et al: Protection of cattle against foot and mouth disease by a synthetic peptide. Science 232:639, 1986
50. Alexander S, Elder JH: Carbohydrate dramatically influences immune reactivity of antisera to viral glycoprotein antigens. Science 226:1328, 1984
51. Dalton JP, Strand M, Mangold BL, Dean DA: Identification of *Schistosoma mansoni* glycoproteins recognized by protective antibodies from mice immunized with irradiated cercariae. J Immunol 136:4689, 1986
52. Sasazuki T, Ohta N, Kaneska R, Kohina S: Association between HLA haplotype and low responsiveness to schistosomal worm antigen in man. J Exp Med 152:3148, 1980
53. Kaji R, Kamijo T, Yano A, Kohima S: Genetic control of immune responses to *Schistosoma japonicum* antigen. Parasitol Immunol 4:25, 1983
54. Jerne NK: Toward a network theory of the immune system. Ann Immunol (Paris) 125c:373, 1974
55. Cosenza H, Augustin A, Julius MH: Induction and characterization of "autologous" anti-idiotypic antibodies. Eur J Immunol 7:273, 1977
56. Brown JG, Rodkey LS: Autoregulation of an antibody response via network induced auto-anti-idiotype. J Exp Med 150:67, 1979
57. Janeway CA: Manipulation of the immune response by anti-idiotype. p. 1150. In Foogerean M, Dausset J (eds): Progress in Immunology. Vol. 4. Academic Press, London, 1981
58. Dreesman GR, Kennedy RC: Anti-idiotypic antibodies: implications of internal image-based vaccines for infectious diseases. J Infect Dis 151:761, 1985
59. Kennedy RC, Melnick JL, Dreesman GR: Anti-idiotypes and immunity. Sci Am July: 48, 1986
60. De St. Groth SF, Scherdeggen D: Production of monoclonal antibodies strategy and tactics. J Immunol Methods 35:1, 1980

61. Kennedy RC, Eichberg JW, Lanford RE, Dreesman GR: Anti-idiotypic antibody vaccine for type B viral hepatitis in chimpanzees. Science 232:220, 1986
62. Grzych JM, Capron M, Lambert PH, et al: An anti-idiotype vaccine against experimental schistosomiasis. Nature 316:74, 1985
63. Reagan KJ, Wunner WH, Wikton TJ, Koprowski H: Anti-idiotypic antibodies induce neutralizing antibodies to rabies virus glycoprotein. J Virol 48:660, 1983
64. McNamara MK, Ward RE, Kohler H: Monoclonal idiotope vaccine against *Streptococcus pneumoniae* infection. Science 226:1325, 1984
65. Sacks DL, Kelsoc GH, Sachs DH: Induction of immune responses with anti-idiotypic antibodies: implications for the induction of protective immunity. Springer Semin Immunopathol 6:79, 1983
66. Ertl HCJ, Homans E, Tournas S, Finberg RW: Sendai virus-specific T cell clones. V. Induction of cytolytic T cells by an anti-idiotypic antibody directed against a helper T cell clone. J Exp Med 159:1778, 1984
67. Eichmann K, Pajewsky K: Induction of T and B cell immunity by anti-idiotypic antibody. Eur J Immunol 5:661, 1975
68. Grove DI: Strongyloidiasis. p. 373. In Warren KS, Mahmoud AAF (eds): Tropical and Geographic Medicine. McGraw-Hill, New York, 1984
69. Ottesen EA: Immunopathology of lymphatic filariasis in man. Springer Semin Immunopathol 2:373, 1980
70. Greene BM: Onchocerciasis. p. 413. In Warren KS, Mahmoud AAF (eds): Tropical and Geographical Medicine. McGraw-Hill, New York, 1984
71. Mahmoud AAF: Schistosomiasis. p. 433. In Warren KS, Mahmoud AAF (eds): Tropical and Geographical Medicine. McGraw-Hill, New York, 1984
72. Ottesen EA, Hiatt RA, Cheever AW, et al: The acquisition and loss of antigen-specific cellular immune responsiveness in acute and chronic schistosomiasis in man. Clin Exp Immunol 33:38, 1978
73. Piessens WP, Partono F, Hoffman SL, et al: Antigen-specific suppressor T lymphocytes in human lymphatic filariasis. N Engl J Med 307:144, 1982
74. Greene BM, Gbakima AA, Albiez EJ, Taylor HR: Humoral and cellular immune responses to *Onchocerca volvulus* infection in humans. Rev Infect Dis 7:789, 1985
75. Ellner JJ, Tweardy DJ, Osman GS, et al: Increased blastogenic responses to worm antigen and loss of adherent suppressor cell activity after treatment for human infection with *Schistosoma mansoni*. J Infect Dis 151:320, 1985
76. Boros DL: Immunoregulation of granuloma formation in murine schistosomiasis mansoni. Ann NY Acad Sci 465:313, 1986
77. Rocklin RE: Factors that modify the cellular immune response in patients infected by *Schistosoma mansoni*. J Immunol 125:1916, 1980
78. Ellner JJ: Suppressor cells of man. Clin Immunol Rev 1(1): 119, 1981
79. Colley DG, Hieny SE, Bartholomew RK, JA Cook: Immune responses during human schistosomiasis mansoni. III. Regulatory effect of patient sera on human lymphocyte blastogenic responses to schistosomal antigen preparations. Am J Trop Med Hyg 26:917, 1977
80. Olds GR, Kresina TF: Network interactions in *Schistosoma japonicum* infection: identification and characterization of a serologically distinct immunoregulatory auto-anti-idiotypic antibody population. J Clin Invest 76:2338, 1985
81. Kamel KA, Higashi GI: Suppression of mitogen-induced lymphocyte transformation by plasma from patients with hepatosplenic schistosomiasis mansoni: role of immune complexes. Parasite Immunol 4:283, 1982
82. Aune TM, Freeman GL, Colley DG: Production of the lymphokine soluble im-

mune response suppressor (SIRS) during chronic experimental schistosomiasis mansoni. J Immunol 135:7768, 1985
83. Salam EA, Ishaac S, Mahmoud AAF: Histocompatibility-linked susceptibility of hepatosplenomegaly in human schistosomiasis mansoni. J Immunology 123:1829, 1979
84. Eichmann K: Expression and function of idiotypes of lymphocytes. Adv Immunol 26:195, 1978
85. Meven, SC, Fitzgerald KA, Hussy RE, et al: Clonotypic structures involved in antigen-specific human T cell function: relationship to the T3 molecular complex. J Exp Med 153:705, 1983
86. Beezley BB, MH Ruddle: A critical analysis of the T cell hybrid technique. J Immunol Methods 52:269, 1982
87. Altman A, Katz DH: The biology of monoclonal lymphokines secreted by T cell lines and hybridomas. Adv Immunol 33:73, 1982
88. Paraskevas F: Pathways of T cell suppression. CRC Crit Rev Immunol 5(2):95, 1984
89. Dorf ME, Benacerraf B: Suppressor cells and immunoregulation. Annu Rev Immunol (2):127, 1984
90. Keller RH, Clavanico NJ: Suppressor macromolecules. CRC Crit Rev Immunol 5(2):149, 1984
91. Nutman TB, Ottesen EA, Fauci AS, Volkman DJ: Parasite antigen-specific T cell lines and clones: MHC restriction and B cell helper function. J Clin Invest 73:1754, 1984
92. Nutman TB, Volkman DJ, Hussain R, et al: Filarial parasite specific T cell lines: induction of IgE synthesis. J Immunol 134:1178, 1985
93. Veith M, Pestel J, Loiseau S, et al: Eosinophil activation by lymphokines and T cell clone products in the rat. Eur J Immunol 15:1244, 1985
94. Lammie PJ, Linette GP, Phillips SM: Characterization of *Schistosoma mansoni* antigen-reactive T cell clones that form granulomas in vitro. J Immunol 134:4170, 1985
95. Mak MK, Sanderson CJ: The T-cell mediated immune response to *Schistosoma mansoni* generation of stage-specific, MHC-restricted proliferative T-cell clones to soluble egg antigens. Immunology 54:625, 1985
96. Pestel J, Dissous C, Dessaint J, et al: Specific *Schistosoma mansoni* rat T cell clones. I. Generation and functional analysis in vitro and in vivo. J Immunol 134:4132, 1985
97. Kresina TF, Olds GR: Concomitant cellular and humoral expression of a regulatory cross-reactive idiotype in acute *S. japonicum* infection. Infect Immun 53:90, 1986
98. Mathew RC, Boros DL: Regulation of granulomatous inflammation in murine schistosomiasis. IV. Recruitment of antigen-specific I-J+ T suppressor cells of the granulomatous responses by an I-J+ soluble suppressor factor. J Immunol 136:1093, 1986
99. Abe T, Colley DG: Modulation of *Schistosoma mansoni* egg-induced granuloma formation. III. Evidence for an anti-idiotypic, I-J positive, I-J restricted, soluble T suppressor factor. J Immunol 132:2084, 1984
100. Lustigman S, Mahmoud AAF, Hamburger J: Glycoproteins in soluble egg antigen of *Schistosoma mansoni:* isolation, characterization and elucidation of their immunochemical and immunopathological relation to the major egg glycoprotein (MEG). J Immunol 134:1961, 1985

101. Wong MM, Guest MF: Filarial antibodies and eosinophilia in human subjects in an endemic area. Trans R Soc Trop Med Hyg 63:796, 1969
102. Piessens WP, McGreeny PB, Ratiwayanto S, et al: Immune responses in human filarial infections with *Prugia malayi:* correlation of cellular and humoral reactions to microfilarial antigens with clinical status. Am J Trop Med Hyg 29:563, 1980
103. Ellner JJ, Olds GR, Osman GS, et al: Dichotomies in reactivity to worm antigen in human schistosomiasis mansoni. J Immunol 126:309, 1981
104. Olds GR, El Kholy A, Ellner JJ: Modulatory and effector function of monocytes in heavy human schistosomiasis mansoni infection. Trans Assoc Am Physicians 45:120, 1982
105. Olds GR, Ellner JJ: Modulation of macrophage activation and resistance by suppressor T lymphocytes in chronic murine *Schistosoma mansoni* infection. J Immunol 133:2720, 1984
106. Dessein AJ, Parker WL, James SL, David JR: IgE antibody and resistance to infection. I. Selective suppression of the IgE antibody response in rats diminishes the resistance and the eosinophil response to *Trichinella spiralis* infection. J Exp Med 153:4233, 1981
107. Damian RT, Roberts ML, Powell MR, et al: *Schistosoma mansoni* egg granuloma size reduction in challenged baboons after vaccination with irradiated cryopreserved schistosomula. Proc Natl Acad Sci USA 81:3552, 1984
108. Klei TR, Enright FM, Blanchard DP, Uhl SA: Effects of presensitization on the development of lymphatic lesions in *Brugia pahangi* infected jirds. Am J Trop Med Hyg 31:280, 1982
109. Ohta N, Ninai M, Sasazuki T: Antigen-specific suppressor T-lymphocytes (Leu 2a+3a−) in human schistosomiasis japonica. J Immunol 131:2524, 1983
110. Ohta M, Nishimura YK, Iuchi M, Sasazuki T: Immunogenetic analysis of patients with post-schistosomal liver cirrhosis in man. Clin Exp Immunol 49:493, 1982
111. King CJ, Lett R, Nanduri J, et al: Isolation and characterization of a M_r 68,000 candiate antigen for schistosomiasis mansoni. Clin Res 34:522A, 1986

6 Drug Action and Drug Resistance: Antifolate Resistance in Parasitic Protozoa

Robin C. Hightower
Daniel V. Santi

Parasitic protozoa are a major cause of human suffering and mortality throughout the world. Among others, they cause debilitating diseases such as malaria, African sleeping sickness, amebic dysentery, and leishmaniasis, which are estimated to afflict hundreds of millions of individuals annually.[1] Recently, *Pneumocystis carinii* pneumonia has emerged as the most common opportunistic infection in patients with acquired immunodeficiency syndrome (AIDS).[2] Currently, there are no effective vaccines for the major protozoan diseases, and the mainstay of treatment is chemotherapy.[3,4] However, there are few effective drugs for treatment of these diseases; most agents are old and for the most part unsatisfactory, and the development of new drugs has been slow and inadequate. Development of effective chemotherapeutic agents against parasitic protozoa has been hindered by similarities in host and protozoan parasite metabolism; most agents used have had a limited specificity for the parasite and have shown toxicity to the host. Ongoing research is attempting to identify differences between host and parasite in the hope of developing antiprotozoan agents that are exquisitely targeted. To compound the problem of limited numbers of drugs, parasitic protozoa that are resistant to the available drugs have been rapidly emerging. Moreover, the mechanisms by which such organisms may become drug-resistant remain unknown. Without alternative means of treatment, the diseases caused by protozoa could become even more prevalent.

We have begun investigations on the molecular basis of drug resistance in pathogenic protozoa. In addition to providing information on fundamental aspects of protozoan biochemistry and biology, we hope such studies will provide insight on how to cope with drug resistance in these organisms. In the following discussion we describe background information on the use of antifolates in protozoan diseases and recent results from our laboratory on the mechanism of antifolate resistance in *Leishmania*.

DIHYDROFOLATE REDUCTASE AS A CHEMOTHERAPEUTIC TARGET

The enzyme dihydrofolate reductase (DHFR) is an important target for chemotherapy of microbial infections and certain neoplastic diseases. DHFR catalyzes the reduction of dihydrofolate (DHF) to tetrahydrofolate (THF), the precursor of folate cofactors required for one-carbon transfer reactions.[5] The enzyme is metabolically linked to thymidylate synthetase (TS), which catalyzes the conversion of uridylate and the folate cofactor 5,10-methylene tetrahydrofolate to thymidylate (dTMP) and DHF. This sequence of reactions, together with that catalyzed by serine transhydroxymethylase, is often referred to as the dTMP cycle (Fig. 6-1). For each mole of dTMP produced, 1 mole of THF is destroyed, and continued reduction of DHF by DHFR is necessary for continued thymidylate synthesis. Therefore, inhibition of either DHFR or TS causes a functional dTMP deficiency, which ultimately results in cell death. Furthermore, in the absence of folate cofactors, purine biosynthesis cannot occur, and additional inhibitory effects on nucleic acid synthesis are observed. These metabolic relationships indicate why inhibition of DHFR can effectively inhibit and/or kill cells, but they do not address the question of why certain DHFR inhibitors show selective toxicity for one cell or one organism versus another, thereby enabling DHFR inhibitors to be effective chemotherapeutic agents.

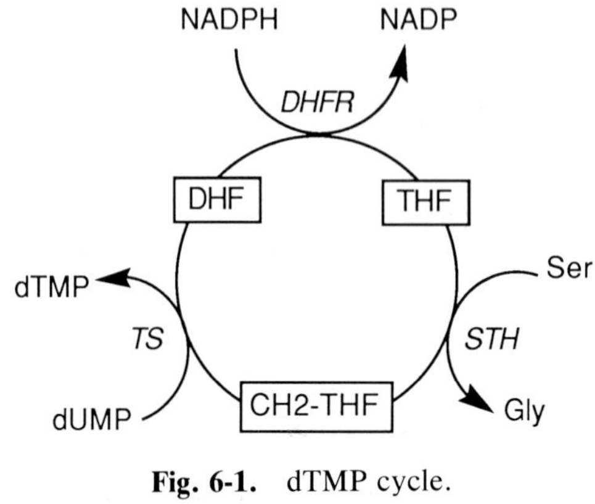

Fig. 6-1. dTMP cycle.

The most important reason for selective toxicity of certain DHFR inhibitors lies in the fact that the structure of the enzyme has diverged greatly throughout evolution.[5] For example, it is difficult to align the nucleotide sequences of the genes (or the predicted amino acid sequences of the proteins) of bacterial DHFRs with those of vertebrate DHFRs. As a result of this sequence divergence, DHFRs from different sources can show dramatic differences in their inhibition by DHFR inhibitors.

The most extensively studied and successful DHFR inhibitors are analogs of 2,4-diaminopyrimidines, which include trimethoprim (TMP) and pyrimethamine (Pyr), and analogs of 2,4-diaminopteridine such as methotrexate (MTX) (Fig. 6-2).[6] Both TMP and Pyr are paradigms of selective enzyme inhibitors. By orders of magnitude they are more potent inhibitors of DHFR from microbes than of DHFR from mammalian hosts; consequently, they are effective in treating numerous infections under conditions that are safe for the host. In contrast, MTX is an extremely potent and equipotent inhibitor of DHFR from all sources. It is used in treatment of neoplasia but shows marginal selective toxicity. DHFR inhibitors used in the treatment of microbial diseases are often combined with sulfonamides. Sulfonamides inhibit the biosynthesis of folates, which is obligatory in some organisms. In such cases these agents

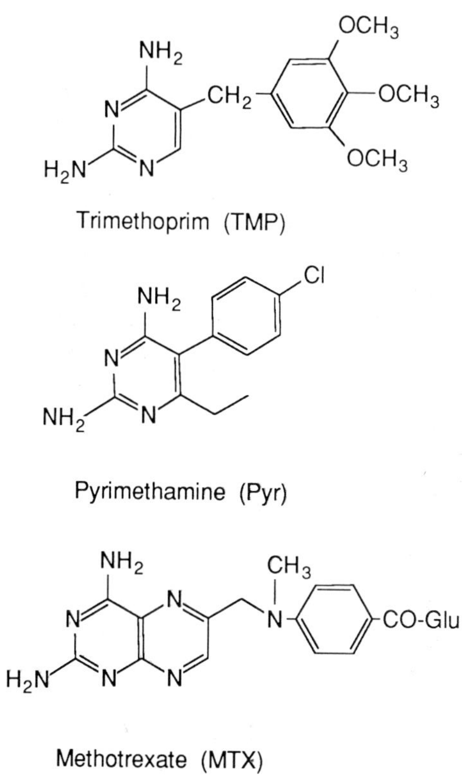

Fig. 6-2. Structures of clinically useful antifolates.

Pyr. The chicken DHFR enzyme is 12-fold less sensitive to Pyr than the *Eimeria* DHFR enzyme from unsporulated oocysts.[9] Pneumonia due to the protozoan parasite *Pneumocystis carinii* often responds favorably to the combination of TMP with sulfamethoxazole. (See Chapters 11 and 12.)

DHFR inhibitors have not been clinically useful in the treatment of other important protozoan diseases such as trypanosomiasis and leishmaniasis. Although the reason for inefficacy in most of these cases is unknown, we have recently shown that TMP and Pyr are very poor inhibitors of the *Leishmania* DHFR (unpublished results). We wish to emphasize that although TMP and Pyr are broad-spectrum DHFR inhibitors, they are not necessarily the most potent nor the most specific for any given organism. This has been well documented in one of the early studies of the effects of 2,4-diamino-5-benzylpyrimidines in various organisms but seems to have been forgotten.[10]

DRUG RESISTANCE IN PROTOZOA

Drug resistance in protozoan parasites was first described early in this century, and numerous instances of drug-resistant protozoa have been reported.[11–13] Because there are relatively few effective chemotherapeutic agents for the treatment of protozoan diseases, the emergence of drug-resistant organisms represents a particularly serious problem. Presumably if we understood the mechanisms of resistance, effective means could be developed for its prevention or circumvention.

The mechanisms by which protozoa may become resistant to drugs remain unknown, owing in part to a lack of basic understanding of the biology of protozoa and the host-parasite relationship. Parasites may show reduced sensitivity to chemotherapy for a variety of reasons. Some general mechanisms of resistance, which are often cited but which are not specific to particular organisms or drugs, include sequestered forms of the organism; differences in susceptibility of the various stages of the protozoan life cycles; dependence of drug efficacy on host immune response; and inherent variations in drug sensitivity among strains or species of parasites.[14] These explanations may all be true; however, they do not address directly the issue of true drug resistance. Truly drug-resistant organisms are stable genotypic variants, selected from a normally sensitive population by drug exposure, which survive and multiply in the presence of normally effective drug concentrations.[15] Our discussion will focus on the molecular basis for true drug resistance.

Drug resistance in protozoa has been studied most extensively in *Plasmodium,* with particular emphasis on the DHFR inhibitor Pyr.[14] Clinical resistance of *Plasmodium* to Pyr is geographically widespread. There are several possible mechanisms of resistance to DHFR inhibitors in *Plasmodium,* which include an altered DHFR, DHFR overproduction, decreased drug uptake, and enhanced uptake of folic acid or products of folate metabolism. Of these possibilities, two have been demonstrated: altered DHFR[16,17] and exogenous uptake of folate cofactors.[14] It has been suggested that an altered DHFR active site might lead to decreased affinity for the natural substrate, resulting in a less fit strain of parasites. In theory, in the absence of drug pressure the less fit strain would eventually be overgrown by sensitive parasites having normal affinity for the natural substrate. Resurgence of drug-sensitive parasites has indeed been observed when drug pressure is removed. However, some Pyr-resistant strains have been observed in geographic areas where Pyr has rarely been used, which indicates that resistant parasites may persist and cause rapid emergence of drug resistance when Pyr is introduced. Resistance to combinations of sulfa drugs and DHFR inhibitors has also been well documented.

A major advance in the study of drug resistance has been the experimental production of drug-resistant lines of *Plasmodium*.[18] These lines provide an important tool for investigating resistance to a particular compound and give insight into the mode of action of a drug. With such lines, new drugs which might circumvent resistance can be evaluated. In vitro studies allow the use of high drug concentrations and chemical mutagens. In the absence of host immunity, even minimal numbers of surviving parasites will be able to grow. Cloning of drug-resistant cells permits genetic analysis of drug resistance, and the use of cultures facilitates biochemical studies on the mechanisms of drug action and drug resistance.

Leishmania as a Model of Drug Resistance in Protozoa

In recent years we have begun investigations on the molecular basis of drug resistance in the pathogenic protozoan *Leishmania*, which may serve as a model for resistance in other protozoa. *Leishmania* was chosen because it can be grown in culture and there is background information regarding the organism's biology and biochemistry.[19] The drug targets studied have been TS and DHFR, which are present as a bifunctional protein in protozoa. Our approach included thoroughly defining the system, selecting drug-resistant mutants, and then characterizing the molecular basis of resistance.

The bifunctional TS-DHFR enzyme from *Leishmania* has been studied extensively in this laboratory; it has been purified to homogeneity and its structural and catalytic properties have been characterized.[20,21] The enzyme consists of two identical subunits with a molecular weight of about 60,000, each of which has both enzyme activities existing on two separate domains, with the DHFR domain on the blocked N-terminal part of the protein. Nucleic acid sequencing of a cDNA and genomic clone of TS-DHFR yielded additional information on the structure of the bifunctional protein.[22,23] The TS and DHFR domains are similar in size to their monofunctional counterparts in nonprotozoan organisms, and the domains are separated by a hydrophilic and unstructured junctional peptide. The *Leishmania* TS sequence is extremely homologous to the corresponding enzyme found in other sources; in contrast, the sequence of DHFR is extremely variable. The bifunctional protein may be maintained in protozoa by a selective advantage over the corresponding monofunctional counterparts. Since the genes encoding the TS and DHFR sequences are contiguous, one advantage could be coordinate regulation of these two sequential reactions in dTMP synthesis. In support of this proposal we have shown that there is substrate channeling in TS-DHFR.[20] The DHF produced by TS is channeled to DHFR faster than it diffuses into solvent, thereby providing optimal substrate utilization in sequential enzymatic reactions. The subunits of TS-DHFR are arranged to give an interesting dumbbell-shaped protein, and all four domains interact with each other (Fig. 6-3).[23] This configuration may explain the substrate channeling and reveal other interesting features of the protein. Finally, we have shown that *Leishmania* DHFR exhibits different drug sensitivities compared with human DHFR. The *Leishmania* DHFR enzyme is not effectively inhibited by TMP or Pyr, which explains why these drugs have not been successful in treatment of leishmaniasis (unpublished results). Recently, we have cloned and expressed *Leishmania* TS-DHFR in *Escherichia coli*. This will provide an abundant source of protein for future studies of the structure, function, and inhibition of the TS-DHFR protein (unpublished results).

Development of Drug-Resistant *Leishmania* Cell Lines

We have developed strains of *Leishmania* that are resistant to MTX (a DHFR inhibitor) and CB3717 (a TS inhibitor).[24,25] These lines are being studied for a better understanding of the mechanism(s) of drug resistance in these organisms. Characterization of the system has shown that some but not all features of antifolate resistance in *Leishmania* are analogous to those observed in drug-resistant mammalian cells that undergo gene amplification, a common process whereby cells become resistant to the action of selective agents.[26] A primary mechanism for resistance to the antifolate MTX in cultured mammalian cells is amplification of the gene coding for DHFR.[27] Amplified genes in mammalian cells occur in two forms: (1) on extrachromosomal double minutes (DMs), which are small acentromeric chromosomes; or (2) integrated into chromosomes as homogeneously staining regions (HSRs), which are expanded chromosomal regions giving uniform cytologic staining.[27] Unstable variants,

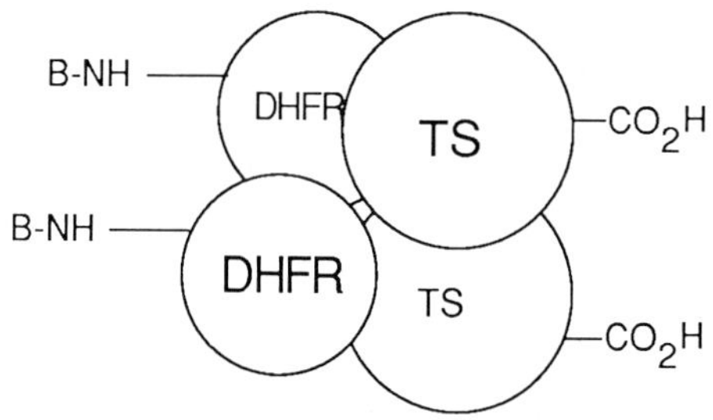

Fig. 6-3. Dimeric structure of TS-DHFR.

which are cells that lose resistance to MTX after removal of the drug from the culture medium, contain DMs, whereas stable variants contain HSRs. Thus far it has been difficult to determine the precise molecular form and organization of the amplified genes because the regions of amplified DNA are generally large and variable.

As in mammalian cells, MTX resistance in *Leishmania* can result from gene amplification, which is exemplified in our studies. The resistant organisms overproduce the drug target, the bifunctional TS-DHFR, and possess amplified regions of DNA. In two mutants these properties were unstable when the selective pressure of the drug was removed but rapidly re-emerged when the organisms were re-exposed to high concentrations of the drug. In another mutant these properties remained even after removal of the drug. Three independent resistant cell lines have been developed in our laboratory.

In our first study promastigotes of *Leishmania* were selected for resistance to MTX.[24] The MTX-resistant cell line overproduced the bifunctional protein TS-DHFR and contained an amplified-region of 30-kilobase (kb) DNA (R-region DNA).[28] The R region originated from the joining of two regions of DNA seperated by roughly 30 kb in chromosome 4 of wild-type cells, which results in a novel "junction" in the amplified DNA. The copy number of the R-region DNA was roughly 100 times that in the wild-type organisms. The conclusions drawn from this study were that cells grown in 1mM MTX for short periods of time (3 months, R10003) contained amplified R-region DNA in the form of 30-kb extrachromosomal, supercoiled circles.[28] When these resistant cells were grown in 1mM MTX for longer periods (over 11 months, R100011), most of the amplified DNA cosedimented with chromosomal DNA on cesium chloride–ethidium bromide gradients. This result, together with restriction map analysis, led us to believe that most of the amplified DNA had been incorporated into chromosomal DNA as a repetitive array of the 30-kb unit. In support of this interpretation and as seen in mammalian cells, R100011 R-region DNA remained in these cells when MTX was withdrawn, whereas R10003 R-region DNA was shown to be unstable when MTX was removed from the culture medium (in analogy with the respective properties of HSR and DM amplified DNA in mammalian cells).[28]

A second resistant cell line (CB cell line) was developed by selecting for resistance to 10-propargyl-5,8-dideazafolate, a potent and specific inhibitor of TS.[25] These cells also overproduced TS-DHFR by R-region DNA amplification. The restriction map of the R-region DNA in these cells was nearly identical to the R1000 map except for a slight increase in the size of the fragment containing the junctional region. After growth in the presence of CB3717 for 2 months, cells were shown to contain unstable R-region DNA when the drug was removed from the culture medium.

A third independent resistant cell line (D7B cell line) was developed, and cells resistant to 1mM MTX were obtained (unpublished results). The amplified R-region is larger (~37 kb) than those of the other two cell lines (~30 kb), and this size difference also involves the junctional region. The R-region DNA in D7B cells is unstable in the absence of MTX.

Demonstration of Extrachromosomal Stable Amplified DNA

The chromosomes of wild-type *Leishmania* and drug-resistant mutants have been directly examined through the technique of orthogonal-field-alternation gel electrophoresis (OFAGE) (Fig. 6-4).[29] This technique is capable of separating very large, chromosome-size pieces of DNA. The amplified DNAs in the resistant cells displayed unusual migration and were clearly extrachromosomal regardless of whether the amplified DNAs were stable or unstable. The observation that R100011 cells contain stable amplified extrachromosomal DNA is in contrast to previously reported results for cultured animal cells and to our knowledge is the first demonstration in eukaryotic cultured cells of stable amplified DNA that is extrachromosomal and circular. We have proposed that the stability observed in the stable amplified R-region DNA involves acquisition of mitotic-stabilizing sequences in DNA by small changes that are not detectable by restriction map analysis. Since transformation is not yet possible in *Leishmania*, such sequences cannot be identified directly. Instead, an assay for mitotic stability in yeast was chosen, as described below.[30]

Analysis for Mitotic-Stablizing Sequences in Stable Amplified DNA from MTX-Resistant *Leishmania*

Recent work has shown that both stable and unstable amplified DNAs in antifolate-resistant *Leishmania* are extrachromosomal circles. As observed in other systems,[31] sequences responsible for autonomous replication (ars) are

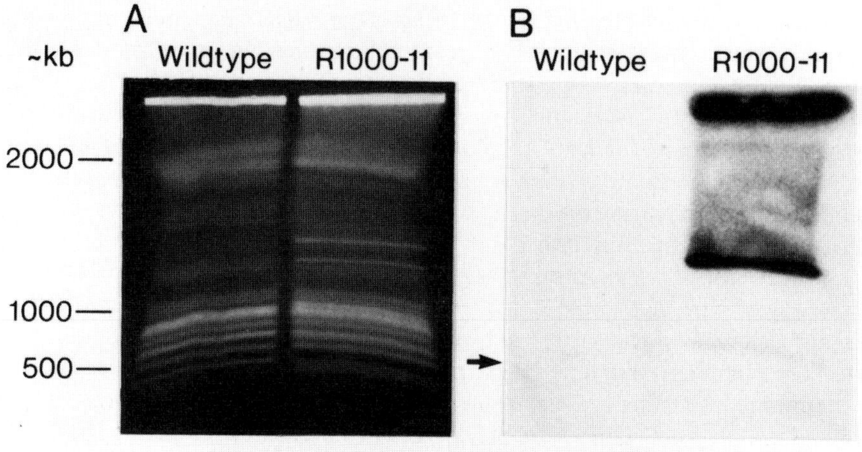

Fig. 6-4. OFAGE of wild-type and MTX-resistant *Leishmania major* DNA. (**A**) Ethidium bromide–stained. Note the two heavy staining bands in the resistant R1000-11 DNA at about 1400 kb; the lower is R-region DNA and the top is H-region DNA. (**B**) Southern blot analysis of the gel shown in A, using *Leishmania* TS-DHFR cDNA as a hybridization probe.

probably present on the extrachromosomal amplified DNAs; the copy number increases during selection and is maintained subsequently through many generations. In other eukaryotic systems the stability of plasmids and chromosomes requires mitotic stabilizing (MS) sequences such as the sequences of centromere DNA (CEN) of *Saccharomyes cerevisiae*,[32] which are responsible for accurate segregation of chromosomes during mitosis and meiosis. Copy number and size also influence the stability of plasmids in some organisms.[33,34] However, since the size and copy number of R-region DNAs are similar in unstable and stable cell lines, stability appears to be independent of these characteristics.

Yeast Studies Because transformation is not yet possible in *Leishmania*, an assay for mitotic stability in yeast was chosen for indirect identification of MS sequences in stable amplified DNA.[30] The procedure is well developed for identification of stabilizing sequences in yeasts and has been used as a heterologous system with *Caenorhabditis elegans* DNA.[35] Although there is no compelling reason to believe that CEN sequences in yeast are the same as in *Leishmania*, it is possible that mitotic-stabilizing sequences from *Leishmania* could be detected by using this heterologous system. The molecular basis of the stability is important because it may involve a common mechanism of drug resistance in parasitic protozoa, and its understanding may make possible rational approaches for "curing" organisms of resistance.

In yeast mitotic stability under nonselective growth conditions is a predictable characteristic of plasmids containing a functional centromere[32]; plasmids that do not contain a functional centromere, even when they are capable of autonomous replication, are not mitotically stable. For example, YRp7, a pBR322 derivative containing the yeast ars1 and TRP1 sequences, segregates randomly and is rapidly lost when yeast cells are grown under nonselective conditions (in a medium supplemented with tryptophan).[31] If CEN sequences are cloned into YRp7, these plasmids segregate accurately, like chromosomes, and are stably maintained under nonselective growth conditions.[30] This assay has been used to identify sequences that enhance the mitotic segregation of autonomously replicating plasmids in *C. elegans*; presumably, this in some way reflects their role in *C. elegans*.[35]

The five BglII fragments encompassing all the stable amplified DNA were cloned into YRp7, and these constructs were transformed into yeast.[36] Transformant colonies were purified and tested in the assay for mitotic stability as described.[30] If CEN sequences were present, then the plasmid construct would be maintained and the yeast transformant would be Trp+ under nonselective growth conditions. If CEN sequences were not present, then the plasmid construct would segregate randomly and be lost, resulting in a yeast transformant that would be Trp^- under nonselective growth conditions. In this experiment, the control CEN-bearing plasmid YcP50 was maintained under nonselective conditions, as expected, whereas YRp7 transformants showed rapid loss of this plasmid after growth under these conditions, also as expected, since they do not contain CEN sequences. Transformants containing constructs YRp7-4, YRp7-7, and YRp7-12, which contained respectively, the 4.1- 7.2-, and 12.8-kb BglII fragments from the R-region amplified DNA, behaved similarly to YRp7, showing rapid loss of these plasmids under nonselective growth conditions (which indicated that these constructs to not contain mitotic-stabilizing sequences). Transformants containing constructs YRp7-3A and YRp7-3B, each containing a distinct 3.3-kb BglII fragment from the R-region amplified DNA, show no apparent loss of these plasmid sequences. Since the frequency of reversion was low in the original transformation experiment, these colonies probably represent either integration or gene conversion events, or they contain extremely stable plasmids. Southern hybridization analysis detected no plasmid sequences in yeast transformed with YRp7-3A or YRp7-3B; therefore a recombination event probably occurred at the trp locus, resulting in transformants with a Trp+ phenotype but containing no pBR322 sequences.

The above results show that the constructs containing the BglII fragments encompassing all the stable amplified R-region DNA do not have sequences that will confer mitotic stability on an unstable circular DNA in yeast. However, this result does not exclude the possibility that the stable amplified DNA contains mitotic-stabilizing sequences that are operative in *Leishmania*.

Structure of Amplified DNA from Antifolate-Resistant *Leishmania*

The OFAGE technique has been used to analyze the amplified DNAs with regard to size, structure, and location in the three resistant cell lines described above.[29] From this analysis the following salient features of the amplified R-region DNAs were determined: (1) The amplified DNAs are extrachromosomal in all cell lines, whether the DNA is unstable or stable. (2) The amplified DNAs appear to be circular on the basis of their resistance to exonuclease III and their migration pattern on OFAGE. From recent experiments, it has been determined that the amplified DNAs are substrates for calf thymus topoisomerase I and T4 topoisomerase II, which shows that they are supercoiled circular DNA molecules (unpublished results). (3) In the three cell lines examined, each cell line contains at least two different species of R-region DNA. Although these species are resolved on OFAGE, the R-region DNAs from each cell line are not distinguishable by restriction map analysis. Therefore, what characteristics of these molecules determine their differential mobility on OFAGE? Several possibilities include: (1) differences in the primary structure (e.g., nucleotide insertions, deletions, or mutations); (2) differences in molecular structure (e.g., circular versus catenated DNAs) or differences in linkage numbers of relaxed state (e.g., DNA isomers); and (3) another component present on the molecule (e.g., RNA or protein).

Analysis of Amplified DNA Patterns in Cell Clones from the Antifolate-Resistant Cell Lines

With respect to the species of R-region DNA, the multiplicity of amplified DNAs in each cell line might reflect heterogeneous populations. Of these cells only the CB cells have been cloned (on agar after 7 months of growth in 50

μM CB3717), and this line has been maintained for nearly a year without subcloning. Therefore, we do not know whether the multiple R regions in a given cell line arise from different cells or are present as a heterogeneous population in the same cell. Initially, we plan to prepare clones of these cell lines by plating on agar.[37] Clones representative of each population will be grown in culture and samples prepared for OFAGE. Amplified DNA patterns from cell clones will be compared with patterns from the respective uncloned populations.

H-Region DNA from Antifolate-Resistant *Leishmania*

Another amplified DNA, referred to as H-region DNA, was found in MTX-resistant cells and has not yet been assigned a function.[29] This DNA was suggested to exist initially as an 80-kb unstable, circular DNA in R10003 cells and was thought to integrate into chromosomes in R100011 cells. No H-region DNA was observed in the other two antifolate-resistant lines, CB and D7B. Using OFAGE we have recently observed that an H-region DNA is present in multiple copy in the parental wild-type *Leishmania* strain (unpublished results). It is an extrachromosomal, circular DNA, which appears to have properties similar to those of to the R-region amplified DNAs. Thus, we now have evidence that wild-type organisms have such elements. We are interested in knowing whether such elements are related to the acquisition of resistance, and if so, how. Studies addressing these questions are now in progress.

CONCLUDING REMARKS

By developing drug-resistant strains of *Leishmania* in the laboratory and studying the molecular mechanisms of resistance, we have observed a previously unreported mechanism of drug resistance in protozoa. Current and future studies will reveal the detailed molecular mechanisms of this phenomenon. It will be important to ascertain how prevalent DNA amplification is in drug-resistant protozoa and whether similar processes occur in nature.

ACKNOWLEDGMENTS

This work was supported by U.S. Public Heath Service grant AI 19358. D. V. Santi is a Burroughs Wellcome scholar in molecular parasitology.

REFERENCES

1. Walsh JA, Warren KS: Selective primary health care. An interim strategy for disease control in developing countries. N Engl J Med 301:967, 1979
2. Morbity Mortality Weekly Rep 34:245, 1985

3. Geary TG, Jensen JB: Malaria. p. 87. In Campbell WC, Rew RS (eds): Chemotherapy of Parasitic Diseases. Plenum Press, New York, 1986
4. Wang CC: Basic principles of antiparasitic chemotherapy. p. 611. In Katzung BG (ed): Basic and Clinical Pharmacology. Lange Medical Publications, Los Altos, California, 1982
5. Blakley RL: Folates and Pterins. p. 191. In Blakley RL, Benkovic SJ (eds): Chemistry and Biology of Folates. Vol. 1. John Wiley & Sons, New York, 1984
6. Hitchings GH, Smith SL: Dihydrofolate Reductases as Targets for Inhibitors Adv Enzyme Regul 18:349, 1980
7. Garrett CE, Coderre JA, Meek TD, et al: A bifunctional thymidylate synthetase-dihydrofolate reductase in protozoa. Mol Biochem Parasitol 11:257, 1984
8. Peters W: Drug combinations. p. 225. In Peters W, Richards WHG (eds): Antimalarial Drugs. Vol. 2. Springer-Verlag, New York, 1984
9. Wang CC, Stotich RL, Poe M: Dihydrofolate reductase from *Eimeria tenella:* rationalization of the chemotherapeutic efficacy of pyrimethamine. J Protozool 22:564, 1975
10. Roth B, Falco EA, Hitchings GH: 5-Benzyl-2,4-diaminopyrimidine as antibacterial agents. I. Synthesis and antibacterial activity in vitro. J Med Pharm Chem 5:1103, 1962
11. Ehrlich P: Experimental Researches on Specific Therapeutics. Paul B. Hoeber, New York, 1909
12. Peters W: Drug resistance in trypanosomiasis and leishmaniasis. p. 309. In Ciba Foundation Symposium 20: Symposium on Trypanosomiasis and Leishmaniasis with Special Reference to Chagas' Disease. Elsevier, New York, 1974
13. Rollo IM: Drugs used in the chemotherapy of malaria. p. 1038. In Gilman AG, Goodman LS, Gilman A (eds): The Pharmacological Basis of Therapeutics. Macmillan, New York, 1980
14. Geary TG, Edgar SA, Jensen JB: Drug resistance in protozoa. p. 209. In Campbell WC, Rew RS (eds): Chemotherapy of Parasitic Diseases. Plenum Press, New York, 1986
15. Bruce-Chwatt LJ: Chemotherapy of Malaria. World Health Organization, Geneva, 1986
16. McCutchen TF, Welsh JA, Dame JB, et al: Mechanism of pyrimethamine resistance in recent isolates of *Plasmodium falciparum.* Antimicrob Agents Chemother 26:656, 1984
17. Sirawaraporn W, Yuthavong Y: Kinetic and molecular properties of DHFR from pyrimethamine sensitive and resistant *P. cabaudi.* Mol Biochem Parasitol 10:355, 1984
18. Peters W: Experimental production of drug resistance. p. 461. In Peters W, Richards WHG (eds): Antimalarial Drugs. Vol. 1. Springer-Verlag, New York, 1984
19. Berens RL, Marr JJ: An easily prepared defined medium for cultivation of *Leishmania donovani* promastigotes. J Parasitol 64:160, 1978
20. Meek TD, Garvey EP, Santi DV: Purification and characterization of the bifunctional thymidylate synthetase-dihydrofolate reductase from methotrexate-resistant *Leishmania tropica.* Biochemistry 24:678, 1985
21. Garvey EP, Santi DV: Limited proteolysis of the bifunctional thymidylate synthase-dihydrofolate reductase from *Leishmania tropica.* Proc Natl Acad Sci USA 82:7188, 1985
22. Beverley SM, Ellenberger TE, Cordingley JS: Primary structure of the gene encoding the bifunctional dihydrofolate reductase-thymidylate synthase of *Leishmania major.* Proc Natl Acad Sci USA 83:2584, 1986

23. Grumont R, Washtien WL, Caput D, Santi DV: Bifunctional thymidylate synthase-dihydrofolate reductase from *Leishmania tropica:* sequence homology with corresponding monofunctional proteins. Proc Natl Acad Sci USA 83:5387, 1986
24. Coderre JA, Beverley SM, Schimke RT, Santi DV: Overproduction of a bifunctional thymidylate synthetase-dihydrofolate reductase and DNA amplification in methotrexate-resistant *Leishmania tropica*. Proc Natl Acad Sci USA 80:2132, 1983
25. Garvey EP, Coderre JA, Santi DV: Selection and properties of *Leishmania tropica* resistant to 10-propargyl-5,8-dideazafolate, an inhibitor of thymidylate synthetase. Mol Biochem Parasitol 17:79, 1985
26. Schimke RT: Gene Amplification. Cold Spring Harbor, NY, 1982
27. Hamlin JL, Milbrandt JD, Heintz NH, Azizkhan JC: DNA sequence amplification in mammalian cells. Int Rev Cytol 90:31, 1984
28. Beverley SM, Coderre JA, Santi DV, Schimke RT: Unstable DNA amplifications in methotrexate-resistant *Leishmania* consist of extrachromosomal circles which relocalize during stabilization. Cell 38:431, 1984
29. Garvey EP, Santi DV: Stable amplified DNA in drug-resistant *Leishmania* exists as extrachromosomal circles. Science 233:431, 1985
30. Fitzgerald-Hayes M, Buhler JM, Cooper TG, Carbon J: Isolation and subcloning analysis of functional centromere DNA (CEN11) from *Saccharomyces cerevisiae* chromosome XI. Mol Cell Biol 2:82, 1982
31. Stinchcomb DT, Struhl K, Davis RW: Isolation and characterization of a yeast chromosomal replicator. Nature 282:39, 1979
32. Clarke L, Carbon J: Isolation of a yeast centromere and construction of functional small circular chromosomes. Nature 287:504, 1980
33. Lusky M, Botchan MR: Characterization of the bovine papilloma virus plasmid maintenance sequences. Cell 36:391, 1984
34. Glass RE: Gene Function. *E. coli* and its Heritable Elements. University of California Press, Los Angeles, 1982
35. Stinchcomb DT, Mello C, Hirsh D: *Caenorhabditis elegans* DNA that directs segregation in yeast cells. Proc Natl Acad Sci USA 82:4167, 1985
36. Ito H, Fukuda Y, Murata K, Kimura A: Transformation of intact yeast cells treated with alkali cations. J Bacteriol 153:163, 1983
37. Iovannisci DM, Ullman B: High efficiency plating method for *Leishmania* promastigotes in semidefined or completely-defined medium. J Parasitol 69:633, 1983

7 The Development of New Compounds for the Treatment of Parasitic Infections

Ching C. Wang

As discussed in Chapter 1, diseases caused by infections with protozoa or worms have historically been classified together as "parasitic diseases" and considered separately from diseases caused by viruses, bacteria, and fungi. This classification has a rather shaky scientific foundation because of the distant phylogenetic relationship between protozoa (single-cell organisms) and worms (multicellular organisms). However, classifying these diseases as parasitic does emphasize that they are caused by well-defined external agents, which invade the host and then live with the host in a highly adapted intimate relationship. Chemotherapeutic control of parasitic infections should in principle rely on exploiting metabolic differences between the host and the parasite, just as the antibacterial actions of many antibiotics rely on inhibiting metabolic pathways unique to bacteria, such as cell wall synthesis. However, the highly adapted relationships between parasites and hosts often make it difficult to identify and exploit such metabolic differences.

Parasites are, by definition, incapable of growing, differentiating, or even surviving in nature without invading a host. Recent advances in culture techniques have, however, permitted cultivation in research laboratories of large numbers of parasites in various rich media.[1] There is no evidence that parasites require any mysterious "growth factors" from the host, but most parasites are simply very deficient in their metabolic activities owing to the long habit of feeding on the host. Protozoa and helminths therefore require a large number of exogenous nutrients, which simpler microorganisms are able to synthesize for themselves. These metabolic pathway deficiencies should constitute the major vulnerabilities of the parasites to chemotherapeutic attack. Attempts at chemotherapeutic controls of parasitic infections can be traced as far back as the beginning of human civilization (antimalarial herbal medicines such as qinghaosu and quinine were discovered long before the Renaissance). In recent years, the prospect of developing vaccines against parasites has been exciting, but parasites have elaborate mechanisms for evading host immunity, and there has not yet been a single clinically successful vaccine. Chemotherapy will thus remain the only way of curing parasitic infections and may provide a necessary alternative to vaccines for prevention of disease.

Although the search for new agents for antiparasitic chemotherapy should have a good chance for success on theoretical grounds, reality has been just the opposite. No new antileishmanial or antitrypanosomal drug has been developed for clinical use in the last 40 years. No cure is yet available for Chagas' disease. In some diseases such as malaria, further difficulties have been presented by the development of drug-resistant parasites. The heart of the problem, however, lies in our lack of understanding of the metabolic deficiencies of parasites, which should be the focus of chemotherapeutic attack. It was not until the last two decades that many parasites began to be cultivated successfully in vitro without contaminating bacteria or host tissues and that intensive and focused biochemical studies were performed on some of the parasites.[1] These investigations have accumulated a wealth of knowledge, which could lead to the identification of new therapeutic targets. Advanced studies on the mechanism of action of new antiparasitic agents have also contributed to identification of new opportunities for antiparasitic chemotherapy.[2] In this chapter a few recent successful examples of antiparasitic drug development based on biochemical knowledge instead of empirical screening will be presented. These positive experiences could provide some guidance for rational approaches to antiparasitic chemotherapy.

COMBINATION OF SALICYLHYDROXAMIC ACID AND GLYCEROL

In the bloodstream forms of African trypanosomes, which are the causative agents of sleeping sickness in humans and nagana in cattle, each trypomastigote contains a single mitochondrion, which lacks both a functioning tricarboxylic acid cycle and a cytochrome chain for electron transport.[3] Thus, the African trypanosomes *Trypanosoma brucei* and *T. rhodesiense* are entirely dependent on glycolysis for energy production. Glycolysis generates only two molecules of ATP and two molecules of pyruvate from each molecule of glucose.[4] This relatively inefficient yield of energy has made it necessary for glycolysis to proceed at a very rapid rate in order to support the rapid cell divisions of *T. brucei,* which has a generation time of 6 to 8 hours.[5] A very rapid rate of glycolysis is apparently made possible by aggregating the first seven enzymes of the glycolytic pathway in membrane-bound, microbody-like organelles, termed the *glycosomes,*[6] which have been detected among all the trypanosomatids examined thus far.[7] The glycosome, which has a protein concentration of 340 mg/ml and steady concentrations of glycolytic intermediates in the millimolar range,[8] regenerates its NAD^+ from NADH by a dihydroxyacetone phosphate–glycerol-3-phosphate shuttle plus a glycerol-3-phosphate oxidase in the mitochondrion. Under anaerobic conditions the oxidase cannot function, and glycerol-3-phosphate cannot be oxidized back to dihydroxyacetone phosphate. Glycerol-3-phosphate therefore accumulates inside the glycosome, which eventually reverses the glycerol kinase–catalyzed reaction ATP + glycerol → ADP + glycerol-3-phosphate, generating ATP plus glycerol and providing the parasite with energy to survive.[9]

Obviously, this delicate and indispensable glycolytic system should be an attractive target for antitrypanosomal chemotherapy. It was recently demonstrated that glycerol-3-phosphate oxidase could be inhibited by salicylhydroxamic acid (SHAM) to bring *T. brucei* under the equivalent of anaerobic conditions. Glycolysis was then stopped by inhibiting the glycerol kinase with glycerol.[10,11] This combination of SHAM and glycerol causes lysis of African trypanosome bloodstream forms readily in vitro[12] and effectively suppresses parasitemia in animal models.[13] However, while glycerol is not particularly toxic to the host, the curative dose of SHAM caused 44 percent animal mortality due to acute toxicity.[14] Replacement of SHAM with a less toxic but more potent inhibitor of trypanosomal glycerol-3-phosphate oxidase is thus necessary if the combination therapy is to have clinical value. A recent finding that *p*(*n*-tetradecyloxy)benzhydroxamic acid inhibited the parasite oxidase 70 times as effectively as SHAM and was 10 to 20 times more active against trypanosomes in vitro is cause for optimism.[15] However, the rational design of a SHAM analog will have to depend on thorough characterization of the *T. brucei* glycerol-3-phosphate oxidase.

The value of viewing the glycosome as a potential target for antitrypanosomal chemotherapy can be further illustrated by the preferential inhibition of glycosomal dehydrogenases by suramin,[16] which is a well-known antitrypanosomal agent. Glycosomal enzymes have a high positive charge compared with mammalian glycolytic enzymes and have two regions rich in basic amino acids that are approximately 40Å apart in their hypothetical three-dimensional structures.[17] This may explain the strong binding of suramin (which has negatively charged sulfonyl groups separated by about 40Å) to the glycosomal enzymes. Glycosomal enzymes have thus fulfilled the criteria of being indispensable for the parasite and different from the host glycolytic enzymes, and they are therefore potential targets for therapy. Another interesting aspect of the glycosome is the aggregated state of the glycolytic enzymes inside the membrane-bound organelle.[18] Membrane-permeable bifunctional cross-linking reagents such as dimethyl suberimidate or dimethyl 3,3′-dithiobispropionimidate can cross-link all the enzymes while they are in the intact glycosome. The cross-linked enzyme complex, still maintaining the individual enzyme activities,[18] can catalyze the glycolytic chain reactions with a shortened transient time.[19] The close proximity among the glycolytic enzymes and the membrane compartmentalization of the glycolytic intermediates[8] suggests the possibility of accumulating dead end inhibitors of glycolytic enzymes to a very high concentration inside the glycosome.[19] Such a strategy might turn a relatively weak enzyme inhibitor such as 2-deoxyglucose-6-phosphate (an inhibitor of phosphoglucoisomerase) into a therapeutically effective compound.

DL-α-DIFLUOROMETHYLORNITHINE

The formation of polyamines, required for cellular proliferation and differentiation in general, is controlled by ornithine decarboxylase among eukaryotes.[20] Putrescine and spermidine, which constitute the major pool of polyamines in trypanosomatids,[21] are synthesized from ornithine but are also taken up much more slowly from extracellular sources by the parasites.[22] DL-α-Difluoromethylornithine (DFMO), a catalytic, irreversible inhibitor of ornithine decarboxylase with known antitumor activities,[23] has good activity against African trypanosomes both in vitro and in vivo.[24] It is currently undergoing clinical trials with encouraging results, especially on *Trypanosoma gambiense* infections.[25]

DFMO has been shown to deplete the intracellular polyamine pool of *T. brucei*,[26] and its antitrypanosomal activity in the experimental murine model is reversible by intraperitoneal injections of polyamines.[27] It thus appears that DFMO acts on *T. brucei* by inhibiting the ornithine decarboxylase of the parasite. This conclusion has not, however, provided an adequate explanation of why the trypanosomes are more susceptible to DFMO than the mammalian host. Apparently, the trypanosomal ornithine decarboxylase has a higher K_i value (130 μM) for DFMO[28] than does the mammalian enzyme (K_i 39 μM),[29] and should be, in theory, less sensitive to DFMO inhibition. A recent discovery of a novel glutathione-spermidine conjugage with the designated name *trypanothione* as cofactor for glutathione reductase in trypanosomatids[30] has raised the interesting suggestion that the trypanosomes may be particularly sensitive to polyamine deficiencies because of their dependence on trypanothione reductase. The oxidative stress resulting from inhibition of such an enzyme should cause lysis of the trypomastigotes, as indicated by the effect of H_2O_2 and heme on *T. brucei*.[31] However, the in vitro as well as in vivo effect of DFMO on the long slender bloodstream form of *T. brucei* is not cellular lysis but rather a transformation from the long, slender to the short, stumpy form,[26] which is presumably a dead end for the parasite in the mammalian host. Feagin et al.[32] observed that DFMO induces transcription of the mitochondrial genes encoding apocytochrome b, cytochrome c oxidase subunits, and NADH dehydrogenase subunits. Silver et al.[33] indicated that the organized packaging of kinetoplast DNA networks in trypanosomes breaks down and becomes swollen when there is a deficiency of polyamines, and this may facilitate the transcription of mitochondrial genes. Phillips and Wang[34] demonstrated that DFMO inhibited the in vitro growth of *T. brucei* procyclic forms. The inhibition was fully reversible by subsequent additions of putrescine. All the evidence thus suggests that the primary effect of DFMO on *T. brucei* is an inhibition of proliferation by the mechanism of induced differentiation to dead end stumpy forms. However, the explanations for DFMO's effect are not entirely satisfactory, and other mechanisms of action may be discovered.

In order to understand the basis of DFMO's therapeutic value, one has to make detailed comparisons between the mammalian and parasite ornithine decarboxylases. This has been difficult owing to the presence of the *T. brucei* enzyme at too low a level (~10 nmoles/hour per milligram protein) for extensive purifications and characterizations. Fortunately, the close homology between the two enzymes allowed the use of a mouse lymphoma S49 cDNA of ornithine decarboxylase as a heterologous probe to identify and clone the *T. brucei* gene encoding ornithine decarboxylase under relatively stringent conditions.[35] The sequence of the gene encoding the parasite enzyme reveals two major differences from that of the Balb/c mouse cDNA (Fig. 7-1) when the two nucleotide sequences are translated into amino acid sequences. The parasite enzyme has an extra 20 amino acid residues at the N terminus but lacks 36 amino acid residues at the C terminus compared with the Balb/c mouse ornithine decarboxylase. There is 61.8 percent homology between amino acid residues 21 to 445 of the *T. brucei* ornithine decarboxylase and residues 1 to 425 of the Balb/c mouse ornithine decarboxylase. When amino acid substitutions that are similar in charge and structure are counted as homologous, the percentage of homology reaches 90 percent. Clearly, the two enzymes are very similar to each other, which explains their similar susceptibilities to DFMO, their similar subunit molecular weights, and the hybridization between the two encoding DNA's under stringent conditions. These high degrees of homology, however, fail to explain the selective susceptibility of trypanosomes toward DFMO.

The biologic significance of the additional N-terminal amino acids in the parasite enzyme remains unclear. However, the deletion of mouse C-terminal 36-amino-acid peptide in the *T. brucei* enzyme is of considerable interest because MaCrea and Coffino[36] were able to make C-terminal deletions of the mouse ornithine decarboxylase by cDNA excision, cloning, and expression; they found that the mouse enzyme C-terminal could be deleted up to 38 amino acid residues without appreciable decrease in enzymatic activity. Furthermore, the C-terminal domain encompassing amino acids 423 to 449 of the mouse enzyme is classified as a (PEST) region of the protein with a PEST score of 5.2.[37] This means that the domain is very rich in proline, glutamic acid, serine, and threonine and is flanked by basic amino acids. Such PEST sequences are commonly found in many eukaryotic proteins that have half-lives less than 2 hours.[37] According to the PEST hypothesis, phosphorylation of the serine residues may generate Ca^{2+} binding sites in the PEST region, which may stimulate intracellular protein degradation by Ca^{2+}-activated proteases such as the cytoplasmic calpain.[37] Since *T. brucei* ornithine decarboxylase does not possess the

```
Tb    1                                                     MTTKSTPSSLSVNCLVAQTE

        21                 40                  60                  80
Tb   21 KSMDIVVNDDLSCRFLEGFNTRDALCKKISMNTCDEGDPFFVADLGDIVRKHETWKKCLPRVTPFYAVKCND
         *       *                *       *  * * *******  **  * * **************
M     1 MSSFTKDEFDCHILDEGFTAKDILDQKINEVSSSDDKDAFYVADLGDILKKHLRWLKALPRVTPFYAVKCND

               100                 120                 140                 160
Tb   93 DWRVLGTLAALGTGFDCASNTEIQRVRGIGVPPEKIIYANPCKQISHIRYARDSGVDVMTFDCVDELEKVAK
              **** ******** **** * * *** *  ******** * * **   **  ****   ** ***
M    73 SRAIVSTLAAIGTGFDCASKTEIQLVQGLGVPAERVIYANPCKQVSQIKYAASNGVQMMTFDSEIELMKVAR

                       180                 200                 220
Tb  165 THPKAKMVLRISTDDSLARCRLSVKFGAKVEDCRFILEQAKKLNIDVTGVSFHVGSGSTDASTFAQAISDSR
         ***** **** **** * *********     *  ** ** ***** ********* **  ** ** ** *
M   145 AHPKAKLVLRIATDDSKAVCRLSVKFGATLKTSRLLLERAKELNIDVIGVSFHVGSGCTDPDTFVQAVSDAR

           240                 260                 280                 300
Tb  237 FVFDMGTELGFNMHILDIGGGFPGTRDAPLKFEEIAGVINNALEKHFPPDLKLTIVAEPGRYYVASAFTLAV
         **** ** ** ** *********  *  ******  *** ** * ** *    * ****************
M   217 CVFDMATEVGFSMHLLDIGGGFPGSEDTKLKFEEITSVINPALDKYFPSDSGVRIIAEPGRYYVASAFTLAV

                   320                 340                 360
Tb  309 NVIAKKVTPGVQTDVGAHAESNAQSFMYYVNDGVYGSFNCILYDHAVVRPLPQREPIPNEKLYPSSVWGPTC
        * ****     *       *** * ********************* *  * *  * * ** * ** *****
M   289 NIIAKKTVWKEQPGSDDEDESNEQTFMYYVNDGVYGSFNCILYDHAHVKALLQKRPKPDEKYYSSSIWGPTC

        381                400                 420                 440
Tb  381 DGLDQIVERYYLPEMQVGEWLLFEDMGAYTVVGTSSFNGFQSPTIYYVVSGLPDHVVRELKSQKS
        **** ****  **** ** * *** ******   * ***** * **** *           *
M   361 DGLDRIVERCNLPEMHVGDWMLFENMGAYTVAAASTFNGFQRPNIYYVMSRPMWQLMKQIQSHGFPPEVEEQ


M   433 DDGTLPMSCAQESGMDRHPAACASARINV
```

Fig. 7-1. Comparison of the amino acid sequences between *Trypanosoma brucei* ornithine decarboxylase and Balb/c mouse lymphoma S49 ornithine decarboxylase. The identical segments between the *T. brucei* sequence (Tb) and the mouse sequence (M) are marked by asterisks (*).

PEST peptide, it may not be so readily subjected to in vivo proteolysis and may have a relatively long half-life. This was confirmed by our recent observation that *T. brucei* procyclic forms, cultured with inhibitors of protein synthesis, maintained a constant level of ornithine decarboxylase activity for at least 6 hours.[35] This lack of turnover of the parasite enzyme, which distinguishes it from the mammalian ornithine decarboxylase, may account for the trypanosome-specific effect of DFMO. While DFMO remains a potent, irreversible inhibitor of mammalian ornithine decarboxylase, metabolism of the drug in vivo coupled with continuous synthesis of new enzyme molecules quickly nullifies the drug's effect on the mammalian enzyme. However, the ornithine decarboxylase activity in *T. brucei* remains inhibited after removal of free drug molecules owing to the absence of newly synthesized ornithine decarboxylase. Thus, inhibition of the parasite's ornithine decarboxylase, reflected by polyamine deficiency in DFMO-treated *T. brucei,* together with the poor uptake of exogenous polyamines by *T. brucei* should result in inhibition of parasite proliferation.

ALLOPURINOL RIBOSIDE

One of the major metabolic deficiencies among all the parasitic protozoa studied to date is the absence of de novo synthesis of purine nucleotides.[1] Protozoa are thus dependent on purine salvage for survival. Although this deficiency may constitute a major vulnerability among the protozoan parasites, its effective exploitation for chemotherapy has not been overwhelmingly successful. This is attributable to the presence in most parasites of multiple salvage pathways, which are difficult to block with a single compound.[1] It is also due to the major roles of purine phosphoribosyl transferases in purine salvage by many of the parasites. Although some of the parasite purine phosphoribosyl transferases demonstrated different substrate specificities from the host enzyme,[38,39] a potent parasite-specific inhibitor of this family of enzymes has not yet been discovered. Other parasites rely on purine nucleoside kinases[40] or phosphotransferases[41] as their main salvage enzymes, and the same lack of specific and effective inhibitors has prevented the use of these enzymes as targets for chemotherapy. The problem can be traced to a lack of in-depth information on the enzymes, which is essential for design of specific inhibitors. Hypoxanthine-guanine-xanthine phosphoribosyl transferase of *Eimeria tenella*[38] and guanine phosphoribosyl transferase of *Giardia lamblia*[39] have been both purified to apparent homogeneity and shown to have unique substrate specificities, making the enzymes suitable as potential therapeutic targets. However, further characterizations have not been made owing to technical difficulties in preparing enough pure enzyme for the purpose. This problem will have to be resolved by gene cloning and expression in the future.

Meanwhile, some of the purine salvage enzymes in protozoan parasites appear to have more relaxed substrate specificities than the host enzymes, which allows incorporation of certain purine analogs into the nucleotide pools and nucleic acids of parasites.[42,43] Some of the purine nucleotide analogues thus formed by the parasites may be harmful to the parasites and thus have antiparasitic potential.[44] One of the most successful examples of this has been the antileishmanial activity of allopurinol, a hypoxanthine analog and a relatively nontoxic anti-gout drug for human use,[45] which was found to be actively incorporated into the RNA of *Leishmania donovani*.[44] Apparently, the hypoxanthine-guanine phosphoribosyl transferase of *L. donovani,* as well as the remaining parasite enzymes involved in converting hypoxanthine to ATP and incorporating it into RNA, all recognize allopurinol as another hypoxanthine,[44] a mistake not committed by the human enzymes. Consequently, allopurinol is converted by *Leishmania* into a series of phosphorylated purine analogs. Allopurinol ribonucleoside monophosphate is an inhibitor of guanosine monophosphate reductase and inosine monophosphate dehydrogenase, two enzymes that catalyze the interconversion of purine nucleotides. Another product of allopurinol metabolism, aminopurinol ribonucleoside triphosphate, is incorporated into RNA, thereby changing the base composition of RNA and accelerating its catabolism.[44] More recently, allopurinol riboside was found to be an even more potent antileishmanial agent.[46] It is incorporated into the leishmanial nucleotide pool by the action of the unique parasite enzyme purine nucleoside phosphotransferase.[46] Encouraging results have been obtained from recent clinical trials of allopurinol and allopurinol riboside on leishmaniasis patients.[47,48] The compound may become the first new antileishmanial agent discovered in the past 40 years. Additional analogs such as formycin B[49] and 9-deazainosine[50] have also been found to be effective antileishmanial as well as antitrypanosomal agents. The eventual future of these compounds for chemotherapy will be determined by their antiparasitic efficacies and host toxicities and by any technical difficulties in their synthesis.

Thus, the exploitation of deficiencies in purine metabolism among parasitic protozoa has succeeded for an interesting reason. The antileishmanial purine nucleosides do not act by inhibiting a crucial purine salvage enzyme and there by interrupting the purine supply for the parasite; rather, they act by being converted to a poisonous metabolite through the action of a parasite enzyme with relaxed substrate specificity compared with the analogous host enzyme. The enzyme involved, such as phosphotransferase, does not have to be of crucial importance for the survival of the parasite, and its relaxed substrate specificity is not necessarily related to the absence of de novo purine nucleotide synthesis in *Leishmania*. The differences in substrate specificity between human and *Leishmania* enzymes could be simply due to the remote phylogenetic relationship between *Leishmania* and man, and the discovery of antileishmanial purine nucleosides may have been fortuitous.

This conclusion is further verified by our recent observations on *Schistosoma mansoni,* which also is incapable of de novo synthesis of purine nucleotides.[51] Its main pathways for purine salvage are by a hypoxanthine-guanine phosphoribosyl transferase and an adenine phosphoribosyl transferase, with little interconversion between adenine and guanine nucleotides.[51] The hypoxanthine-guanine phosphoribosyl transferase has been purified to apparent homogeneity; partial characterization of the pure enzyme revealed significant differences from the mammalian enzyme.[52] Since tubercidin (7-deaza-adenosine) has long been recognized as a powerful antischistosomal drug,[53] it was a natural assumption that the active form of the drug could be either 7-deaza-adenine, which may be incorporated into RNA after salvage by adenine phosphoribosyl transferase, or 7-deazahypoxanthine, incorporated after salvage by hypoxanthine-guanine phosphoribosyl transferase. However, neither 7-deaza-adenine nor 7-deazahypoxanthine has antischistosomal activity, and 7-deaza-adenine is not a substrate of *S. mansoni* adenine phosphoribosyl transferase.[53] Instead, tubercidin is incorporated into the schistosomal nucleotide pool by the action of a very low level of adenosine kinase in the parasite.[53] The kinase apparently plays no major role in schistosomal purine salvage; its presence has no apparent correlation with the absence of de novo purine synthesis (i.e., it is not needed for the survival of *S. mansoni*). Dependence of drug action on such a dispensable enzyme may predict ready development of drug resistance. The formation of tubercidin mono-, di-, and triphosphate and its incorporation into schistosomal nucleic acids have been demonstrated,[53] but this does not prove that incorporation of the analog into RNA is the mechanism of tubericidin's antiparasitic action. Similar incorporation of formycin A into *S. mansoni* was also observed, but formycin A has no antischistosomal activity even when found in parasite nucleic acids in an amount equal to the lethal dose of tubercidin.[53] In fact, formycin A can reverse the antischistosomal activity of tubercidin,[53] which suggests that the presence of foreign purine nucleotides and their incorporation into nucleic acids are not always lethal to the parasite. For a purine nucleoside to be a potential antiparasitic agent, it must either be a transport inhibitor, or it must first be recognized as a substrate by a phosphotransferase or kinase and then its nucleotide derivatives must inhibit important biologic functions of the parasite.

In spite of the complexities of the purine salvage networks of some parasites that were described above, the concept of exploiting metabolic differences between parasites and their hosts remains valid. When the metabolism of a parasite becomes simplified to the point of depending on a single enzyme to fulfill a vital need, an effective inhibitor of such an enzymic function should kill the parasite. We have found in recent years many examples that confirm this concept among the anaerobic protozoan parasites *Tritrichomonas foetus, Trichomonas vaginalis,* and *Giardia lamblia*. These organisms are totally incapable of de novo synthesis of either purine nucleotides or pyrimidine nucleotides.[40,54–58] They obtain a particular purine or pyrimidine nucleotide with a single major salvage enzyme. For instance, *G. lamblia* acquires essentially all its adenine nucleotides by a functioning adenine phosphoribosyl transferase and all its guanine nucleotides by guanine phosphoribosyl transferase.[56] However, *T. vaginalis* has adenosine kinase and guanosine kinase to fulfill its needs.[40] *T. foetus* relies on one major enzyme, hypoxanthine-guanine-xanthine phosphoribosyl transferase to supply most of the purine nucleotides.[55] *T. vaginalis* cannot convert ribonucleotides to deoxyribonucleotides but depends on a membrane-bound enzyme, deoxyribonucleoside phosphotransferase, to provide all the four deoxyribonucleotides for DNA synthesis.[41] All these enzymes can be classified as excellent targets for antiparasitic controls. Design of specific inhibitors of these enzymes will require extensive structural characterizations, which will only be accomplished when their genes are cloned and expressed.

CONCLUSION

We have discussed only three potential antiparasitic drugs, which are either at a very preliminary stage of investigation or at the early phases of clinical trials. It is uncertain if any of them will succeed clinically. However, they share the distinction of being the first group of drugs to be discovered by some prior understanding of the metabolism of the parasites. Through further studies on the mechanisms of action of these drugs we are identifying valuable targets for antiparasitic chemotherapy. Perhaps even more importantly, the information gained by these studies has helped us to learn how to search for a therapeutic target in a parasite. There is certainly more than one way to approach such a problem. The metabolic deficiencies ordinarily associated with a parasite can provide a good starting point to look for an indispensable and unique enzyme for inhibition studies. However, such a single ideal target does not always exist; instead, there may be several alternative enzymes involved with the simplified metabolism of the parasite, which means that there is no special advantage in exploiting such metabolic defects. The antileishmanial purines and purine nucleosides thus do not owe their activities to the lack of de novo purine nucleotide synthesis in the parasite, but to the relaxed substrate specificity of the parasite's enzymes. On the other hand, the action of SHAM and glycerol on African trypanosomes is a good example of the exploitation of simplified parasite metabolism without requiring that the host and parasite enzymes have different substrate specificities. The simple glycolysis in trypanosomes makes it necessary to aggregate the glycolytic enzymes within membrane-bound microbodies in order to accelerate the glycolytic rate. The aggregation of the enzymes can be treated as an opportunity for therapeutic attack even without demonstrated differences in enzyme substrate specificities between parasite and host. The trypanosomal ornithine decarboxylase is another example demonstrating that a parasite enzyme does not have to have different substrate specificities in order to be a therapeutic target. This enzyme's lack of turnover compared with the mammalian ornithine decarboxylase makes it susceptible to DFMO. A take-home lesson from the DFMO story is that it might be worthwhile to identify all the mammalian enzymes known to have relatively short half-lives in vivo and to search for these same enzymes in parasites and examine their half-lives. Those parasite enzymes with very long half-lives may be a potential target for irreversible inhibition.

Despite the therapeutic opportunities unrelated to unique, essential enzymes in parasites discussed above, it is the unique, essential enzymes that remain the most interesting and perhaps the most challenging targets for antiparasitic chemotherapy. As discussed previously, the design of specific inhibitors will have to rely on thorough characterizations of the target enzyme, x-ray crystallography, and, eventually, design of inhibitors by computer graphics. Gene cloning and gene expression for yielding large quantities of pure, native enzyme appear to be the only means of approaching the goal. Since the goal of this endeavor is to find differences between host and parasite enzymes, cDNA's encoding the mammalian enzyme are often unsuitable as a heterologous probe for identifying the gene for the parasite enzyme. The parasite enzyme must usually be purified to homogeneity in modest quantities in order to provide some amino acid sequence data or specific antibodies before identification of the gene can be attempted. Future approaches to antiparasitic chemotherapy must thus be a combination of intensive biochemical and molecular biologic studies.

REFERENCES

1. Wang CC: Enzymes as potential targets for antiparasitic chemotherapy. J Med Chem 27:1, 1984
2. Wang CC, Pong S-S: Actions of avermectin B_{1a} on GABA nerves. p. 373. In Shep-

pard JR, Anderson VE, Eaton JW (eds): Membranes and Genetic Disease. Alan R. Liss, New York, 1982

3. Bowman IBR, Flynn IW: Oxidative metabolism of trypanosomes. p. 436. In Lumsden WHR, Evans DA (eds): The Biology of the Kinetoplastida. Vol. 1. Academic Press, New York, 1976
4. Grant PT, Sargent JR: Properties of L-glycerol-3-phosphate oxidase and its role in respiration of *Trypanosoma rhodesiense*. Biochem J 76:229, 1960
5. Brohn FH, Clarkson AB: *Trypanosoma brucei brucei:* patterns of glycolysis at 37°C in vitro. Mol Biochem Parasitol 1:291, 1980
6. Opperdoes FR, Borst P: Localization of nine glycolytic enzymes in a microbody-like organelle in *Trypanosoma brucei:* the glycosome. FEBS Lett 80:360, 1977
7. Cannata JJB, Valle E, Docampo R, Cazzulo JJ: Subcellular localization of phosphoenolcarboxykinase in trypanosomatids *Trypanosoma cruzi* and *Crithidia fasciculata*. Mol Biochem Parasitol 6:151, 1982
8. Visser N, Opperdoes FR, Borst P: Subcellular compartmentation of glycolytic intermediates in *Trypanosoma brucei*. Eur J Biochem 118:521, 1981
9. Visser N, Opperdoes FR: Glycolysis in *Trypanosoma brucei*. Eur J Biochem 103:623, 1980
10. Clarkson AB, Brohn FH: Trypanosomiasis: an approach to chemotherapy by the inhibition of carbohydrate metabolism. Science 194:204, 1976
11. Fairlamb AH, Opperdoes FR, Borst P: New approach to screening drugs for activity against African trypanosomes. Nature 265:270, 1977
12. Brohn FH, Clarkson AB: Quantitative effects of salicylhydroxamic acid and glycerol on *Trypanosoma brucei* glycolysis in vitro and in vivo. Acta Trop (Basel) 35:23, 1978
13. Evans DA, Brightman CJ, Holland MF: Salicylhydroxamic acid/glycerol in experimental trypanosomiasis. Lancet 2:769, 1977
14. van der Meer C, Versluijs-Broers JAM, Opperdoes FR: *Trypanosoma brucei:* trypanocidal effect of salicylhydroxamic acid plus glycerol in infected rats. Exp Parasitol 48:126, 1979
15. Grady RW, Bienen EJ, Clarkson AB Jr: p-Alkyloxybenzhydroxamic acids, effective inhibitors of the trypanosome glycerol-3-phosphate oxidase. Mol Biochem Parasitol 19:231, 1986
16. Fairlamb AH, Bowman IBR: Uptake of the trypanocidal drug suramin by bloodstream forms of *Trypanosoma brucei* and its effect on respiration and growth rate in vivo. Mol Biochem Parasitol 1:315, 1980
17. Borst P: How proteins get into microbodies (peroxisomes, glyoxysomes, glycosomes). Biochem Biophys Acta 866:179, 1986
18. Aman RA, Kenyon GL, Wang CC: Cross-linking of the enzymes in the glycosomes of *Trypanosoma brucei*. J Biol Chem 260:6966, 1985
19. Aman RA, Wang CC: Absence of substrate channeling in the glycosome of *Trypanosoma brucei*. Mol Biochem Parasitol 19:1, 1986
20. Pegg AE, McCann PP: Polyamine metabolism and function. Am J Physiol 243:212, 1982
21. Bacchi CJ: Content, synthesis and function of polyamines in trypanosomatids: relationships to chemotherapy. J Protozool 28:20, 1980
22. Bacchi CJ, Vergara C, Garofalo J, et al: Synthesis and content of polyamines in bloodstream *Trypanosoma brucei*. J Protozool 26:484, 1979
23. Sjoerdsma A, Schechter PJ: Commentary: chemotherapeutic implications of polyamine biosynthesis inhibition. Clin Pharmacol Ther 35:287, 1984

24. Bacchi CJ, Nathan HC, Hutner SH, et al: Polyamine metabolism: a potential therapeutic target in trypanosomes. Science 210:332, 1980
25. van Nieuwenhove S, Schechter PJ, Declercq J, et al: Treatment of gambiense sleeping sickness in the Sudan with oral DFMO (DL-α-difluoromethylornithine), an inhibitor of ornithine decarboxylase; first field trial. Trans R Soc Trop Med Hyg 79:692, 1985
26. Giffin BF, McCann PP, Bitonti AJ, Bacchi CJ: Polyamine depletion following exposure to DL-α-difluoromethylornithine both in vivo and in vitro initiates morphological alterations and mitochondrial activation in a monomorphic strain of *Trypanosoma brucei brucei*. J Protozool 33:238, 1986
27. Bacchi CJ, Nathan HC, Hutner SH, et al: Novel combination chemotherapy of experimental trypanosomiasis by using bleomycin and DL-α-difluoromethylornithine: reversal by polyamines. Biochem Pharmacol 31:2833, 1982
28. Bitonti AJ, Bacchi CJ, McCann PP, Sjoerdsma A: Catalytic irreversible inhibition of *Trypanosoma brucei brucei* ornithine decarboxylase by substrate and product analogs and their effects on murine trypanosomiasis. Biochem Pharmacol 34:1773, 1985
29. Bey P: Substrate-induced irreversible inhibition of α-amino acid decarboxylase: application to glutamate, aromatic-L-amino acid and ornithine decarboxylases. p. 27. In Seiler N, Jung MJ, Koch-Weser J (eds): Enzyme-Activated Irreversible Inhibitors. Elsevier/North Holland Biomedical Press, Amsterdam, 1978
30. Fairlamb AH, Blackburn P, Ulrich P, et al: Trypanothione: a novel bis(glutathionyl)spermidine cofactor for glutathione reductase in trypanosomatids. Science 227:1485, 1985
31. Meshnick SR, Chang K-P, Cerami A: Heme lysis of the bloodstream forms of *Trypanosoma brucei*. Biochem Pharmacol 26:1923, 1977
32. Feagin JE, Jasmer DP, Stuart K: Differential mitochondrial gene expression between slender and stumpy blood forms of *Trypanosoma brucei*. Mol Biochem Parasitol 20:207, 1986
33. Silver LE, Torri AF, Hajduk SL: Organized packaging of kinetoplast DNA networks. Cell 47:537, 1986
34. Phillips MA, Wang CC: A *Trypanosoma brucei* mutant resistant to α-difluoromethylornithine. Mol Biochem Parasitol 22:9, 1987
35. Phillips MA, Coffino P, Wang CC: Cloning and sequencing of the ornithine decarboxylase gene from *Trypanosoma brucei*: implications for enzyme turnover and selective difluoromethylornithine inhibition. J Biol Chem 262:8721, 1987
36. MaCrea M, Coffino P: Complementation of a polyamine-deficient *Escherichia coli* mutant by expression of mouse ornithine decarboxylase. Mol Cell Biol 7:564, 1987
37. Rogers S, Wells R Rechsteiner M: Amino acid sequences common to rapidly degraded proteins: the PEST hypothesis. Science 234:364, 368, 1986
38. Wang CC, Simashkevich PM: Purine metabolism in a protozoan parasite *Eimeria tenella*. Proc Natl Acad Sci USA 78:6618, 1981
39. Aldritt SM, Wang CC: Purification and characterization of guanine phosphoribosyltransferase from *Giardia lamblia*. J Biol Chem 261:8528, 1986
40. Heyworth PG, Gutteridge WE, Ginger CD: Purine metabolism in *Trichomonas vaginalis*. FEBS Lett 141:106, 1982
41. Wang CC, Cheng H-W: The deoxyribonucleoside phosphotransferase of *Trichomonas vaginalis*. J Exp Med 160:987, 1984
42. Marr JJ, Berens RL: Mini Review: pyrazolopyrimidine, metabolism in the pathogenic trypanosomatidae. Mol Biochem Parasitol 7:339, 1983

43. Rainey P, Santi DV: Metabolism and mechanism of action of formycin B in *Leishmania*. Proc Natl Acad Sci USA 80:288, 1983
44. Looker DL, Marr JJ, Berens RL: Mechanisms of action of pyrazolopyrimidines in *Leishmania donovani*. J Biol Chem 261:9412, 1986
45. Hitchings GH: Pharmacology of allopurinol. Arthritis Rheum 18:863, 1975
46. Nelson DJ, LaFon SW, Tuttle JV, et al: Allopurinol ribonucleoside as an antileishmanial agent. J Biol Chem 254:11544, 1979
47. Kager PA, Rees PH, Wellde PT, et al: Allopurinol in the treatment of visceral leishmaniasis. Trans R Soc Trop Med Hyg 75:556, 1981
48. Saenz RE, Paz H, Johnson CM, et al: Efficacy and safety of allopurinol riboside in the treatment of American cutaneous leishmaniasis. Ninth International Congress on Infectious and Parasitic Diseases, Munich, July 20–26, 1986
49. Carson DA, Chang K-P: Phosphorylation and antileishmanial activity of formycin B. Biochem Biophys Res Commun 100:1377, 1981
50. Fish WR, Marr JJ, Berens RL, et al: Inosine analogs as chemotherapeutic agents for African trypanosomes: metabolism in trypanosomes and efficacy in tissue culture. Microb Agents Chemother 27:33, 1985
51. Dovey HF, McKerrow JH, Wang CC: Purine salvage in *Schistosoma mansoni* schistosomules. Mol Biochem Parasitol 11:157, 1984
52. Dovey HF, McKerrow JH, Wang CC: Purification and characterization of hypoxanthine-guanine phosphoribosyltransferase from *Schistosoma mansoni:* a potential target for chemotherapy. J Biol Chem 261:944, 1986
53. Dovey HF, McKerrow JH, Wang CC: Action of tubercidin and other adenosine analogs on *Schistosoma mansoni* schistosomules. Mol Biochem Parasitol 16:185, 1985
54. Wang CC, Verham R, Tzeng S-F, et al: Pyrimidine metabolism in *Tritrichomonas foetus*. Proc Natl Acad Sci USA 80:2564, 1983
55. Wang CC, Verham R, Rice A, Tzeng S-F: Purine salvage by *Tritrichomonas foetus*. Mol Biochem Parasitol 8:325, 1983
56. Wang CC, Aldritt SM: Purine salvage networks in *Giardia lamblia*. J Exp Med 158:1703, 1983
57. Wang CC, Cheng H-W: Salvage of pyrimidine nucleosides by *Trichomonas vaginalis*. Mol Biochem Parasitol 10:171, 1984
58. Aldritt SM, Tien P, Wang CC: Pyrimidine salvage in *Giardia lamblia*. J Exp Med 161:437, 1985

8 The Biology of *Cryptosporidium*

William L. Current

Protozoans of the genus *Cryptosporidium* are small (2 to 6 μm, depending on stage in life cycle) coccidian parasites, which may infect the mucosal epithelium of a variety of animals, including humans.[1–3] Infections with *Cryptosporidium* spp. were considered rare in animals, and in humans they were thought to be the result of an opportunistic pathogen of immunodeficient persons outside its normal range.[4–8] Our concept of this intracellular protozoan parasite has changed within the past five years to that of an important, widespread cause of gastrointestinal illness in several animal species, especially calves, lambs, and humans.[1–3]

At least one species of this protozoan genus may produce mild to severe diarrhea, lasting from several days to more than a month,[9,10] in immunocompetent human beings. In immunodeficient persons, especially those with the acquired immune deficiency syndrome (AIDS), cryptosporidiosis may cause a prolonged, life-threatening, cholera-like illness.[9,11] Diarrhea in immunodeficient patients often becomes irreversible, and the fluid loss may be excessive; 3 to 6 L/day is common, and as much as 17 L of watery feces per day has been reported.[12] Recent reports of respiratory[13] and biliary[14] infections demonstrate that this intracellular protozoan is not confined to the gastrointestinal tract of immunodeficient persons. To date, no effective therapy has been found[12]; thus, the finding of cryptosporidiosis in the immunodeficient host often carries an ominous prognosis.

No attempt has been made in this chapter to discuss all the data contained in the numerous publications on *Cryptosporidium* that have appeared since 1982; however, it does address much of our present understanding of the biology of this protozoan parasite and the diseases it produces in immunocompetent and immunodeficient hosts.

TAXONOMY OF *CRYPTOSPORIDIUM* SPECIES

The taxonomy of *Cryptosporidium parvum,* the species thought to be responsible for diarrheal illness in several mammalian hosts, and its relationship to some other protozoans that may infect man is shown in Table 8-1. Clarke[15] may have been the first to observe a species of *Cryptosporidium*—the minute organisms he called *swarm spores* lying free upon the gastric epithelium of mice may have been motile merozoites of *C. muris,* the type species named and then described 15 years later by Tyzzer.[16,17] During the ensuing 75 years approximately 18 other species of *Cryptosporidium* were named,[18] primarily on the assumption that they were host-specific like the closely related coccidia assigned to the genus *Eimeria*.

Cross-transmission studies[18] demonstrating little or no host specificity for isolates of this protozoan obtained from calves, lambs, and humans prompted several investigators to consider *Cryptosporidium* as a single-species genus.[2,19] More recently, Levine[18] consolidated the 19 named organisms into four species, one each for those infecting fish (*C. nasorum*), reptiles (*C. crotali*), birds (*C. meleagradis*), and mammals (*C. muris*). The validity of this consolidation should be questioned for several reasons. The original description of *C. crotali*[20] was based on oocysts in the feces of a snake. However, from the standpoint of morphology, these resistant stages were probably sporocysts of a *Sarcocystis* sp.[21,22] Also, oocysts indistinguishable from those of *C. muris* and *C. parvum,* both originally described from mice by Tyzzer,[17,23] have been recovered from calves.[24] On the basis of oocyst morphology it is *C. parvum,* not *C. muris,* that is associated with all the previously well-documented cases of cryptosporidiosis in mammals.[24] Thus, at the present time the species producing clinical illness in man and other mammals should be referred to as *C. parvum,* or as *Cryptosporidium* sp. if there is not enough morphologic and/or life cycle data to relate it to Tyzzer's description.[23] This conservative approach is used in the present communication; however, the author realizes that careful studies of the proposed differences in host specificity, sites of infection, and pathogenicity among mammalian isolates[1-3] may result in the validation of additional species. Along with this conservative approach, it is preferable to designate a particular parasite as an isolate rather than a strain.

LIFE CYCLE OF *CRYPTOSPORIDIUM*

Just 3 years after his 1907 report[16] of *C. muris* in the gastric glands of laboratory mice, Tyzzer presented much of its life cycle in amazing detail.[17] The most remarkable features of this classic investigation, as well as his subsequent report[23] of *C. parvum* infecting the small intestine of laboratory mice, included detailed descriptions of excystation, a single generation of schizogony, micro- and macrogametogony, fertilization, oocyst wall formation, sporogony, and experimental transmission by oocysts. Approximately 60 years later Tyzzer's comment,[17] "It is remarkable that an organism so minute

Table 8-1. Taxonomic Relationships among Some Parasitic Protozoa Infecting Human

Taxon	*Giardia lamblia*	*Entamoeba histolytica*	*Toxoplasma gondii*	*Cryptosporidium parvum*	*Plasmodium vivax*
Phylum	Sarcomastigophora	Sarcomastigophora	Apicomplexa	Apicomplexa	Apicomplexa
Subphylum	Mastigophora	Sarcodina	—	—	—
Class	Zoomastigophorea	Lobosea	Sporozoasida	Sporozoasida	Sporozoasida
Subclass	—	Gymnamoebia	Coccidiasina	Coccidiasina	Coccidiasina
Order	Diplomonadida	Amoeba	Eucoccidiorida	Eucoccidiorida	Eucoccidiorida
Suborder	Diplomonadina	Tubulina	Eimeriorina	Eimeriorina	Haemospororina
Family	Hexamitidae	Entamoebidae	Sarcocystidae	Cryptosporidiidae	Plasmodiidae

(Adapted from Lee, Hunter, and Bovee,[104] with permission.)

should show so great structural variation and present modes of propagation analogous to those found in organisms very much larger,'' was confirmed by an ultrastructural study of *C. wrairi* in the guinea pig.[25] Vetterling et al.[22,25] did not find oocysts in the feces of infected guinea pigs; thus, they suggested that the oocysts described by Tyzzer were second-generation meronts containing four merozoites. This discrepancy was resolved in part when Pholenz et al.[26] studying naturally infected calves, and Iseki[27] investigating naturally infected cats, found sporulated oocysts free in the feces and within enterocytes. In a more recent study Angus et al.[28] reported that their isolate of *Cryptosporidium* sp. produced oocysts in experimentally infected guinea pigs. They suggested that the extended, incomplete, endogenous development of *C. wrairi* reported by Vetterling et al.[22] was the behavior of an aberrant strain of the parasite in a species that is perhaps not the natural host. Although the existence of oocysts was no longer questioned by these authors, they could not agree on the number of generations of meronts.

The studies discussed above, along with recent investigations of the development of human and calf isolates of *C. parvum* in mice,[3,29] chicken embryos,[30] and cell culture[31] have revealed that, like the other true coccidia (Eimeriorina), the life cycle of *Cryptosporidium* sp. can be divided into six major developmental events: excystation (release of infective sporozoites from oocysts), merogony (asexual replication), gametogony (gamete formation), fertilization, oocyst wall formation, and sporogony (sporozoite formation). The life cycle of *C. parvum* is illustrated in Figure 8-1, and photomicrographs and transmission electron micrographs of developmental stages of this parasite in the mucosal epithelium of the ileum of experimentally infected mice are shown in Figures 8-2 through 8-16. More complete accounts of the life cycle of *C. parvum* in experimentally infected suckling mice have been published,[32–34] and a discussion of the life cycle events that have been confused or misinterpreted in the literature is presented in a review paper.[35]

EPIDEMIOLOGY OF *CRYPTOSPORIDIUM*

Our knowledge of the epidemiology of *Cryptosporidium* is somewhat limited and is confined to information relative to its mode of transmission, potential sources of infection, and prevalence in humans and domesticated animals. Investigations of experimental infections in farm and laboratory animals have clearly shown that cryptosporidiosis in mammals may be transmitted by (thick-walled) oocysts of *C. parvum*[24] that are fully sporulated and infective at the time they are passed in the feces.[3,9,29] Oocysts of *C. parvum,* like those of other coccidian species, are resistant to most disinfectants used in hospitals and laboratories.[2] Infectivity of *Cryptosporidium* sp. oocysts was reported to be destroyed by ammonia, formal saline,[36] freezedrying, and exposure (30 minutes) to temperatures below freezing (−20°C) and above 65°C.[2] Full-strength commercial bleach is used as a disinfectant in our laboratory. Exposure of oocysts to full-strength bleach (5.25 percent sodium hypochlorite) for 30 minutes or longer at room temperature usually destroys their infectivity for suck-

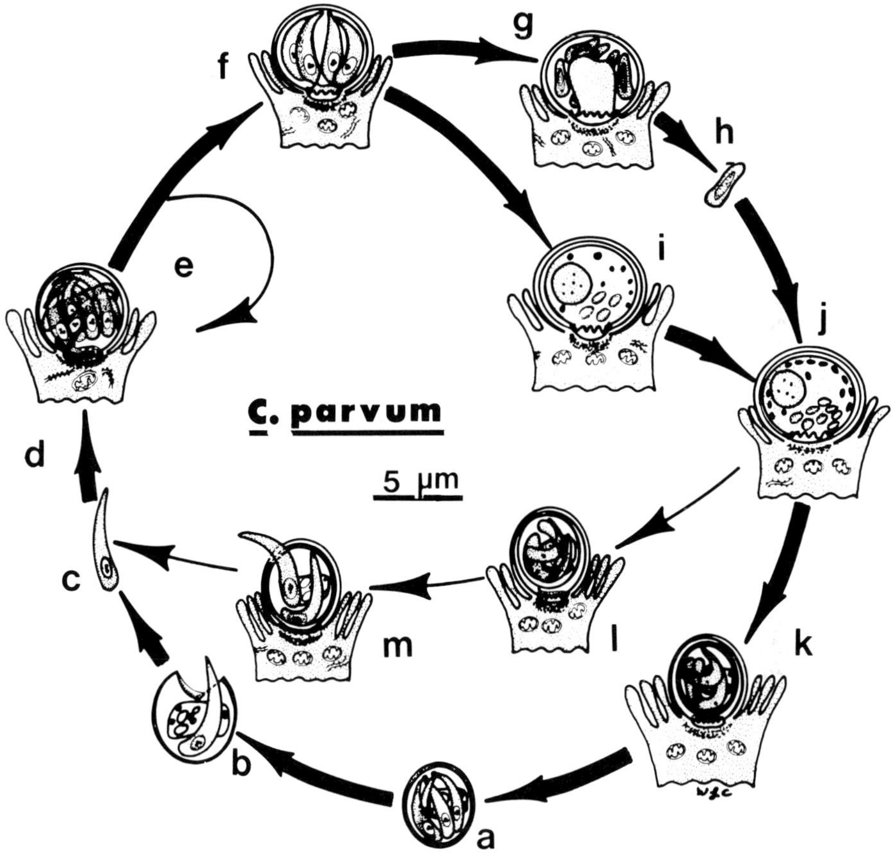

Fig. 8-1. Life cycle of *Cryptosporidium parvum* in experimentally infected mice. (a) Sporulated oocyst in feces. (b) Excystation within intestine. (c) Free sporozoite in intestine before penetration of the microvillous region of an ileal enterocyte. (d) Type 1 meront (six or eight merozoites). (e) Recycling of type 1 merozoite to form more type 1 meronts. (f) Type 2 meront (four merozoites). (g) Microgamont, with approximately 16 microgametes. (h) Microgamete fertilizes macrogamete (i) to form zygote (j). Approximately 80 percent of the zygotes form thick-walled oocysts (k), which sporulate within the host cell. Almost all thick-walled oocysts pass unaltered in the feces; they are the resistant forms that transmit the infection to another host. About 20 percent of the zygotes do not form an oocyst wall, their sporozoites being surrounded only by a unit membrane (l). Sporozoites within autoinfective, thin-walled oocysts (l) are released into the intestinal lumen (m) and reinitiate the endogenous cycle (at c). (Adapted from Current,[3] with permission.)

ling mice (unpublished data). However, if one uses bleach as a disinfectant, the final concentration should be above 70 percent. Incubation of oocysts in solutions of 20 percent commercial bleach (1.05 percent sodium hypochlorite) for 12 minutes in an ice bath did not prevent subsequent release of viable sporozoites under conditions of in vitro excystation[37]; thus, routine chlorination of drinking water should have no effect on the infectivity of *Cryptospori-*

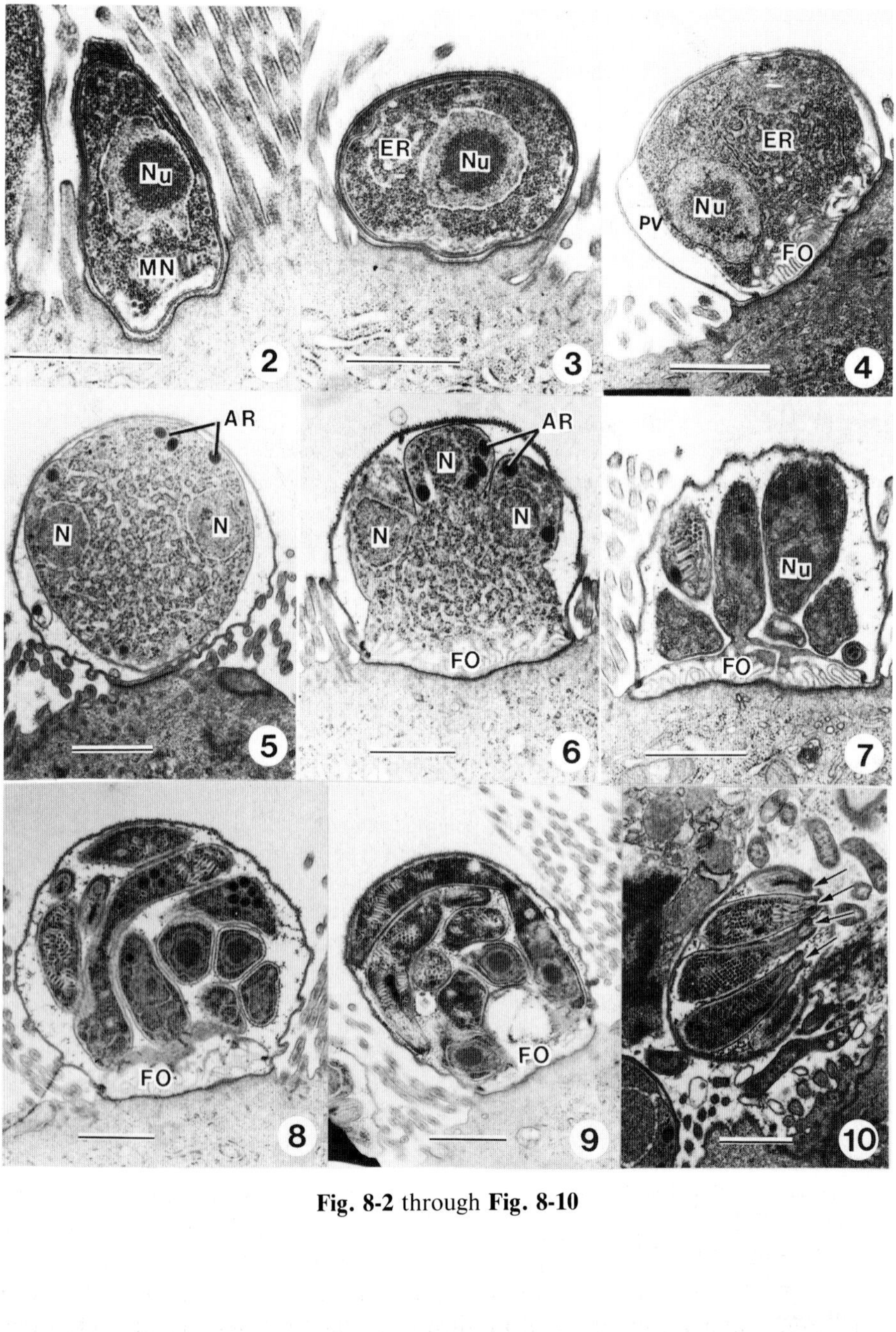

Fig. 8-2 through **Fig. 8-10**

Fig. 8-2. Transmission electron micrograph of *C. parvum* merozoite in final stages of penetrating into microvillus region of the ileal mucosal epithelium of experimentally infected mouse. Note the nucleus with a large nucleolus (Nu) and the vacuolated cytoplasm previously occupied by micronemes (MN). Bar represents 1μm. (Modified from Current,[29] with permission.)

Fig. 8-3. Transmission electron micrograph showing early *C. parvum* uninucleate meront, with dilated endoplasmic reticulum (ER) and a nucleus with a large nucleolus (Nu), in ileal mucosal epithelium of experimentally infected mouse. Bar represents 1 μm. (Modified from Current,[29] with permission.)

Fig. 8-4. Transmission electron micrograph showing late-stage *C. parvum* uninucleate meront in ileal mucosal epithelium of experimentally infected mouse. This meront has extensive endoplasmic reticulum (ER) and an eccentric nucleus with a nucleolus (Nu) that is less prominent than that of the previous stage. The plasma membrane of the parasite has folded extensively to form the feeder organelle (FO) at the base of the parasitophorous vacuole (PV). Bar represents 1 μm. (Modified from Current,[29] with permission.)

Fig. 8-5. Transmission electron micrograph of *C. parvum* meront in ileal mucosal epithelium of experimentally infected mouse. This meront has two nuclei (N) without nucleoli and has anlagen of the rhoptries or micronemes (AR) near the periphery. Bar represents 1 μm. (Modified from Current,[29] with permission.)

Fig. 8-6. Transmission electron micrograph of type 2 *C. parvum* meront in ileal mucosal endothelium of experimentally infected mouse. Meront shows three of four merozoites budding from the surface opposite the feeder organelle (FO). Within each budding merozoite are a nucleus (N) and anlagen of rhoptries or micronemes (AR). Bar represents 1 μm. (Modified from Current,[29] with permission.)

Fig. 8-7. Transmission electron micrograph of *C. parvum* meront in ileal mucosal epithelium of experimentally infected mouse. This nearly mature type 2 meront has three merozoites free in the PV and one in the final stages of budding from the feeder organelle (FO). Merozoite nuclei have prominent nucleoli (Nu). Bar represents 1μm. (Modified from Current,[29] with permission.)

Fig. 8-8. Transmission electron micrograph of *C. parvum* type 1 meront in ileal mucosal epithelium of experimentally infected mouse. This meront has eight merozoites, two of which are in the final stages of budding from the residuum. The basilar portion of the residuum is modified into a feeder organelle (FO). Bar represents 1 μm. (Modified from Current,[29] with permission.)

Fig. 8-9. Transmission electron micrograph of *C. parvum* type 1 meront with six merozoites and a feeder organelle (FO) within the parasitophorous vacuole in ileal mucosal epithelium of experimentally infected mouse. Bar represents 1 μm. (Modified from Current,[29] with permission.)

Fig. 8-10. Transmission electron micrograph showing section through anterior of the four *C. parvum* merozoites (arrows) of a type 2 meront in ileal mucosal epithelium of experimentally infected mouse. Bar represents 1 μ. (Modified from Current,[29] with permission.)

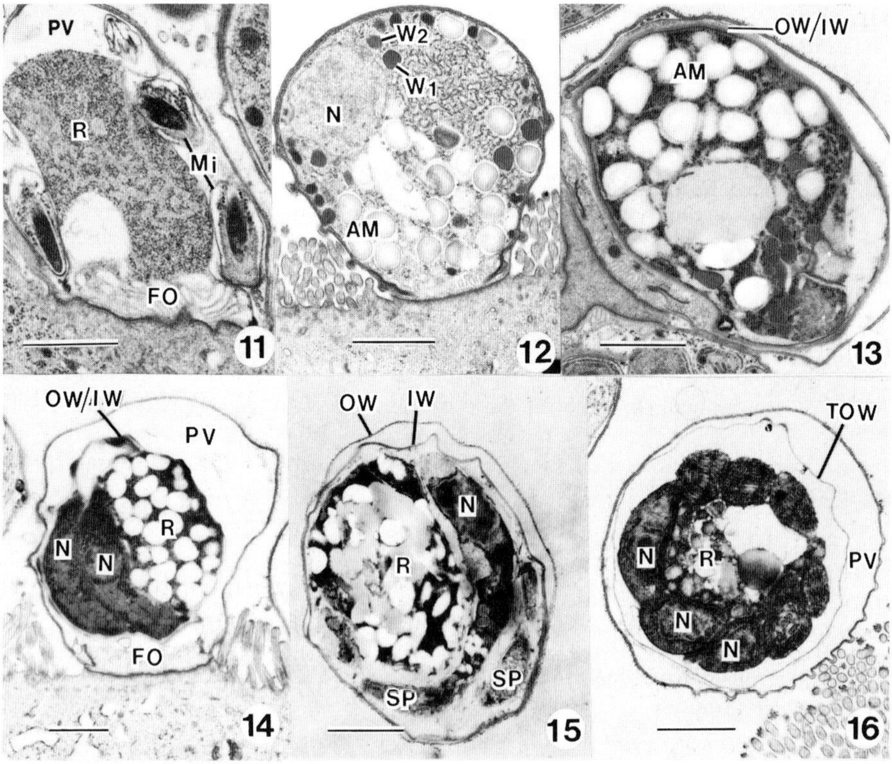

Fig. 8-11. Transmission electron micrograph of nearly mature *C. parvum* microgamont in ileal mucosal enterocyte of experimentally infected mouse. Note microgametes (Mi) free in the parasitophorous vacuole (PV) and budding from the residuum (R). The parasite membrane nearest the host cell has folded extensively to form the feeder organelle (FO). Bar represents 1 μm. (Modified from Current,[29] with permission.)

Fig. 8-12. Transmission electron micrograph of *C. parvum* macrogamete in ileal mucosal enterocyte of experimentally infected mouse. Note the an eccentric nucleus (N) and accumulation of amylopectin-like bodies (AM) near the feeder organelle and the wall-forming bodies (W_1, W_2) near the periphery. Bar represents 1 μm. (Modified from Current,[29] with permission.)

Fig. 8-13. Transmission electron micrograph of unsporulated, thick-walled *C. parvum* oocyst within a parasitophorous vacuole (PV) in ileal mucosal enterocyte of experimentally infected mouse. Amylopectin-like granules (AM) are numerous, and the sporont is surrounded by a two-layered oocyst wall (OW, outer wall; IW, inner wall). Bar represents 1 μm. (Modified from Current,[29] with permission.)

Fig. 8-14. Transmission electron micrograph of sporulated, thick-walled *C. parvum* oocyst within a parasitophorous vacuole (PV) of ileal mucosal enterocyte of experimentally infected mouse. Two of the four sporozoites with posteriorly located nuclei (N) and a residuum (R) with amylopectin-like granules are seen enclosed within the outer and inner oocyst wall (OW/IW). The feeder organelle (FO) is still firmly attached to the base of the PV. Bar represents 1 μm. (Modified from Current,[29] with permission.)

dium sp. oocysts. Although heat (hot water above 70°C or autoclaving) and full-strength bleach may destroy infectivity of *Cryptosporidium* sp. oocysts, a disinfectant is needed for medical instruments that cannot tolerate such harsh treatments.

Studies within the past four years have clearly shown that calves are a source of human infection,[9,38,39] and it has been suggested that companion animals such as rodents, puppies, and kittens are also reservoir hosts.[9,10] This, coupled with a large list[18,35] of animals reported to be infected with what is believed to be a protozoan that readily crosses species barriers, led to the view that zoonotic transmission accounts for most human infections. This view is probably correct for persons living and working in environments where they are exposed to fecal contamination from potential reservoir hosts. Zoonotic transmission cannot, however, explain the large number of infections among urban dwellers whose exposure to animal feces is minimal.

Evidence has been accumulating rapidly that person-to-person transmission of cryptosporidiosis is common. An accidental infection of a researcher demonstrated that a human isolate of *C. parvum* could be transmitted from one person to another.[40] Outbreaks of cryptosporidiosis are being reported among children in day care centers[41,42]; several hospital-acquired infections have been investigated[10,43]; at least one large waterborne outbreak has been documented[44]; and this protozoan appears to be a cause of travelers' diarrhea.[45,46]

After the waterborne outbreak in San Antonio, Texas[44] was investigated, a preliminary study in conjunction with Dr. F. W. Shaefer of the Health Effects Research Laboratory of the Environmental Protection Agency demonstrated that oocysts of *C. parvum* can be recovered from water samples by the high-volume orlon filters[47] used to trap cysts of *Giardia lamblia* (unpublished data). Similar water filtration methods, coupled with an immunofluorescence detection technique, resulted in the recovery and identification of *Cryptosporidium* sp. oocysts from the secondary effluent of a sewage treatment plant in Tucson, Arizona.[48] *Cryptosporidium* sp. oocysts have also been identified by an immunofluorescence detection procedure in materials filtered from several rivers in western Washington.[49]

Fig. 8-15. Transmission electron micrograph of thick-walled *C. parvum* oocyst shed in feces of experimentally infected mouse. The outer (OW) and inner (IW) oocyst wall surrounds the sporozoites (SP) and residuum (R) both of which contain amylopectin-like granules. Note the posterior position of the sporozoite nucleus (N). Bar represents 1 μm. (Adapted from Current,[29] with permission.)

Fig. 8-16. Transmission electron micrograph of thin-walled, autoinfective C. parvum oocyst within a parasitophorous vacuole (PV) of ileal mucosal enterocyte of experimentally infected mouse. The thin oocyst wall (TOW) consists of a single unit membrane surrounding the four sporozoites (three of their nuclei [N] are labeled) and the residuum (R) containing many amylopectin-like granules. Bar represents 1 μm. (Modified from Current,[29] with permission.)

Many epidemiologic features of cryptosporidiosis emphasized above, such as transmission by an environmentally resistant cyst (oocyst), identification of numerous potential reservoir hosts for zoonotic transmission, demonstration of person-to-person transmission, and documentation of waterborne transmission, are similar to those of human giardiasis that came to light during the past decade. The importance of *Giardia lamblia* as a widespread cause of diarrheal illness in man has been recognized for several years, and *Cryptosporidium* is now ascending a similar recognition curve. Studies conducted recently in selected areas of Australia,[50] Costa Rica,[51,52] the United Kingdom,[53] the United States,[54,55] Brazil,[56] Peru,[57] South Africa,[58] Bangledesh,[59] Spain,[60] Denmark,[61] Central Africa,[62] Liberia,[63] and Haiti[64] have provided some data on the importance of *Cryptosporidium* as a cause of diarrheal illness in man. In most of these studies, as well as some others not listed here, *Cryptosporidium* sp. was the most common parasite found. In several of the studies listed above, this protozoan was considered to be the most significant of all known enterpathogens causing diarrheal illness. Other findings common to the studies cited were that children had a significantly higher prevalence of cryptosporidiosis than did adults and that infections were often seasonal, with a higher prevalence during the wetter, warmer months. From the standpoint of infection control, another interesting finding was that oocysts may be present in the feces for up to 2 weeks following resolution of diarrhea. The prevalence data outlined above suggest that *Cryptosporidium* is a major cause of diarrheal illness in man worldwide.

In light of the information just reviewed, physicians, veterinarians, and others involved in informing the public of risk factors associated with the transmission of infectious diseases should be encouraged to broaden their educational role to include cryptosporidiosis. This role should be approached aggressively because of the apparent common occurrence of the disease, because of the large number of potential reservoir hosts, and because persons with compromised immune systems may develop life-threatening cryptosporidiosis (as discussed below). Physicians should become proficient in recognizing when the disease is present in their patients, and veterinarians should train themselves to recognize when the infectious agent is present in farm and companion animals so that persons at high risk of developing serious illness can be warned. The typical clinical features in humans are reviewed below, as well as techniques used to diagnose cryptosporidiosis. Typical clinical signs of cryptosporidiosis in animals have been reviewed.[1,2,35]

HOST DEFENSE MECHANISMS

Most of our knowledge of host defense mechanisms as it applies to cryptosporidiosis can be discussed from the standpoint of age resistance of the host or the development of acquired immunity. It is not easy, however, to separate these two factors, and future studies are likely to show that they often operate in conjunction to protect the host from clinical illness.

It has been our experience that all suckling rodents tested (i.e., mice, rats, cotton rats, guinea pigs and hamsters) may develop heavy intestinal infections following oral inoculation with oocysts of calf and human isolates of *C. parvum*.[3,9,29] However, adults of these species were not infected or developed only mild infections, with just a few parasites scattered through the mucosa of the ileum, following oral inoculation of oocysts.[38] Our attempts to develop an adult, immunosuppressed mouse–*C. parvum* model using cyclophosphamide therapy was disappointing. The immunosuppressive therapy regimen used did not increase the percentage of adult mice that developed infections nor did it result in heavier infections following challenge with *C. parvum*. Several of the immunosuppressed mice did, however, shed a small number of oocysts for several days beyond the normal patent period (unpublished data). Similar results (i.e., heavy infections in all neonates and very light infections in about half of the adults) were obtained following oral inoculation of oocysts of *C. parvum* into athymic nude mice and their immunocompetent heterozygous littermates.[65] The reasons for the apparent decrease in susceptibility of older rodents is unknown, and its occurence in other animals has not been sufficiently investigated. The apparent absence of *C. parvum* infections in adult cattle has been attributed to age resistance; however, it may also be due to acquired immunity since most calves are probably exposed to the parasite during the first month of life. Age resistance does not appear to be a significant factor in human cryptosporidiosis because infections occur both in children and in adults.

In humans a major factor controlling the susceptibility to and severity of cryptosporidiosis appears to be the immune status of the host. Immunocompetent persons have a short-term (less than 2 weeks) gastrointestinal illness following oral exposure to oocysts whereas individuals with immune deficiencies may develop a prolonged life-threatening gastrointestinal, respiratory, or hepatic infection.[3] Such prolonged, life-threatening infections have been reported in patients undergoing immunosuppressive chemotherapy and persons with congenital (e.g., hypogammaglobulinemia) and acquired immune deficiencies (see section on clinical features for additional details and references). Since at least one of the persons with hypogammaglobulinemia and prolonged cryptosporidiosis was reported to have normal T-cell function[9] and since some AIDS patients with prolonged infections had high antibody titers to *Cryptosporidium* sp.,[66] one may conclude that both humoral and cell-mediated immunity is involved in the clearance of a gastrointestinal infection.

Our previous study has demonstrated that most immunocompetent persons have serum antibodies specific to *C. parvum* that are detectible for several months following recovery from gastrointestinal cryptosporidiosis.[66] One of these individuals had an indirect immunofluorescent antibody titer greater than 1 : 80 approximately 2 years after recovery from cryptosporidiosis. Serum from this individual obtained 2 to 3 months following recovery recognized more than 20 sporozoite and/or oocyst antigens of *C. parvum* separated by SDS-PAGE electrophoresis (unpublished data). Since *C. parvum* is apparently confined to the microvillous region of the mucosal epithelium of immunocompetent persons, it is difficult to support the concept that serum antibodies may play a major role in acquired immunity, especially since such a role has not been well established by extensive laboratory investigations of the development of immunity of a variety of animals to other coccidia species.[67] It is more probable that local antibodies (intestinal immunoglobulins A and G) coupled with cell-mediated immune mechanisms are required for the clearance of parasites from the gut.

The importance of T cells for recovery from gastrointestinal cryptosporidiosis was suggested recently by a study[65] monitoring the course of experimentally induced *C. parvum* infections in suckling, athymic nude mice and their heterozygous immunocompetent littermates. The immunocompetent white mice did not develop diarrhea and stopped shedding oocysts 21 to 30 days after inoculation whereas their T-cell–deficient nude littermates developed diarrhea and shed oocysts in their feces until they died or until the experiment was terminated on day 56. It is doubtful that the immune mechanisms responsible for recovery from a primary infection and for resistance to subsequent oocyst challenge will be revealed until an immunocompetent adult rodent–*Cryptosporidium* sp. model is developed.

PATHOGENESIS OF CRYPTOSPORIDIOSIS

Much of our limited knowledge of the pathology and pathogenesis of human cryptosporidiosis has been obtained from histologic studies of intestinal tissues obtained from immunodeficient persons with the disease. In these patients developmental stages of the parasite have been found in the pharynx, esophagus, stomach, duodenum, jejunum, ileum, appendix, colon, and rectum.[4–7,11–14] Postmortem examination of three patients revealed that the jejunum was the most heavily infected region of the gut.[7,8,68]

Histologic lesions in heavily infected regions of the small intestine obtained from humans included villous atrophy, an increase in crypt length, and mild to moderate mononuclear cell infiltration of the lamina propria.[4–8] Similar microscopic lesions have been reported in the small intestine of experimentally infected mice,[65] pigs,[69] and lambs,[70] and in the small[71] and large[72] intestines of germ-free calves monoinfected with *C. parvum*. Heine et al.[71] proposed that malabsorption due to villous atrophy of the small intestine was the basis for cryptosporidial-induced diarrhea in these germ-free calves. The subsequent report of Pholenz et al.[72] demonstrated that gnotobiotic calves monoinfected with *Cryptosporidium* sp. also had extensive colonization of the spiral colon by the parasite, and that infected regions had marked erosion of epithelium. It appears, therefore, that malabsorption and impaired digestion in the small intestine coupled with malabsorption in the large intestine are major factors responsible for diarrhea in calves with cryptosporidiosis. Malabsorption has also been reported in immunosuppressed humans with cryptosporidiosis.[8,11] However, the secretory (often described as cholera-like) diarrhea common to many immunodeficient persons with cryptosporidiosis would suggest hypersecretion into the gut. Slow marker intestinal profusion tests of a patient with acquired immune deficiency syndrome (AIDS) and a *Cryptosporidium* infection of the entire small bowel indicated profuse fluid secretion into the duodenum and proximal jejunum and normal reabsorption of water and sodium in the ileum and colon.[73] Presently, the pathophysiologic mechanism(s) of *Cryptosporidium*-induced diarrhea are poorly defined. Definitive, systematic studies of the mechanisms by which *Cryptosporidium* and its metabolites or toxins may alter normal intestinal function of a susceptible animal model are needed.

CLINICAL FEATURES OF CRYPTOSPORIDIOSIS

Much of the published literature portrays cryptosporidiosis as a short-term, often cholera-like, diarrheal illness in immunocompetent persons or as a prolonged, life-threatening, cholera-like illness in immunodeficient persons.[1–9] However, the clinical presentation of gastrointestinal cryptosporidiosis in immunocompetent and immunodeficient persons does not always fit within one of these two divergent categories. Persons with the laboratory and clinical features of AIDS have been known to clear *Cryptosporidium* infections after several months of diarrhea, and persons reported to be immunocompetent have had prolonged infections lasting for more than a month.[10] Mild and even asymptomatic infections may occur in immunocompetent[9] as well as in immunodeficient persons.[74]

Immunodeficient Persons

In most immunodeficient persons diarrheal illness resulting from a *Cryptosporidium* infection of the gastrointestinal tract becomes progressively worse and may be a major factor leading to death. Life-threatening cryptosporidiosis has been documented in individuals on immunosuppressive chemotherapy,[4,7,75,76] persons with congenital immunodeficiencies such as hypogammaglobulinemia,[5,8,9] and patients with AIDS.[9,11,13,14,77–79] Of the gastrointestinal pathogens identified in AIDS patients, *Cryptosporidium* is perhaps the most ominous in its effects on morbidity and its contributions to mortality.[80] Fluid loss by patients with AIDS and cryptosporidiosis is often extensive; as noted above, 3 to 6 L of diarrheic stool per day is common, and as much as 17 L of watery feces per day has been reported.[12]

In immunodeficient persons *Cryptosporidium* infection is not always confined to the gastrointestinal tract. Acute and gangrenous cholecystitis in AIDS patients has been attributed to *Cryptosporidium* infections of the biliary tree and gallbladder epithelium.[14,18,82] Infections of the respiratory tract have been associated with chronic coughing, dyspnea, bronchiolitis, and pneumonitis in immunodeficient persons.[13,83,84] The importance of *Cryptosporidium* sp. as a cause of pulmonary and hepatic disease in immunodeficient and perhaps in immunocompetent persons merits further investigation.

Immunocompetent Persons

In most of the 18 case reports of cryptosporidiosis in immunocompetent humans published prior to 1983[38,39,85–89] and in the numerous case reports since then[40–46,50–64] a self-limiting cholera-like illness or a short-term, flu-like gastrointestinal illness is described. The most commonly reported symptoms in immunocompetent individuals with cryptosporidiosis include profuse, watery diarrhea (cholera-like) and abdominal cramping, nausea, vomiting, low-grade fever, anorexia, and headache (flu-like).

In most well-nourished persons diarrheal illness due to cryptosporidiosis usually lasts 3 to 12 days. Occasionally, fluid replacement therapy may be required, especially in patients whose diarrheal illness last for more than 2 weeks. In poorly nourished persons, especially children less than 2 years old, oral parenteral rehydration therapy is often needed because of extensive fluid loss. It is not unusual for young malnourished children with cryptosporidiosis to have diarrhea lasting for more than 3 weeks. Diarrheal illness is a major cause of morbidity and mortality, especially in young children living in developing countries. Estimates of Walsh and Warren indicate that in Asia, Africa, and Latin America there are as many as 5 billion episodes of diarrhea and 5 to 10 million diarrheal-associated deaths annually.[90] Although recent surveys demonstrate that cryptosporidiosis is a major cause of diarrheal illness worldwide,[50–64] it is not clear to what extent this protozoan disease contributes to morbidity and mortality. Additional detailed studies employing the proper diagnostic tools should define more clearly the impact of cryptosporidiosis on human health in developing and developed countries.

DIAGNOSIS OF CRYPTOSPORIDIOSIS

Prior to 1980 the diagnosis of human cryptosporidiosis required identification of small spherical endogenous stages of *Cryptosporidium* sp. obtained by biopsy of the microvillous region of the intestinal mucosa and processed subsequently for examination by light or electron microscopy (Figs. 8-17,8-18). Such time-consuming, invasive procedures are no longer warranted since a variety of techniques have been developed for identifying *Cryptosporidium* oocysts in fecal specimens.[9,91–97] Intestinal biopsy may, however, still be useful to determine the region of the gut infected with *Cryptosporidium* and to ascertain histopathologic changes that may occur in the affected tissues.

Fecal specimens obtained from most hosts (animal and human) with cryptosporidiosis will contain large numbers of oocysts, and use of most published concentration[9,91] or staining[92–97] techniques should result in a positive diagnosis. However, some fecal samples may contain only a few oocysts which makes it difficult for the medical microbiologist or the veterinary diagnostician to decide if one or two *Cryptosporidium*-like bodies seen in a stained fecal smear warrant a positive diagnosis. This may be especially true for some of the modified acid-fast staining procedures because of the small spherical objects

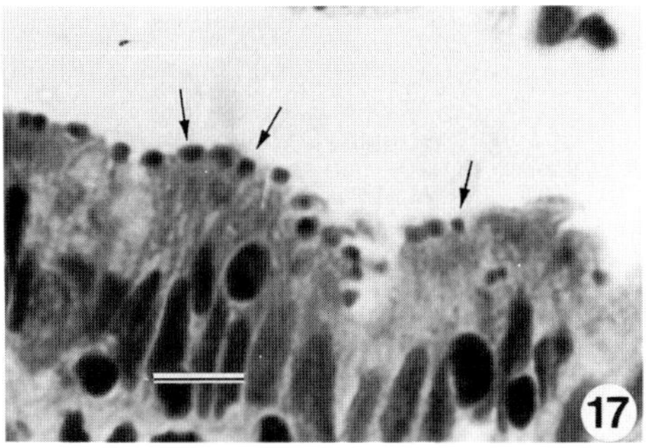

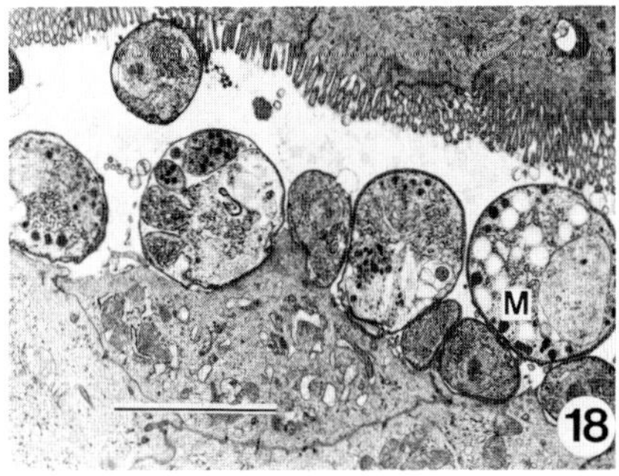

Fig. 8-17. Histologic section of a small bowel biopsy of a human stained with hematoxylin and eosin showing numerous developmental stages of *C. parvum* in the microvillous region of the ileal mucosal enterocytes. Arrows point to three of the parasites. Bar represents 20 μm.

Fig. 8-18. Transmission electron micrograph showing developmental stages of *C. parvum* in ileal mucosal enterocytes. One macrogamete (M) is evident; the remainder of the parasites are meronts in various stages of development. Bar represents 5 μm.

other than *Cryptosporidium* oocysts that can appear acid-fast in some stool samples. Increased sensitivity can be achieved by using oocyst concentration techniques such as Sheather's sugar flotation.[91] Material concentrated from stool samples can be examined prior to[9] or after staining.[92]

Several widely used techniques for demonstrating *Cryptosporidium* oocysts in fecal specimens from animals and humans are modified acid-fast staining,[92–94] negative staining,[95,96] and Sheather's sugar flotation[9,91] (Figs. 8-19 through 8-21.) The last two procedures are used in our research laboratory because they are rapid, relatively simple, and inexpensive, and they allow one to distinguish *Cryptosporidium* oocysts from the yeasts commonly found in stool specimens. Most clinical microbiology laboratories use acid-fast staining techniques because these procedures are incorporated more easily into the stool examination protocols that are normally used.

Any laboratory faced with the task of diagnosing cryptosporidiosis should have one or more persons become familiar with two stool detection techniques, one technique to be used as the primary diagnostic procedure and the other as backup for specimens that give confusing results with the first method. Good-quality, *Cryptosporidium*-positive fecal specimens should be available while laboratory personnel are becoming familiar with the techniques of choice and as a reference source while the diagnostic procedures are being used. Many laboratories may obtain good quality reference specimens through routine submissions. If stool samples containing *Cryptosporidium* oocysts are stored cold (4°C) in either 2.5 percent potassium dichromate or 10 percent formalin, they should remain useful for at least 12 months.[3]

Since several rapid, inexpensive, and reliable techniques for identifying *Cryptosporidium* oocysts in fecal specimens are now available, cryptospori-

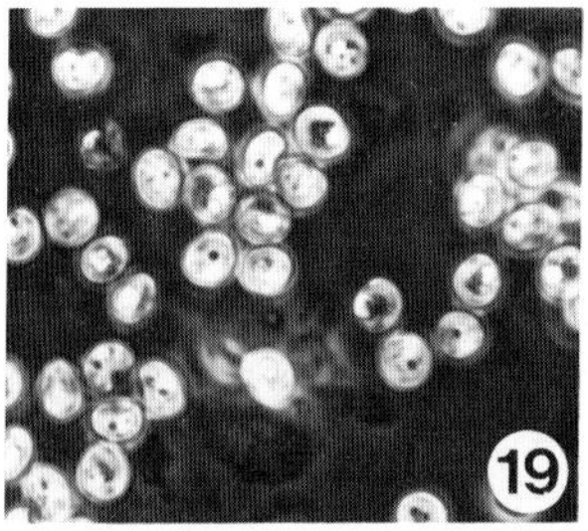

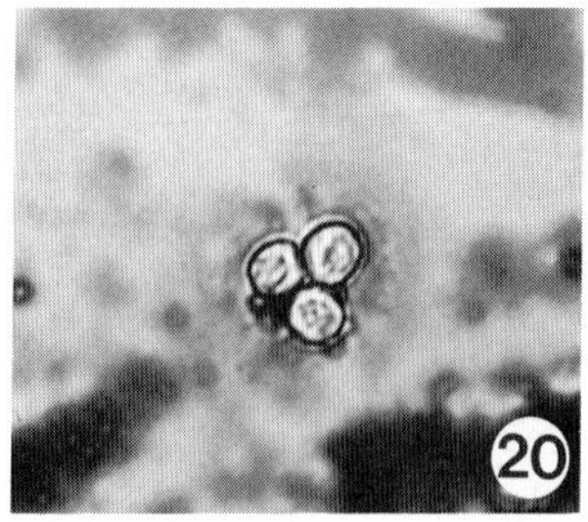

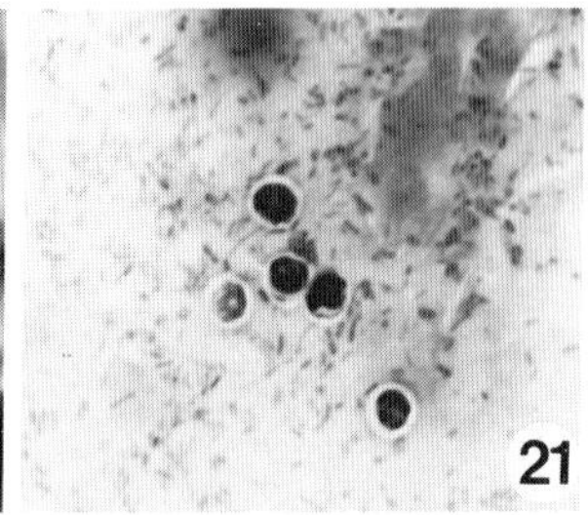

Fig. 8-19. Oocysts of *C. parvum* (4 to 5 μm) demonstrated by Sheathers sugar flotation of stool suspension. Oocysts are bright and refractile, with one to four dark bodies when viewed by phase contrast microscopy.

Fig. 8-20. Kinyouin's carbol fuchsin negative stain of *C. parvum* oocysts (4 to 5 μm) in a fecal smear. Background material, including yeasts, stain darkly. The oocysts do not stain and are bright and refractile.

Fig. 8-21. Acid-fast stain (modified Kinyouin carbol fuchsin method) showing red-staining *C. parvum* oocysts (4 to 5 μm) in a fecal smear.

diosis should be considered in the routine diagnosis of diarrheal illness in animals and humans. Veterinarians and veterinary diagnosticians may consider incorporating such diagnostic procedures into health monitoring programs for pets, especially if the pet owners are immunocompromised. Physicians may consider the use of these diagnostic procedures prior to placing patients on immunosuppressive chemotherapy. Delaying immunosuppressive chemotherapy until after a mild or subclinical *Cryptosporidium* infection is resolved may avoid a life-threatening diarrheal illness.

TREATMENT OF CRYPTOSPORIDIOSIS

Treatment of cryptosporidiosis, especially in immunodeficient persons, has been unsuccessful and frustrating in most cases. To date there have been no controlled studies, and all therapeutic information is based on isolated reports. The number of unsuccessful attempts to treat cryptosporidiosis in immunodeficient persons is growing rapidly. Many of these attempts have been reviewed in recent papers[11,98,99] and are listed in Table 8-2. Some therapies reported to be of value in the treatment of cryptosporidiosis in immunodeficient persons are briefly discussed below.

Antimicrobial and Antiparasitic Agents

Of the numerous antimicrobial and antiparasitic drugs administered to immunodeficient persons with intestinal cryptosporidiosis, spiramycin is the only one reported to have some efficacy. Spiramycin administered orally at 3 g/

Table 8-2. List of Antimicrobial/Antiparasitic Agents and Preventive Modalities Used for *Cryptosporidium* Infections.

Amphotericin B[m]
Ampicillin[m,a]
Amprolium[m,a]
Arpinocin[a]
Bismuth salicylate[m]
Bleomycin[a]
Bovine transfer factor[m,c]
Cabenicillin[m]
Cefamandole[m]
Chloramphenicol[a]
Chloroquine[m]
Cholestyramine[m]
Cimetadine[m]
Clindamycin[m]
Clondine[m]
Clopidol[a]
Cloxacillin[m]
Colistin[m]
Cotrimoxazole[m]
Decoquinate[a]
Difluoromethyl-ornithine[m,a]
Diloxanide furoate[m]
Dimetridazole[a]
Dinitolmide[a]
Diphenoxylate HCl[m]
Doxycycline[m]
Emtryl[a]
Enterolyte N[a]
Erythromycin[m]
Ethopabate[a]
Furaltadone[a]
Furazolidone[m,a]
Gamma globulin[m]
Gentamicin[m,a]
Glucose + amino acids[m]
Gluten-free diet[m]
Halofuginone[a]
Indomethacin[m]
Interferon[m]
Interleukin-2[m]
Iodoquinol[m]
Ipronidazole[a]
Ivermectin[a]
Kaolin-oectin[m,a]
Ketoconazole[m]
Lactose-free diet[m]
Lasalocid[a]
Levamisol[m]
Lincomycin[a]
Loperamide[m]
Mepacrine[m]
Methylbenzoquate[a]
Metronidazole[m,a]
Monensin[a]
Naproxyn[m]
Neomycin[a]
Nicarbazin[a]
Nystatin[a]
Paragoric[m]
Paramomycin[m]
Penicillin[m]
Pentamidine[m]
Phenamidine[a]
Piperazine[m]
Primaquine[m]
Pyrimethamine[m]
Quinacrine[m,a]
Quinine[m]
Robenidine[a]
Salinomycin[m,a]
Septrin[m]
Spectinomycin[a]
Spiramycin[m,b]
Streptomycin[a]
Sulfonamides[m,a]
Transfer factor[m,c]
Tetracycline[m]
Thiabendazole[m]
Trimethoprim[m,a]
Trimethoprim-sulfamethoxazole[m,a]
Tincture of opium[m]
Trinamide[a]
Vancomycin[m]
Zoaquin[a]

[m] = Use reported in man
[a] = Use reported in other animals
[b] Some have reported that spiramycin may control diarrhea in some AIDS patients. (see Treatment and Portnoy.[100])
[c] Bovine transfer factor therapy was recently reported to result in resolution of diarrhea in six of seven patients with cryptosporidiosis and AIDS (see Treatment and Louie.[103])
(Data from Navin,[11] Current,[35] Soave,[98] and Hart.[99])

day was reported to control diarrhea in nine patients with AIDS and cryptosporidiosis.[100] However, some of these AIDS patients continued to shed *Cryptosporidium* oocysts in their feces. Other physicians have reported to me that therapy with this macrolide antibiotic is of little value in the treatment of cryptosporidiosis in persons with AIDS. These conflicting views may be explained, in part, by the observation that spiramycin therapy may control diarrhea in some patients treated for cryptosporidiosis early in the progression of AIDS; however, it does not appear to have a noticeable effect on the course of clinical cryptosporidiosis in patients who have had AIDS for several months.[101] Carefully controlled studies are needed to determine if spiramycin therapy is effective in the treatment of cryptosporidiosis in immunodeficient persons.

Immunomodulation

A major factor determining the severity and duration of a *Cryptosporidium* infection appears to be the immune status of the host. Discontinuing immunosuppressive chemotherapy, thereby allowing restoration of immune function, has resulted in clearance of cryptosporidiosis from the intestinal tract of several patients.[4,75,76] These findings suggest that immunomodulation, or passive transfer of antibodies or lymphocytes, may be of value in the treatment of cryptosporidiosis in immunodeficient patients. The author is aware of at least one patient who has been given serum from three persons with high antibody titers (determined by immunofluorescence procedures[66]) to *C. parvum*. In addition, lymphocytes obtained from the immune donors were irradiated and given to the patient with hypogammaglobulinemia and cryptosporidiosis. Neither passive transfer of immune serum nor that of lymphocytes had an effect on the course of cryptosporidiosis in this immunodeficient patient.

Mata et al.[52] reported a lower incidence of cryptosporidiosis in breast-fed babies compared with infants fed artificial diets and suggested that lactogenic immunity may be of some value in preventing cryptosporidiosis in neonates. Lactogenic immunity does not appear to play a role in altering the course of cryptosporidiosis in suckling calves or mice. We routinely infect calves by mixing oocysts of *C. parvum* with the first liter of colostrum fed. The calves then receive an additional 1 to 2 L of colostrum during the next 36 h. High antibody titers (primarily IgG) were found by indirect immunofluorescence[10,66] in three of four the colostrum samples examined. The presence of colostral antibodies *C. parvum* had no apparent effect on the course of cryptosporidiosis in these calves (unpublished data). Similarly, female mice that recovered from neonatal cryptosporidiosis and that were challenged orally with *C. parvum* oocysts during gestation did not confer protective lactogenic immunity to their offspring that were challenged with *C. parvum* oocysts.[102] Bovine colostrum containing antibodies (IgG) to *C. parvum* administered orally for several days was of no apparent value in the treatment of cryptosporidiosis in one patient with AIDS (unpublished data). Additional studies are needed to determine the role of lactogenic immunity in preventing cryptosporidiosis in neonates.

Transfer factor prepared from lymphoid cells obtained from calves that had recovered from cryptosporidiosis and were resistant to challenge with *C. parvum* oocysts was recently reported to be effective in the treatment of cryptosporidiosis in several AIDS patients.[103] Oral administration of the bovine transfer factor resulted in the resolution of diarrhea in six of seven patients with cryptosporidiosis and AIDS. Four of these patients also stopped shedding *Cryptosporidium* oocysts in their feces. One patient showed no symptomatic or parasitologic improvement during or following bovine transfer factor therapy. More extensive studies are needed to confirm the results obtained from this small number of AIDS patients and to determine if transfer therapy is of any value in the treatment of cryptosporidiosis in persons with AIDS and other forms of immunodeficiency.

Supportive Therapy

Antidiarrheal compounds may provide little symptomatic relief from cryptosporidiosis in immunodeficient persons; however, they often lessen the severity of diarrhea in immunocompetent persons.

Oral or parenteral rehydration therapy is often required by both immunodeficient and immunocompetent persons with severe cryptosporidial diarrhea, especially young children with prolonged infections. Parenteral nutrition may also help sustain the nutritional status of some immunodeficient patients with persistent cryptosporidiosis; however, this procedure has not been sucessful in sustaining many AIDS patients with cryptosporidiosis. Until an effective drug is found to treat cryptosporidiosis, supportive therapy is the only avenue available to most clinicians.

REFERENCES

1. Angus KW: Cryptosporidiosis in man, domestic animals and birds, a review. J R Soc Med 76:62, 1983
2. Tzipori S: Cryptosporidiosis in animals and humans. Microbiol Rev 47:84, 1983
3. Current WL: Cryptosporidium and cryptosporidiosis. p. 355. In Gottlib MS, Groopman JE (eds): Acquired Immune Deficiency Syndrome. Vol. 16. Univ. Calif. Los Angeles Symp. on Molecular and Cellular Biology, New Series, 1984
4. Meisel JL, Perera DR, Meligro C, Rubin CE: Overwhelming watery diarrhea associated with *Cryptosporidium* in an immunosuppressed patient. Gastroenterology 70:1156, 1976
5. Lasser KH, Lewin KJ, Ryning FW: Cryptosporidial enteritis in a patient with congential hypogammaglobulinemia. Hum Pathol 10:234, 1979
6. Stemmerman GN, Hayasaki T, Glober GA, et al: Cryptosporidiosis: report of a fatal case complicated by disseminated toxoplasmosis. Am J Med 69:637, 1980
7. Weisburger WR, Hutcheon DF, Yardley JH, et al: Cryptosporidiosis in an immunosuppressed renal-transplant recipient with IgA deficiency. Am J Clin Pathol 72:473, 1979

8. Sloper KS, Dourmashkin RR, Bird RB, et al: Chronic malabsorption due to cryptosporidiosis in a child with immunoglobulin deficiency. Gut 23:80, 1982
9. Current WL, Reese NC, Ernst JV, et al: Human cryptosporidiosis in immunocompetent and immunodeficient persons: studies of an outbreak and experimental transmission. N Engl J Med 308:1252, 1983
10. Koch KL, Phillips DJ, Aber RC, Current WL: Cryptosporidiosis in hospital personnel: evidence for person-to-person transmission. Ann Intern Med 102:593, 1985
11. Navin TR, Juranek DD: Cryptosporidiosis: clinical, epidemologic, and parasitologic review. Rev Infect Dis 6:313, 1984
12. Centers for Disease Control: Cryptosporidiosis: assessment of chemotherapy of males with acquired immune deficiency syndrome (AIDS). MMWR 31:589, 1982
13. Forgacs P, Tarshis A, Ma P, et al: Intestinal and bronchial cryptosporidiosis in an immunodeficient homosexual man. Ann Intern Med 99:793, 1983
14. Guarda LA, Stein SA, Cleary KA, Ordonez NG: Human cryptosporidiosis in the acquired immune deficiency syndrome. Arch Pathol Lab Med 107:562, 1983
15. Clarke JJ: A study of coccidia met with in mice. J Microsc Sci 37:277, 1895
16. Tyzzer EE: A sporozoan found in the peptic glands of the common mouse. Proc Soc Exp Biol Med 5:12, 1907
17. Tyzzer EE: An extracellular coccidium *Cryptosporidium muris* (gen. et sp. nov.) of the gastric glands of the common mouse. J Med Res 23:487, 1910
18. Levine ND: Taxonomy and review of the coccidian genus *Cryptosporidium* (Protozoa: Apicomplexa). J Protozool 31:94, 1984
19. Tzipori S, Angus KW, Campbell I, Gray EW: *Cryptosporidium:* evidence for a single-species genus. Infect Immun 30:884, 1980
20. Triffit MJ: Observations on two new species of coccidia parasitic in snakes. Protozoology 1:19, 1925
21. Hoare CA: Studies on some new ophidian and avian coccidia from Uganda, with a revision of the classification of the *Eimeriidae*. Parasitology 25:359, 1933
22. Vetterling JM, Harvis HR, Merrill TG, Sprinz H: *Cryptosporidium wrairi* sp. n. from the guinea pig *Cavia porcellus,* with an emendation of the genus. J Protozool 18:243, 1971
23. Tyzzer EE: *Cryptosporidium parvum* (sp. nov.), a coccidian found in the small intestine of the common mouse. Arch Protistenkd 26:394, 1912
24. Upton SJ, Current WL: The species of *Cryptosporidium* (Apicomplexa:Cryptosporidiidae) infecting mammals. J Parasitol 71:625, 1985
25. Vetterling JM, Takeuchi A, Madden PA: Ultrastructure of *Cryptosporidium wrairi* from the guinea pig. J Protozool 18:248, 1971
26. Pholenz J, Bemrick WJ, Moon HW, Cheville NF: Bovine cryptosporidiosis: a transmission and scanning electron microscopic study of some stages in the life cycle and of the host-parasite relationship. Vet Pathol 15:417, 1978
27. Iseki M: *Cryptosporidium felis* sp. n. (Protozoa: Eimeriorina) from the domestic cat. Jpn J Parasitol 28:285, 1979
28. Angus KW, Hutchison G, Munro HMC: Infectivity of a strain of *Cryptosporidium* found in the guinea pig (*Cavia porcellus*) for guinea pigs, mice and lambs. J Comp Pathol 95:151, 1985
29. Current WL, Reese NC: A comparison of endogenous development of three isolates of *Cryptosporidium* in suckling mice. J Protozool 33:98, 1986
30. Current WL, Long PL: Development of human and calf *Cryptosporidium* in chicken embryos. J Infect Dis 148:1108, 1983

31. Current WL, Haynes TB: Complete development of *Cryptosporidium* in cell culture. Science 224:603, 1984
32. Reduker DW, Speer CA, Blixt JA: Ultrastructure of *Cryptosporidium* oocysts and excysting sporozoites as revealed by high resolution scanning electron microscopy J Protozool 32:708, 1985
33. Brandler U: Licht-und elektronenmikroskopische Untersuchungen der Entwicklung von *Cryptosporidium* sp. im Darm experimentell infizierter Mäuse. Vet Med Dissertation, Munich, 1982
34. Goebel E, Brandler U: Ultrastructure of microgametogenesis, microgametes, and gametogony of *Cryptosporidium* sp. in the small intestine of mice. Protistologica 18:331, 1982
35. Current WL: *Cryptosporidium:* its biology and potential for environmental transmission. CRC Crit Rev Environ Control 17:21 1987
36. Campbell I, Tzipori S, Hutchison G, Angus KW: The effect of disinfectants on survival of *Cryptosporidium* oocysts. Vet Rec 111:414, 1982
37. Reduker DW, Speer CA: Factors influencing excystation in *Cryptosporidium* oocysts from cattle. J Parasitol 71:112, 1985
38. Reese NC, Current WL, Ernst JV, Bailey WS: Cryptosporidiosis of man and calf: a case report and results of experimental infections in mice and rats. Am J Trop Med Hyg 31:226, 1982
39. Anderson BC, Donndelinger T, Wilkins RM, Smith J: Cryptosporidiosis in a veterinary student. J Am Vet Med Assoc 180:408, 1982
40. Blagburn BL, Current WL: Accidental infection of a researcher with human *Cryptosporidium.* J Infect Dis 148:772, 1983
41. Alpert G, Bell LM, Kirkpatrick CE, et al: Cryptosporidiosis in a day care center. N Engl J Med 311:860, 1984
42. Centers for Disease Control: Cryptosporidiosis among children attending day care centers—Georgia, Pennsylvania, Michigan, California, New Mexico. MMWR 33:599, 1984
43. Baxby D, Hart CA, Taylor C: Human cryptosporidiosis: a possible case of hospital cross infection. Br Med J 287:1760, 1983
44. D'Antonio RG, Winn RE, Taylor JP, et al: A waterborne outbreak of cryptosporidiosis in normal hosts. Ann Intern Med 103:886, 1986
45. Soave R, Ma P: Cryptosporidiosis travelers diarrhea in 2 families. Arch Intern Med 145:70, 1985
46. Jokipii L, Pohjola S, Jokipii AMM: Cryptosporidium: a frequent finding in patients with gastrointestinal symptoms. Lancet 1:358, 1983
47. Jakubowski W, Erikson TH: Methods for detection of *Giardia* cysts in water supplies. In Jakubowski W, Hoff JC (eds): Waterborne Transmission of Giardiasis. U. S. Environmental Protection Agency EPA-60019-79-001. National Technical Information Service, Springfield, VA, 1979
48. Sterling CR, Arrowood MJ: Detection of *Cryptosporidium sp.* infections using a direct immunofluorescent assay. Pediatr Infect Dis 5:5139, 1986
49. Stibbs HH, Ongreth J: Immunofluorescent detection of *Cryptosporidium* oocysts in fecal smears and river water. Abstr. No. 100. 60th Am Soc Parasitol Annu Meeting, Athens, GA, Aug. 4–8, 1985
50. Tzipori S, Smith M, Birch C, et al: Cryptosporidiosis in hospital patients with gastroenteritis. Am J Trop Med Hyg 32:931, 1983
51. Mata L, Bolaños H, Pizarro D, Vives M: Cryptosporidiosis in children from some highland Costa Rican rural and urban areas. Am J Trop Med Hyg 33:24, 1984

52. Mata L, Bolaños H, Pizarro D, Vives M: Cryptosporidiosis en niños de Costa Rica: estudio transversal y longitudinal. Rev Biol Trop 32:129, 1984
53. Hart CA, Baxby D, Blundell N: Gastroenteritis due to *Cryptosporidium:* a prospective survey in a children's hospital. J Infect 9:264, 1984
54. Holley P, Westphal M, Dover C: Cryptosporidiosis—a common cause of parasitic diarrhea in children. Pediatr Res 19:296, 1985
55. Richter JM, Wolfsen JS, Waldron MA, McCarthy DM: Cryptosporidiosis in immunocompetent patients. Gastroenterology 88:1555, 1985
56. Weikel CS, Johnson LI, DeSousa MA, Guerrant RL: Cryptosporidiosis in northeastern Brazil: association with sporadic diarrhea. J Infect Dis 151:963, 1985
57. Seegar JK, Gilman RH, Galarza T, et al: *Cryptosporidium*—an important agent of infantile diarrhea in Peru. Abstr No. 369. 33rd Am Soc Trop Med Hyg Annu Meeting, Boston, 1984
58. Smith G: *Cryptosporidium* in association with diarrheal disease in South Africa. S Afr Med J 67:442, 1985
59. Shahid NS, Rahaman ASMH, Anderson BC, et al: Cryptosporidiosis in Bangladesh. Br Med J 290:114, 1985
60. Portus M, Serra T, Botet J, et al: Cryptosporidiosis humama en España. Med Clin (Barc) 84:462, 1985
61. Holten-Andersen W, Gerstoft J, Henriksen SA, Pedersen NS: Prevalence of *Cryptosporidium* among patients with acute enteric infections. J Infect 9:277, 1984
62. Bogaerts J, Lepage P, Rouvony D, Vandepitte J: *Cryptosporidium* spp., a frequent cause of diarrhea in Central Africa. J Clin Microbiol 20:874, 1984
63. Hojlyny N, Molbak K, Jepsen S, Hansson AP: Cryptosporidiosis in Liberian children. Lancet 1:734, 1984
64. Pape JW, Levine E, Marshall F, et al: Cryptosporidiosis in Haitian children. Clin Res 33:414, 1985
65. Heine J, Moon HW, Woodmansee DB: Persistent *Cryptosporidium* infection in congenitally athymic (nude) mice. Infect Immun 43:856, 1984
66. Campbell PN, Current WL: Demonstration of serum antibodies to *Cryptosporidium* sp. in normal and immunodeficient humans with confirmed infections. J Clin Microbiol 18:165, 1983
67. Rose ME: Host immune responses. p. 329. In Long PL (ed): The Biology of the Coccidia. University Park Press, Baltimore, 1982
68. Boothe CC, Slavin G, Dourmashkin RR: Immunodeficiency and cryptosporidiosis. Demonstration at the Royal College of Physicians of London. Br Med J 281:1123, 1983
69. Moon HW, Bemrick WJ: Fecal transmission of calf cryptosporidia between calves and pigs. Vet Pathol 18:248, 1981
70. Angus KW, Tzipori S, Gray EW: Intestinal lesions in specific pathogen-free lambs associated with a *Cryptosporidium* from calves with diarrhea. Vet Pathol 19:587, 1982
71. Heine J, Pholenz JFL, Moon HW, Woode GN: Enteric lesions and diarrhea in gnotobiotic calves monoinfected with *Cryptosporidium* species. J Infect Dis 150:768, 1984
72. Pholenz JFL, Woode GN, Woodmansee D: Typhlitis and colitis in gnotobiotic calves experimentally infected with 10^8-10^9 chemically purified *Cryptosporidium* oocysts. Conference of Research Workers in Animal Diseases, Chicago, Nov. 12–13, Abstract No. 273, 1984
73. Andrean T, Modigliani R, Charpentier Y, et al: Acquired immunodeficiency with

intestinal cryptosporidiosis: possible transmission by Haitian whole blood. Lancet 1:1187, 1983

74. Zar F, Geiseler PJ, Brown VA: Asymptomatic carriage of *Cryptosporidium* in the stool of a patient with acquired immune deficiency syndrome. J Infect Dis 151:195, 1985
75. Miller RA, Holmberg RE, Clausen CR: Life-threatening diarrhea caused by *Cryptosporidium* in a child undergoing therapy for acute lymphocytic leukemia. J Pediatr 103:256, 1983
76. Lewis IJ, Hart CA, Baxby D: Diarrhoea due to *Cryptosporidium* in acute lymphoblastic leukaemia. Arch Dis Child 60:60, 1985
77. Pitilka SD, Fainstein V, Garza D, et al: Human cryptosporidiosis: spectrum of disease. Report of six cases and reviews of the literature. Arch Intern Med 143:2269, 1983
78. Malebranche R, Arnoux E, Guérin JM, et al: Acquired immunodeficiency syndrome with severe gastrointestinal manifestations in Haiti. Lancet 2:873, 1983
79. Koch KL, Shankey TV, Weinstein GS, et al: Cryptosporidiosis in a patient with hemophilia, common variable hypogammaglobulinemia, and the acquired immunodeficiency syndrome. Ann Intern Med 99:337, 1983
80. Weinstein WM: The gastrointestinal tract as a target organ. In Gottlieb MS, Moderator: The Acquired Immunodeficiency Syndrome Ann Intern Med 99:208, 1983
81. Pitlik S, Fainstein V, Rios A, et al: Cryptosporidial cholecystitis. N Engl J Med 308:976, 1983
82. Blumberg RS, Kelsey P, Perrone T, et al: Cytomegalovirus- and *Cryptosporidium*-associated acalculous gangrenous cholecystitis. Am J Med 76:1118, 1984
83. Ma P, Villanueva TG, Kaufman D, Gillooley JF: Respiratory cryptosporidiosis in the acquired immune deficiency syndrome. J Am Med Assoc 252:1298, 1984
84. Kocoshis SA, Cibull ML, Davis TE: Intestinal and pulmonary cryptosporidiosis in an infant with severe combined immune deficiency. J Pediatr Gastroenterol Nutr 3:149, 1984
85. Nime FA, Burek JD, Page DL, et al: Acute enterocolitis in a human being infected with the protozoan *Cryptosporidium*. Gastroenterology 70:592, 1976
86. Tzipori S, Angus KW, Gray DW, Campbell I: Vomiting and diarrhea associated with cryptosporidial infection. N Engl J Med 303:818, 1980
87. Fletcher A, Sims TA, Talbot IC: Cryptosporidial enteritis without general or selected immune deficiency. Br Med J 285:22, 1982
88. Babb RR, Differding JT, Trollope ML: Cryptosporidia enteritis in a healthy professional athlete. Am J Gastroenterol 77:833, 1982
89. Centers for Disease Control: Human cryptosporidiosis—Alabama. MMWR 31:252, 1982
90. Walsh JA, Warren KS: Selective primary care. An interim strategy for disease control in developing countries. N Engl J Med 301:967, 1979
91. Anderson BC: Patterns of shedding of cryptosporidial oocysts in Idaho calves. J Am Vet Med Assoc 178:982, 1981
92. Garcia LS, Bruckner DA, Brewer TC, et al: Techniques for the recovery and identification of *Cryptosporidium* oocysts from stool specimens. J Clin Microbiol 18:185, 1983
93. Ma P, Soave R: Three step stool examination for cryptosporidiosis in ten homosexual men with protracted watery diarrhea. J Infect Dis 147:824, 1983
94. Payne P, Lancaster LA, Heinzman M, et al: Identification of *Cryptosporidium* in

patients with the acquired immunodeficiency syndrome. N Engl J Med 309: 614, 1983
95. Heine J: Eine einfache Nachweismethode fur Kryptosporidien in Kot. Zentralbl Veterinaermed [B] 29:324, 1982
96. Current WL: Human cryptosporidiosis. N Engl J Med 309:1326, 1983
97. Baxby D, Blundell N, Hart CA: The development and performance of a simple, sensitive method for detection of *Cryptosporidium* oocysts in faeces. J Hyg (Camb) 93:317, 1984
98. Soave R: Therapy and prevention of coccidiosis. p. 232. In Leive L, Schlessenger D (eds): Microbiology—1984. Am Soc Microbiol, Washington, 1984
99. Hart A, Baxby D: Management of cryptosporidiosis. J Antimicrob Chemother 15:3, 1985
100. Portnoy D, Whiteside ME, Buckley E, MacLeod CL: Treatment of intestinal cryptosporidiosis with spiramycin. Ann Intern Med 101:202, 1984
101. Soave R: Diagnosis, management, and prognosis of human cryptosporidiosis. Abstr. No. 135. 34th Am Soc Trop Med Hyg Annu Meeting. Miami, Nov. 3–7, 1985
102. Moon HW: Intestinal cryptosporidiosis: pathogenesis and immunity. 10th Int. Symp. on Intestinal Microecology, Minneapolis, Oct. 2–3, 1985
103. Louie E, Borkowsky W, Klesius PH, et al: Treatment of cryptosporidiosis with oral bovine transfer factor. Interscience Conference on Antimicrobial Agents and Chemotherapy Abstr. 817. Minneapolis, Sept. 29–Oct. 2, 1985
104. Lee JL, Hunter SH, Bovee EC (eds): An illustrated guide to the protozoa. Society for Protozoology, Lawrence, KS 1985

9 Biologic Differences among Isolates of *Giardia lamblia*

Theodore E. Nash

Giardia lamblia is a protozoan that inhabits the small intestines of humans and other animals. After ingestion of the relatively resistant cyst stage, the parasite excysts in the small intestine, and the resulting motile trophozoites multiply. After about 1 week, cysts, sometimes 5 to 10 million per gram, are excreted in the feces. *Giardia* is one of the most common parasitic infections.[1–3] In the United States infections occur frequently in children, particularly those attending day care centers,[4,5] and in travelers,[6] backpackers,[7] and homosexuals[8]. Epidemics involving large communities have been noted after contamination of water supplies. In some developing countries, infection with *Giardia* in young children is practically universal.[2,3] Although most infected persons are asymptomatic, others may complain of diarrhea with or without malabsorption, nausea, vomiting, flatus, and abdominal cramping and discomfort.

Giardia morphologically identical to those infecting humans have been found in an increasing variety of mammals, including beavers,[9,10] dogs,[10] cats,[11] muskrats,[12] cattle,[10] and coyotes.[10] Although experiments have shown that cysts obtained from humans can infect animals,[10] it is not known if humans commonly acquire *Giardia* from animals. Infected beavers have been implicated in contaminating water supplies and causing epidemics.[9] It is not clear if the *Giardia* of these animals are similar to those commonly infecting humans.

We have recently developed methods to characterize *G. lamblia* and found that a majority of isolates are biochemically unique and some are also biologically different as well. Major differences among *Giardia* isolates have broad biologic implications and may account for the variability of the host's immune responses, the presence or absence of symptoms, the chronicity of infection, and the host's ability to resist reinfection.

A major impetus to the study of *Giardia* was the development of techniques that allowed in vitro culture and growth.[13,14] Since 1981 axenization of *Giardia* has become an easier and more certain endeavor.[15,16] (*Axenization* refers to cultures performed in the absence of other metabolizing cells.) In the present experiments 19 isolates were axenized and analyzed.[15,16] Table 9-1 is a summary of the origin and/or method of isolation of the *Giardia,*[15,16] which included 15 human and 4 animal isolates (two from beaver and one each from a cat and a guinea pig). Trophozoites for culture were obtained after in vitro excystation or from the small intestines of suckling mice inoculated with purified cysts. The *Giardia* isolates had been maintained in culture for varying periods of time before study, but generally they were analyzed as soon as possible or cryopreserved until used.

ENDONUCLEASE RESTRICTION ANALYSIS OF DNA

Our first major indication of the extent of the variability of *Giardia* was obtained by endonuclease restriction analysis of the DNA of 15 *Giardia* isolates.[15] In these studies the DNA of various isolates was extracted, digested with endonuclease restriction enzymes, subjected to electrophoresis in agarose, transfered to nitrocellulose, and hybridized to nondefined *Giardia*-specific probes. The four possible combinations from two different probes and restriction enzymes were used and, except in rare instances, yielded the same results. An autoradiograph is shown in Figure 9-1, and a schematic representation of the banding patterns of 15 isolates using restriction enzyme Hind III and probe G6A10 is shown in Figure 9-2. Six isolates showed identical patterns (WB, Isr, RS, LT, Be-2, and CAT-1); two were from animals and four from humans. The rest of the isolates were unique but six showed at least one band in common with the WB isolate (GP-1, P-1, N, AB, JH, and DH) and the remaining three [two from humans (CM and GS/E) and one from a beaver (Be-1)] had no bands in common with WB and dramatically differed from the WB-like *Giardia*. No particular pattern was characteristic of isolates derived from animals. These studies introduced a valid way to characterize or type *Giardia* isolates and demonstrated marked diversity among the isolates.

SURFACE ANTIGEN STUDIES

Although these studies suggested general differences in the DNA sequences of the various *Giardia* isolates, it was not known if these differences would be reflected in changes of important protein antigens. Earlier studies showed that the surface of *Giardia* could be radiolabeled with iodine and then analyzed by polyacrylamide electrophoresis followed by autoradiography.[17] In addition, when viable, surface-labeled *Giardia* are maintained in culture, the surface antigens are released into the medium and these excretory-secretory (E-S) products react with anti-isolate antisera.[17] Analysis of the surface antigens of 19 isolates revealed a wide spectrum of sizes and patterns (Fig. 9-3).[16] Of the six isolates with identical DNA banding patterns after endonuclease restriction, four had an identical 170,000-molecular-weight (170-kd) antigen, one had a similar but not identical antigen, and the other had a unique pattern (Fig. 9-4).

The E-S products of these 19 isolates were immunoprecipitated with antisera to a number of *Giardia* isolates.[16] As judged by the amount of radiolabeled E-S products precipitated by the various antisera, *Giardia* isolates could be loosely placed into three related groups, which roughly correlated with the groups identified by restriction enzyme analysis of DNA, as seen in Table 9-2. Group 1 (WB-like) antisera reacted primarily with Group 1 E-S products. In contrast, Group 3 antisera reacted moderately to weakly only with group 3 E-S products. Group 2 consisted of a number of isolates whose antisera and E-S products reacted moderately.

Variability of the surface antigens of *Giardia* was further demonstrated by using monoclonal antibodies that reacted only with the 170-kd antigen of WB.[18] These monoclonals (4G3E4, 6E7E10, and 4F9H3) bound to the surface of only those isolates containing the 170-kd antigen (WB and Isr) (Table 9-3).[18] A surprising finding was that monoclonals that reacted with the 170-kd antigen were cytotoxic only to this subset of *Giardia*. Cytotoxicity occurred within minutes and was complement-independent (Table 9-4).[18] Although the manner of killing is not known, it is possible that the same or a similar mechanism may be responsible for killing of *Giardia* within the gut.

These studies demonstrate that differences in restriction enzyme patterns of DNA from different isolates of *G. lamblia* may be associated with variability in surface antigens. When *Giardia* isolates were disrupted and then allowed to react with the same panel of anti-isolate sera used in the previous experiment, few differences in reactivity were noted, suggesting that the internal antigens of these isolates are similar.[19] The defined antigenic differences among *Giardia* seem to reside primarily on their surface.

EVALUATION OF BIOLOGICAL DIFFERENCES

Next, to determine whether there were biologic differences among *Giardia* isolates, experimental infections were studied in both gerbils and humans. When gerbils were infected by gavage with trophozoites of two unique isolates, GS/E and WB, the patterns of infection were different (Fig. 9-5).[20] The WB-infected gerbils were rapidly self-cured following peak infection at 14 days after inoculation. In contrast, GS/E-infected gerbils tended to remain infected. The responses to challenge infections with either homologous of heterologous isolates also differed. Primary infection with WB induced almost complete resistance to WB and GS/E, while prior GS/E infection induced partial but definite resistance to GS/E and at best limited resistance to WB. Humoral, comple-

Table 9-1. Origin and/or Method of Isolation of 19 *Giardia lamblia* Isolates

Isolate	Geographic Origin	Source	Method of Isolation	Comments[a]
Portland-1 (P-1) (Human)	Oregon	Dr. G. S. Visvesvara	Culture of small intestinal contents	Originally isolated by Dr. E. A. Meyer
WB (Human)	Afghanistan	National Institutes of Health (NIH)	Culture of small intestinal contents	—
RS (Human)	Ecuador	Dr. M. Wittner	Culture of small intestinal contents	—
LT (Human)	Puerto Rico	Dr. M. Wittner	Culture of small intestinal contents	—
CM (NIH:0883:2)	Florida	NIH	Trophozoites from neonatally infected mice	Patient with common variable hypogammaglobulinemia
AB (NIH:0883:1) (Human)	Peru	NIH	Trophozoites excysted in vitro	—
CAT-1 (cat)	Oregon	Dr. G. S. Visvesvara	Culture of small intestinal contents	Originally isolated by Dr. E. A. Meyer
Guinea pig-1 (GP-1)	Oregon	Dr. G. S. Visvesvara	Culture of small intestinal contents	Originally isolated by Dr. E. A. Meyer
JH (NIH:1182) (Human)	West Virginia	NIH	Trophozoites from neonatally infected mice	—
N (NIH:0782) (Human)	New Orleans	NIH	Trophozoites from neonatally infected mice	—

Beaver-1 (Be-1) (IP-0482:1)	Banff National Park, Canada	Dr. G. Faubert and M. Belosevic	Trophozoites from infected Mongolian jirds	Cysts obtained from feces of a beaver found in pond mud
Beaver-2 (Be-2) (IP-0583:1)	Calgary, Canada	Dr. G. Faubert and M. Belosevic	Trophozoites from infected Mongolian jirds	Cysts obtained from colon and rectum of a beaver
DH (Human) (NIH:0284-2)	West Virginia	NIH	Trophozoites excysted in vitro	—
DH/M (Human)	West Virginia	NIH	Trophozoites from neonatally infected mice	—
GS/E (Human) (NIH:1083-1)	Alaskan wilderness	NIH	Trophozoites excysted in vitro	—
GS/M (Human) (NIH:1083-2)	Alaskan wilderness	NIH	Neonatally infected mice	—
Isr (Human) (NIH:1183)	Maryland	NIH	Neonatally infected mice	—
Nat (Human) (NIH:0284-1)	Wisconsin	NIH	Neonatally infected mice	—
Erin (Human) (NIH:0384-1)	Wisconsin	NIH	Trophozoites from infected mice	—
Sug (Human) (NIH:0784-1)	Maryland	NIH	Excysted in vitro	—
AC (Human) (NIH 0484-1)	Dominican Republic	NIH	Excysted in vitro	—

[a] The first 15 isolates were used for DNA studies.

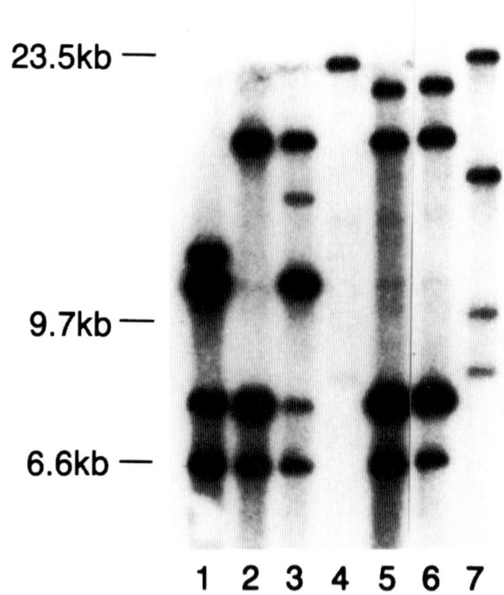

Fig. 9-1. Autoradiograph of a Southern blot of DNA from seven isolates of *G. lamblia* that were restricted with Hind III and hybridized to probe G6A10. Lane 1, JH; 2, N; 3, AB; 4, CM; 5, WB; 6, Be-2; and 7, Be-1. There are obvious differences in the number and size of the bands, indicating marked diversity among isolates.

ment-independent cytotoxicity developed during the infection and appeared to be the best indicator of subsequent resistance to homologous or heterologous challenge. Therefore, the biologic behavior of two distinct *Giardia* isolates differs and suggests that the previously defined or other biochemical differences alter the host-parasite relationship.

Although alteration in biologic behavior could be clearly demonstrated in animal models, it was not known whether differences could also be seen in human infections. To answer this question, five human volunteers were inoculated enterally with trophozoites from two distinct *Giardia* isolates, GS/M and Isr.[21] GS/M originated from patient GS, but trophozoites for initial axenization were obtained after suckling mouse inoculation instead of in vitro excystation (GS/E). Isr originated from an infant with diarrhea and biochemically appears similar, if not identical, to WB. The design of the experiment is shown in Table 9-5. All five of the GS/M-inoculated volunteers became infected. Two developed an illness typical of giardiasis, and one also developed fever and headache. None of the Isr-inoculated volunteers became infected, and this group therefore serves as a control group. As shown in Table 9-6, there were more symptoms in the infected group as compared with the Isr control group; there were nine episodes of diarrhea in two patients in the infected group compared a single episode of diarrhea in the control group.

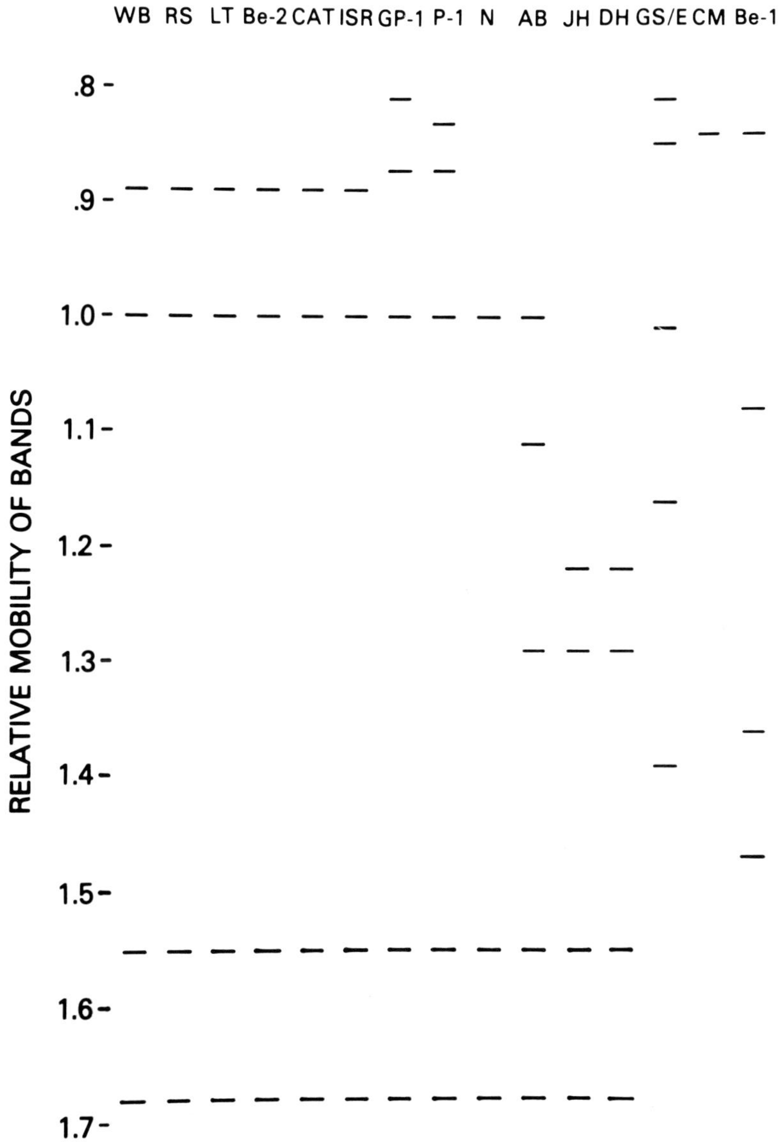

Fig. 9-2. Schematic representation of the banding patterns of 15 isolates of *Giardia* after endonuclease restriction with Hind III and hybridization to probe G6A10. Since WB was present on all blots, bands are drawn as a ratio, calculated by dividing the distance traveled by each band by the distance traveled by the second WB band from the top of the gel. There are three major groups: group 1 (WB, RS, LT, Be-2, CAT-1, and Isr), isolates identical to the WB; group 2 (GP-1, P-1, N, AB, JH, and DH), isolates with at least one band in common with WB; group 3 (GS/E, CM, and Be-1), isolates with no bands in common with WB.

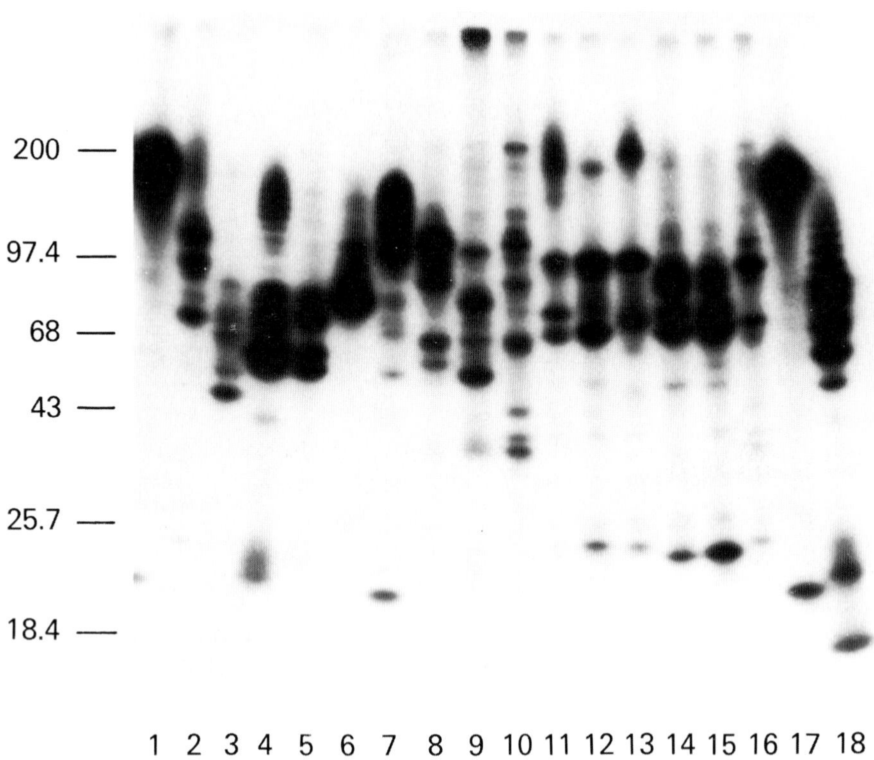

Fig. 9-3. Autoradiograph of a 5 to 15 percent acrylamide gel of surface-labeled *Giardia* run under nonreducing conditions. Lane 1, WB; 2, N; 3, GP-1, 4, CAT-1; 5, CAT-1 (labeled at another time); 6, AB; 7, Be-2; 8, Be-1; 9, GS/M; 10, CM; 11 ES/M; 12, Nat; 13, Sug; 14, JH; 15, DH; 16, Ac; 17, Isr; and 18, P-1. There are obvious differences among many of the isolates.

Table 9-2. Percent Precipitation of E-S Preparations of Various *Giardia* Isolates

	Group 1					Group 2			
Antisera to	WB	RS	LT	Isr	Be-2	ES/M	Nat	AB	CAT-1
WB	67.8	65.9	82.4	76.0	70.2	44.7	15.1	9.6	46.7
RS	66.8	64.6	83.6	74.0	69.5	18.5	7.3	6.4	33.1
LT	65.8	61.5	81.0	72.2	62.0	—	2.0	5.5	4.7
Isr	65.1	65.2	81.8	74.8	65.0	30.9	2.4	4.1	12.0
JH	0.3	−4.9	9.1	1.1	2.0	34.9	45.2	44.6	39.7
N	3.3	−0.7	5.5	5.0	3.0	20.2	20.2	11.1	22.8
GP-1	12.8	14.5	18.8	13.8	15.9	49.8	27.9	8.5	63.5
CM	1.1	−3.9	2.6	0.4	1.2	−0.9	1.2	2.8	4.7
GS/E	−0.4	−0.7	−0.5	3.1	−4.2	−2.2	0.4	0.4	1.7
P-1	−0.6	0.6	—	—	—	14.6	—	—	—

Radiolabeled E-S products of 19 *Giardia* isolates were allowed to react with specific anti-isolate antisera and the amount of radiolabel bound to antibody determined and expressed as the percent of added radiolabeled E-S precipitated. Major differences in reactivity are present and roughly correlate with the groupings noted in Fig. 9-2.

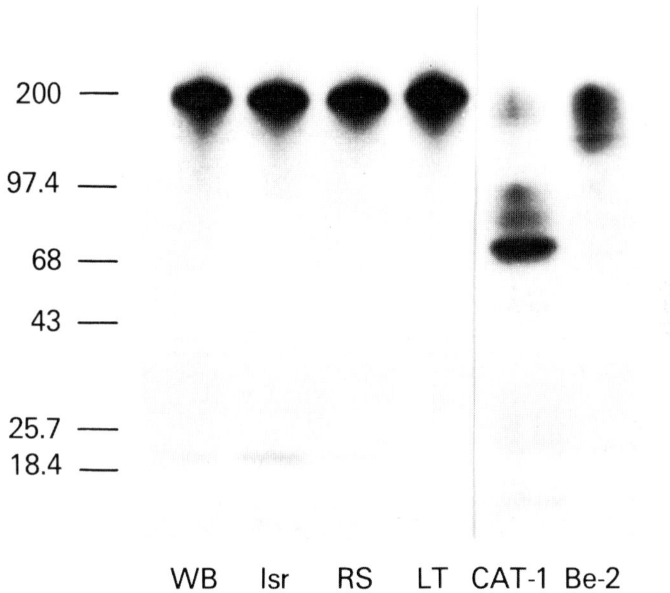

Fig. 9-4. Autoradiograph run under nonreducing conditions, of a 5 to 15 percent acrylamide gel of surface-labeled *Giardia* with identical DNA banding patterns. WB, Isr, RS, and LT have identical surface labeling patterns. The major surface antigen of Be-2 is similar to but not identical with WB, and the surface antigens of CAT-1 are dissimilar in comparison with WB.

Group 2							Group 3		
DH/M	JH	N	Sug	Ac	GP-1	P-1	CM	Be-1	GS/E
13.7	17.3	23.7	20.9	8.0	14	34.8	2.3	2.4	3.0
6.6	8.8	22.1	12.1	10.9	6.0	14.7	2.4	3.9	1.9
−1.6	3.1	18.9	4.7	−1.5	−2.3	4.7	−0.8	−0.6	5.6
0.2	3.4	18.7	4.6	0.3	−3.2	6.1	−2.3	−1.2	3.3
39.1	56.8	34.3	39.0	25.7	0.2	8.6	−1.2	−4.9	−1.1
3.0	21.9	48.6	21.0	5.9	−3.9	10.0	−4.8	−2.0	7.8
41.2	33.7	35.4	41.5	15.4	23.8	26.9	5.8	2.5	4.5
−2.7	3.1	8.7	2.4	10.2	−9.4	2.7	29.2	25.9	16.2
−3.5	2.7	4.8	3.7	2.7	−3.6	5.8	10.2	3.6	33.9
25.8	—	—	—	—	—	—	—	—	—

Table 9-3. Binding of a Reactive McAb to the Surface of WB and other *Giardia* Isolates

	Fluorescence (Arbitrary Units)	
Isolates	4G3E4 (Reacting McAb)	4G3H1 (Nonreacting McAb)
WB[a]	29.038 ± 13.34[b]	0.100 ± 0.141
DH/M	4.057 ± 8.076	2.017 ± 4.023
GS/M	4.400 ± 5.637	3.000 ± 3.880
Isr[a]	32.157 ± 8.673	3.075 ± 2.161
GS/E	3.543 ± 8.019	7.714 ± 11.368
N	7.886 ± 8.336	8.833 ± 4.744
ES/M	3.867 ± 5.009	0.480 ± 2.081
AC	2.180 ± 4.875	0.00 ± 0.00

[a] WB and Isr are the only isolates significantly reacting with 4G3E4 ($p \leq 0.001$).
[b] Mean ± SD.

These studies fulfill Koch's postulates in humans and confirm the pathogenicity of *G. lamblia*. The finding that one isolate easily induced infection and disease while another failed to do so indicates that the described differences among isolates may be biologically important in humans.

To summarize, using a number of complementary but different techniques we analyzed the genetic makeup, the surface antigens and E-S products, and infectivity and host responses to *Giardia* in gerbils and humans. Despite the variety of approaches, each series of experiments revealed differences between many of the isolates, indicating a diversity among *Giardia* isolates. The mechanism(s) responsible for this diversity remain obscure.

Table 9-4. Number of *Giardia* Surviving after Exposure to McAb

Isolate	Media	6E7E10	4F9H3
Expt. 1			
WB	14,060 ± 2,311	1,500 ± 1,206	2,680 ± 841
Isr	17,740 ± 1,906	2,540 ± 904	3,410 ± 1,754
RS	18,560 ± 1,796	4,080 ± 2,051	3,350 ± 483
CM	8,300 ± 1,092	9,100 ± 2,482	8,300 ± 1,079
GS/M	16,700 ± 3,969	18,060 ± 3,680	13,430 ± 2,743
Expt. 2			
WB	58,640 ± 2,582	9,420 ± 657	5,031 ± 2,066
Ac	25,500 ± 2,012	21,370 ± 2,801	23,770 ± 1,112

Monoclonal antibodies were allowed to react with *Giardia* for 1 hour in wells of microtiter plates. After cooling, a constant volume of the reaction mixture containing both surviving and dead *Giardia* was transferred to tubes containing culture medium, and the number of surviving organisms was ascertained 24 hour later. The number of *Giardia* obtained was directly proportional to the size of the original inoculum. 6E7E10 and 4F9H3 are monoclonals antibodies that react with the 170-kd antigen of WB. 6E7E10 and 4F9H3 were cytotoxic for WB, Isr, and RS ($P \leq 0.001$), and only WB, Isr, and RS possess the 170-kd antigen. Mean ± SD.

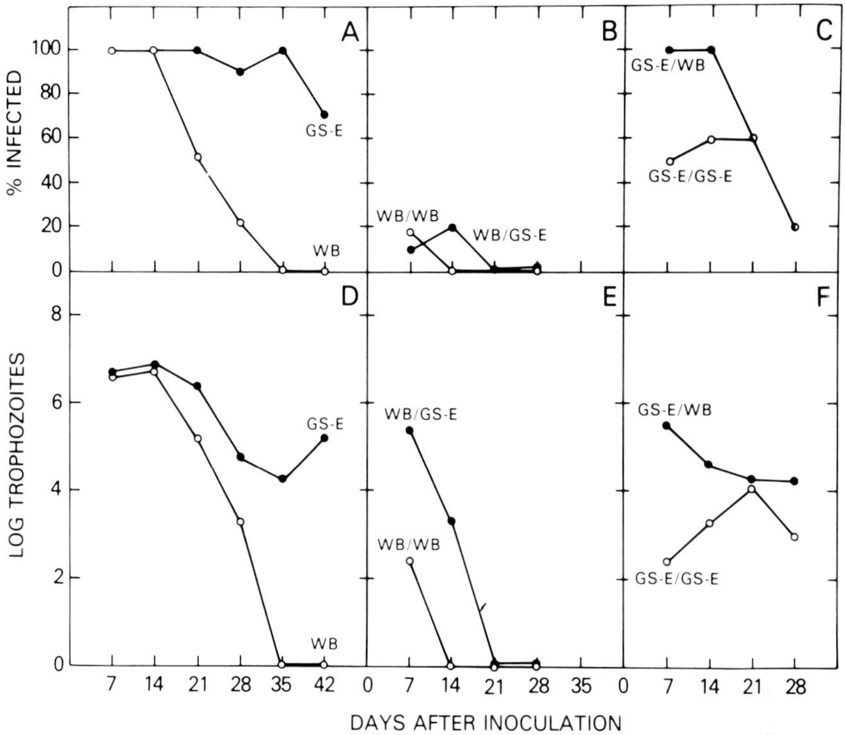

Fig. 9-5. The lower half of the graph shows the number of trophozoites in the small intestines of gerbils, and the upper half shows the percent of animals infected on different days after inoculation with WB or GS-E isolates. Each point represents the logarithm of the mean trophozoite counts from 10 to 15 gerbils. WB, GS-E: panels A and D represent infection with the WB or GS-E isolate. WB/WB: panels B and E, primary WB infection challenged with WB. WB/GS-E: panels B and E, primary WB infection challenged with GS-E. GS-E/WB: panels C and F, primary GS-E infection challenged with WB. GS-E/GS-E: panels C and F, primary GS-E infection challenged with GS-E.

Table 9-5. Summary of Protocol

Pre	Selection of subjects, history, physical examination, psychological testing Stools—ova and parasitology, culture and sensitivity, chest x-ray, electrocardiogram, urinalysis Serum glutomic-oxaloacetic transaminase (SGOT), serum glutamic-pyruvic transaminase (SGPT) amylase, complete blood count (CBC), blood urea nitrogen (BUN), creatinine, fasting glucose, VDRL, hepatitis B antigen, immunoglobulins, HTLV III
Day 0	Jejunal aspirate and culture for aerobic bacteria and fungi
Daily	Stool for *Giardia,* stool for culture and sensitivity, stool grade and volume recorded, stool frozen, and stool placed in formaldehyde Symptoms scored and physical examination if necessary
Day 5	String test
Day 10	String test
Day 14	Jejunal aspirate and culture for aerobic bacteria, fungi, and *Giardia;* CBC, SGOT, SGPT, amylase, BUN, creatinine
Day 15	Treatment with atabrine
Day 19	Jejunal aspiration for presence of *Giardia*
Day 20	Discharge
Day 28	Stool for ova and parasites, stool for culture and sensitivity

Table 9-6. Comparison of GSM-versus Isr-Inoculated Volunteers

	Symptoms and Signs	
	GS/M-Inoculated	Isr-Inoculated
Group 1 Symptoms	66[a] (31, 21, 8, 4, 2)	29 (23, 3, 2, 1, 0)
Loose Stools (grade 3 stools)	11 (9, 2, 0, 0, 0)	1 (0, 0, 0, 1, 0)

[a] Symptoms score is the numerical sum of the symptoms that occurred from day 1 to day 14 (see text). The numbers in parentheses are the values for each patient.

REFERENCES

1. Craun GR: Waterborne outbreaks of giardiasis. p. 117. In Jakubowski W, Hoff JC (eds): Waterborne Transmission of Giardiasis. Washington, U.S. Environmental Protection Agency, 1979
2. Mata LJ: The Children of Santa Maria Cauque: A Prospective Field Study of Health and Growth. MIT Press, Cambridge, MA 1978
3. Dupont HL, Sullivan PS: Giardiasis: the clinical spectrum, diagnosis and therapy. Pediatr Infect Dis 5:S131, 1986
4. Black RE, Dykes AC, Sinclair SP, Wells JG: Giardiasis in day-care centers: evidence of person-to-person transmission. Pediatrics 360:486, 1977
5. Keystone JS, Krajden S, Warren MR: Person-to-person transmission of *Giardia lamblia* in day-care nurseries. Can Med Assoc J 119:241, 1978
6. Brodsky RE, Spencer HC Jr, Schultz MG: Giardiasis in American travelers to the Soviet Union. J Infect Dis 130:319, 1974
7. Barbour AG, Nichols CR, Fukushima T: An outbreak of giardiasis in a group of campers. Am J Trop Med Hyg 25:384, 1976
8. Schmerin MJ, Jones TC, Klein H: Giardiasis: association with homosexuality. Ann Intern Med 88:801, 1978
9. Juranek D: Waterborne giardiasis. p. 150. In Jakubowski W, Hoff JC (eds): Waterborne Transmission of Giardiasis. U.S. Environmental Protection Agency, Washington, 1979
10. Davies RB, Hibler CP: Animal reservoirs and cross-species transmission of *Giardia*. p. 104. In Jakubowksi W, Hoff JC (eds): Waterborne Transmission of Giardiasis. U.S. Environmental Protection Agency, Washington, 1979
11. Kirkpatrick CE, Farrell JP: Feline giardiasis: observations on natural and induced infection. Am J Vet Res 4:2182, 1984
12. Pacha RE, Clark GW, Williams EA: Occurrence of *Campylobacter jejuni* and *Giardia* species in muskrat (*Ondatra zibethica*). Appl Environ Microbiol 50:177, 1985
13. Meyer EA: *Giardia lamblia:* isolation and axenic cultivation. Exp Parasitol 39:101, 1976
14. Keister DB: Axenic cultivation of *Giardia lamblia* in TYI-S-33 medium supplemented with bile. Trans R Soc Trop Med Hyg 77:487, 1983
15. Nash TE, McCutchan T, Keister DB, et al: Endonuclease restriction analysis of DNA from 15 *Giardia* isolates obtained from man and animals. J Infect Dis 152:64, 1985
16. Nash TE, Keister DB: Differences in excretory-secretory products and surface antigens among 19 isolates of *Giardia*. J Infect Dis 152:1166, 1985
17. Nash TE, Gillin FD, Smith PD: Excretory-secretory products of *Giardia lamblia*. J Immunol 131:2004, 1983

18. Nash TE, Aggarwal A: Cytotoxicity of monoclonal antibodies to a subset of *Giardia* isolates. J Immunol 136:2628, 1986
19. Ungar BLP, Nash TE: Cross-reactivity of *Giardia lamblia* isolates using immunofluorescent antibody and enzyme immunoassay techniques. Am J Trop Med Hyg 37:283, 1987
20. Aggarwal A, Nash TE: Comparison of two antigenically distinct *Giardia lamblia* isolates in gerbils. Am J Trop Med Hyg 36:325, 1987
21. Nash TE, Herrington DA, Losonsky GA, Levine NM: Experimental human infections with *Giardia lamblia*. J Infect Dis 156:974, 1987

10 Amebiasis and Giardiasis in Homosexual Men

Paul M. Sullam

Amebiasis and giardiasis have been viewed traditionally as uncommon illnesses in developed countries. Disease outbreaks were known to occur in unusual settings, such as psychiatric institutions, or during lapses in public sanitation, but such epidemics were considered exceptional.[1] In recent years, however, both *Entamoeba histolytica* and *Giardia lamblia* have been recognized as sexually transmitted pathogens among homosexual men.[2] The emergence of these organisms within this population has been associated with novel modes of transmission as well as unique clinical syndromes, and has raised new issues with regard to public health measures and optimal therapy.

To understand fully the controversies surrounding protozoan infections among homosexual men it is best first to examine the biology of these organisms, their complex interactions with the host, and their epidemiology in this new disease setting.

AMEBIASIS

Microbiology and Life Cycle

E. histolytica is a protozoan parasite in the subphylum Sarcodina, class Lobosea, order Amoebida. A member of the family Entamoebidae, it is distinguished from other species (such as *Entamoeba coli*) primarily on the basis of its morphology. Like all amebas except *Dientamoeba fragilis, E. histolytica* has two stages in its life cycle, a motile trophozoite form and a cyst. Trophozoites have an average diameter of 25 μm (range 10 to 60 μm) and contain a single 3- to 5-μm nucleus with a distinct central nucleolus.[3] The cytoplasm is finely granular and may contain ingested red blood cells. The cysts are somewhat smaller (12 μm in average diameter) and have one to four nuclei that are identical in morphology to those seen in trophozoites. Their cytoplasm can have visible chromatoidal bars and, on occasion, glycogen vacuoles.[4]

While both forms may be shed by infected persons, trophozoites can survive only a few hours outside the host. In contrast, cysts remain viable in a moist environment for weeks or months. For this reason, transmission in usually dependent on the ingestion of cysts from a fecally contaminated source. After passage through the stomach, trophozoites emerge from the cysts (excystation) in the intestine. Depending on incompletely understood host and parasite factors, trophozoites may either remain as commensals in the colon, produce disease by invading the gut mucosa, or revert to the cyst form (encystation). With shedding of both cysts and trophozoites in the stool, the life cycle is completed.

Pathogenesis and Host Response

Infection with *E. histolytica* may be a totally asymptomatic or a life-threatening event. Both clinical and laboratory investigations have indicated that strains vary greatly in their virulence.[5] While numerous mechanisms have been proposed as pathogenetic determinants, their importance in mediating the outcome of infection has not been delineated.

One clue has been the observation that different strains can be distinguished by phenotypic isoenzyme patterns called *zymodemes*. Working with lysates of whole trophozoites, Sargeaunt et al. have examined the electrophoretic motility of four enzymes synthesized by *E. histolytica* (glucose phosphate isomerase, L-malate–NADP+ oxidoreductase, phosphoglucomutase, and hexokinase).[6,7] Depending on which isoenzymes are present, all strains may be stratified into one of at least 20 distinct zymodeme groups. Amebas have remarkable stability in their zymodeme characteristics; only recently have investigators been able to induce a shift in zymodeme pattern by the repeated passage of organisms.[8]

Surveys performed in several diverse locations have demonstrated that only strains belonging to certain zymodemes are capable of producing invasive amebiasis. For example, of 125 isolates from patients in Mexico City, merely 11.2 percent were associated with dysentery or hepatic abcesses.[9,10] These pathogenic strains belonged to a limited number of zymodemes (II, VI, VII, and XI). In subsequent South African studies, all amebas cultured directly from 38 hepatic abcesses and 48 patients with dysentery belonged to zymodemes II and XI.[11] Seropositivity for antibodies to *E. histolytica,* which is highly correlated with tissue invasion, was present in 94 to 100 percent of persons infected with these zymodemes.[12,13] In contrast, organisms isolated from asymptomatic carriers belonged to numerous zymodemes, of which only 4 percent were considered virulent. Unlike patients harboring invasive strains, only 2 to 4 percent of individuals infected with nonvirulent strains were seropositive.

Recent experiments with an animal model of amebic colitis confirm that only a few zymodemes can produce invasive disease.[14] However, since none of the enzymes evaluated by zymodeme analysis are directly involved with known pathogenetic processes, this association of zymodemes with invasion remains an intriguing but unexplained observation.

Numerous pathogenetic mechanisms have been proposed for disease due to *E. histolytica*. It is difficult to unite these processes under a single hypothesis because several studies have produced conflicting results, and many basic steps in pathogenesis remain undelineated. However, putative mechanisms may be classified broadly as those involving; (1) secretory enzymes; (2) soluble or trophozoite-free products (enterotoxins or cytotoxins); and (3) contact-dependent cytolysis.

Several enzymes that may directly produce tissue destruction, such as trypsin, pepsin, amylase, and hyaluronidase, have been isolated from trophozoites.[15] While they may be important in the initial disruption of the intestinal endothelium, both virulent and nonpathogenic strains produce these enzymes. Thus, their synthesis is probably not a crucial determinant of invasion.

Gadasi and Kessler have decribed collagenolytic activity in lysates of whole trophozoites, which was correlated with the reported virulence in vivo of three amebic strains.[16] Collagenolytic activity is associated with the plasma membrane fraction of lysed trophozoites. However, activity can be removed from the membrane by elution and is present in the supernatant from cultured trophozoites, suggesting that collagenolytic activity is not an integral part of the plasma membrane.

Several studies indicate a role for extracellular products in mediating amebic disease. McGowan et al. have found that lysates of whole trophozoites are cytotoxic for baby hamster kidney cells, HeLa cells, and adrenal cells in vitro.[17] Cytotoxic activity in vitro is correlated with virulence in an animal model. Purification of the trophozoite lysates by ammonium sulfate precipitation and gel filtration produces a cytolytic fraction containing four proteins (25,000 to 68,000 molecular weight). Lushbaugh et al. have isolated a 25,000- to 35,000-molecular-weight protein that has enterotoxic properties and is cytotoxic for cell monolayers.[18] More recently, Feingold et al. have partially purified two distinct proteins produced in vitro by intact trophozoites; both proteins are enterotoxins and lyse baby hamster kidney cells in tissue culture.[19]

E. histolytica can also cause tissue injury by direct contact with target cells. Contact-dependent cytolysis is a complex event, which may proceed by multiple mechanisms. The initial event in this process is the attachment of the trophozoite to the cell surface by means of two lectin-like adhesions on the parasite.[20,21] Subsequent cell lysis appears to require microfilament function, since it can be blocked by cytochalasin B[22,23] and may be mediated by calcium ion flux in both the ameba and host cells.[24] In addition, cytolysis may be induced in part by a calcium-dependent phospholipase A on the trophozoite membrane.[25,26] How these different aspects of contact-dependent cytolysis are interrelated has not been determined.

In addition to their ability to directly produce tissue destruction and invasion, virulent strains are resistant to several host defense mechanisms. Unlike nonvirulent strains, which are killed by polymorphonuclear cells (PMNs), pathogenic strains can lyse and ingest PMNs.[27] Similarly, while *E. histolytica* activates complement via both the classical and alternative pathways, only nonvirulent strains are susceptible to lysis by complement.[28–30] Thus, not only are pathogenic amebas resistant to two major host defense mechanisms (PMNs and complement), but it has been proposed that the local activation of complement and lysis of PMNs may further contribute to tissue injury.

Several host factors may determine the outcome of infection with *E. histolytica,* including intestinal mucus production, dietary content, and immunity. Leitch et al. have shown recently that intestinal mucus limits trophozoite motility, which may prevent contact with gut endothelial cells and subsequent invasion.[31] Important dietary factors include protein and iron. Low protein intake has been associated both clinically and in animal models with increased tissue destruction.[32,33] In contrast, diets extremely low in iron may limit trophozoite growth, thus restricting disease.[34]

Infection with *E. histolytica* induces both a humoral and cellular immune response. The importance of these host defense mechanisms in preventing or limiting disease has not been fully characterized. Some epidemiologic surveys have demonstrated that the frequency of infection declines with age, suggesting that resistance is acquired.[35] However, invasive disease may occur in patients with high circulating immunoglobulin G antibodies specific for *E. histolytica,* which indicates that humoral immunity is not protective.[36]

In contrast, the importance of cell-mediated immunity in limiting amebic disease is demonstrated by several studies. Depression of cell-mediated immunity by steroids, radiation, or antimacrophage antiserum is associated with more invasive disease in animals.[37,38] In addition, protection against infection, either by vaccination or by prior exposure to organisms, is correlated with enhanced peripheral blood lymphocyte cytotoxicity against amebic trophozoites.[39,40] Lymphocytes from patients with treated amebic liver abscesses have a greater proliferative response to amebic antigens and enhanced cytotoxicity for trophozoites, as compared with lymphocytes from uninfected controls. Lymphokine production, as measured by the killing of trophozoites by monocyte-derived macrophages, is also increased.[41] Thus, these results indicate that the cell-mediated immune response is the major host defense mechanism against invasive amebiasis.

Epidemiology

To better comprehend the unique aspects of amebiasis in homosexual men, it is worthwhile to first examine the epidemiology and clinical features of this disease in more traditional settings. An estimated 10 percent of the world's population is thought to have *E. histolytica* infection.[42] A recent survey of rural and urban inhabitants of Bangladesh showed that 15 to 34 percent were infected[43] and 80 percent had serum antibodies against *E. histolytica,* indicating high levels of past exposure to invasive strains. Similar high rates of infection have been demonstrated among South East Asian refugees, U.S. Peace Corps volunteers returning from service abroad, and American missionaries overseas.[44–46]

In western countries the prevalence of *E. histolytica* is far lower. As for the United States, most authors cite a prevalence of 1 to 4 percent.[47–49] Such estimates are usually based on surveys performed during the 1950s and 1960s in southeastern communities.[50] These studies did not always differentiate *E. histolytica* from the nonpathogen *Entamoeba hartmanni.*[35] In addition, the surveys examined predominantly lower income groups, which often had poor levels of sanitation. As a result, these studies may have overestimated the prevalence of infection. Recent surveys indicate that a prevalence of 0.2 to 1.0 percent is a more accurate figure.[51,52] Similar frequencies have been noted in western Europe.[53] Certain groups are known to have exceptionally high rates of infection, such as persons in psychiatric institutions (26 to 70 percent), North American Indians living on reservations (15 to 33 percent), and sewage workers.[54,55]

Within the past decade homosexual men have been identified as an additional high-risk population.[56–59] By 1977 health officials in both New York and San Francisco had detected a marked change in the epidemiology of amebiasis.[60,61] Previously, the few cases reported each year occurred with equal frequency in men and women and were often associated with overseas travel. In contrast, 89 percent of cases reported to the San Francisco Department of Public Health in 1977 were in male homosexuals 20 to 39 years of age with no history of recent travel or common food exposure.[62] Not only were these demographic changes observed, but the total number of cases had risen from 17 in 1969 to 98 in 1976.[2] In subsequent years the incidence of amebiasis has continued to increase; in 1983 alone, 1026 cases were reported to the Department of Public Health (Fig. 10-1). Despite recent changes in sexual practices among homosexual men in San Francisco,[63] the number of new cases remains high (766 cases in 1985). In part, this high incidence is due to newer screening and contact investigation programs enacted by the city. Nonetheless, it is apparent that amebiasis remains endemic among homosexuals in San Francisco, as well as other cities in the United States and western Europe.

The exact prevalence of *E. histolytica* is difficult to assess, owing to problems in sampling techniques (Table 10-1). Among homosexual men evaluated at a clinic for sexually transmitted diseases in New York, 19.6 percent were found to carry *E. histolytica*. Similar results were reported by clinics in Sweden (21 percent) and Scotland (10 percent).[64,65] Kean et al. noted a higher prevalence (31.7 percent) in a homosexual screening clinic in New York,[58] as did Junod et al. in Paris (52 percent).[66] Ortega et al. found a prevalence of 36 percent in homosexual men seeking medical care from a San Francisco physician in private practice.[67] While these data may be representative of certain sectors of the

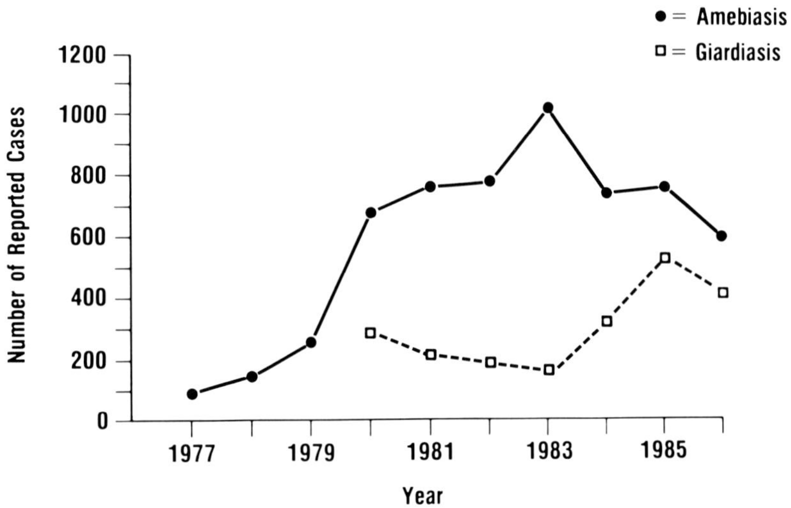

Fig. 10-1. Incidence of amebiasis and giardiasis in San Francisco, 1977–1986. Prior to 1980 no data were available for giardiasis.

homosexual population, they cannot be applied to the group as a whole because of biases in sampling methods. In some studies (e.g., Kean and Junod), infected persons were detected because they sought medical attention for gastrointestinal complaints. Moreover, patients attending a sexually transmitted diseases clinic differ from the overall population in terms of sexual behavior and socioeconomic level.

For these reasons investigators in Toronto, Berlin, and the San Franscisco area have attempted to survey more accurately their homosexual populations.[68–71] Volunteers were obtained by contacting homosexual community groups and by advertisement. One survey screened participants at a health fair for homosexuals. In all three studies a high prevalence of infection, ranging

Table 10-1. Prevalence of Protozoan Infection in Homosexual Men

Study	Date	Location	Number of Patients Evaluated	*Entamoeba histolytica*, %	*Giardia lamblia*, %
William	1978	New York	89	20	12
Kean	1979	New York	126	32	18
Keystone	1980	Toronto	200	27	13
Phillips	1981	New York	163	20	4
Junod	1983	Paris	200	52	13
Hankansson	1984	Göteborg	133	21	8
McMillan	1984	Edinburgh	350	10	3
Markell	1984	San Francisco	508	29	5
Bienzle	1984	Berlin	197	23	9
Allason-Jones	1986	London	225	20	3

from 23 to 29 percent, was detected. In contrast, only 1 percent of heterosexual controls were infected.

Shortly after an increase in amebic infection was noted in several U.S. cities, it was evident that amebiasis in homosexual men was predominantly a sexually transmitted disease. Not only were the usual settings for foodborne infection lacking, but several new risk factors, all implicating sexual transmission, were identified. Prevalence of infection was correlated directly with a high number of sexual partners, anal intercourse, and anilinction.[71,72] In addition, infected persons were more likely to have past histories of other sexually transmitted diseases.[73,74] Finally, coinfection with other enteric pathogens such as *Giardia lamblia,* as well as nonpathogenic protozoa, was very common, further indicating a high prevalence of fecal contact.[65] Thus, these data implicated sexual activity as the major mechanism for transmission of amebiasis in the homosexual population.

Several factors have contributed to the spread of amebiasis.[75] First, the sexual practices of homosexuals are probably efficient modes of transmission because of exposure to a high concentration of organisms during oral-genital contact or of direct intrarectal inoculation. Second, the large number of sexual contacts reported by many homosexual men facilitates transmission. Homosexuals attending the Denver Metro Clinic averaged 5.5 to 7.9 sexual partners per month, as compared with 2.3 contacts in heterosexual men.[72] Quin, et al. have noted similar findings in homosexuals with proctitis.[76] Further contributing to spread is the frequent anonymity of homosexual encounters, which renders ineffective disease control measures such as contact investigation. Finally, the frequent absence of symptoms in infected persons, their reluctance to seek medical attention, and physicians' unfamiliarity or discomfort in dealing with sexually transmitted diseases in this population may all perpetuate endemicity.

Despite the high prevalence of amebiasis, recent data suggest that this and other sexually transmitted diseases may soon decline in frequency as homosexual men modify their sexual practices in response to the acquired immunodeficiency syndrome (AIDS). In San Francisco the incidence of both rectal gonorrhea and amebiasis have declined since 1983. Moreover, a decrease in multiple sexual partners, anilinction, and other high-risk sexual practices is reported by homosexual men, while use of protective measures during receptive anal intercourse has risen.[63] If widely practiced, these behavioral changes may limit the spread of amebic infection.

Clinical Features

In less developed countries infection with *E. histolytica* is usually asymptomatic. However, 10 to 20 percent of infected persons will develop gastrointestinal complaints ranging from mild diarrhea to severe dysentery.[77] Intestinal disease may be complicated by stricture formation, amebomas, or peritonitis, which is often fatal. In addition, approximately 10 percent of patients develop amebic liver abscesses.

In contrast, amebic infection in homosexual men produces relatively mild symptoms and few sequelae.[65,78] Many patients are asymptomatic or have only intermittent complaints. Symptomatic individuals may report nausea, abdominal cramps, acute or chronic diarrhea, blood or mucus in their stools, flatulence, or tenesmus. Frank dysentery is seen only rarely. Less specific complaints, such as weight loss or fatigue, are also common. None of these symptoms is pathognomonic for amebiasis in homosexual men; giardiasis, shigellosis, herpes simplex, and numerous other infections may have similar presentations.

The true frequency of symptoms attributable to amebic infection is difficult to determine in homosexual men. While 50 to 72 percent of infected men have gastrointestinal complaints, a similar prevalence occurs in men without amebiasis.[64,70,71] This extraordinarily high frequency of symptoms is often due to infection with other pathogens; for many men, however, their complaints are idiopathic.

The failure in several studies to correlate amebic infection with symptoms has led some investigators to suggest that *E. histolytica* is not a pathogen in this population.[74,79] However, the high prevalence of intestinal complaints due to other etiologies may make it more difficult to detect an association between symptoms and amebic infection. In fact, some investigations have noted a correlation between amebiasis and gastrointestinal complaints.[65] Moreover, the increased frequency of bowel mucosal abnormalities[78] and the symptomatic response to specific antiamebic therapy[80] both suggest that *E. histolytica* is a true pathogen in the homosexual population.

One striking aspect of amebic infection among homosexual men is the rarity of invasive disease. Only five cases of amebic liver abscess have been reported, including one man receiving steroids and sulfadiazine for presumed inflammatory bowel disease.[81-83] Complications of colitis, such as perforation or stricture formation, are equally uncommon, even in patients with AIDS. Unlike amebiasis in less developed countries, disease in homosexual men almost never produces seropositivity, which further indicates a lack of tissue invasion.[53,68,78] Zymodeme analysis on strains isolated from homosexuals in both Great Britain and the United States has detected only nonvirulent strains.[53,79,84] Thus, the rarity of severe colitis, extraintestinal involvement, and antiamebic antibodies in homosexuals is probably due to an absence or a very low prevalence of invasive strains in the population.

Diagnosis

The diagnosis of intestinal amebiasis requires the isolation of *E. histolytica* from stool specimens or tissue biopsies. In most laboratories this is done by microscopic examination of fecal samples for cysts and trophozoites. When possible, fresh specimens should be obtained and evaluated within 2 hours of collection. Wet mount preparations should be made and examined for motile trophozoites. If more than 2 hours will elapse before processing, fresh specimens should be stored at 4°C.[85]

At the time of collection a portion of the sample should be placed in a separate vial containing polyvinylchloride (PVC), a fixative that preserves both cysts and trophozoites. A third part of the specimen should be fixed in 10 percent formalin and then concentrated by flotation or sedimentation. This technique is valuable for detecting cysts in stools with a low concentration of parasites.[86] Permanent stain smears of the fixed samples are made and examined by light microscopy.

The sensitivity of microscopy is highly dependent on several factors. Yield increases with the number of specimens collected. Since a single sample will miss 12 to 70 percent of cases detected by repeated sampling, collection of three specimens on separate days is recommended.[85] If possible, patients should not have received bismuth, barium, kaolin, antimicrobials, or soap enemas 10 to 14 days prior to testing, since these agents may obscure results. Phosphate purgatives enhance the diagnostic yield of microscopy in some patients. Phillips et al. reported that 55 percent men with nonpathogenic protozoa on their initial stool evaluation, had *E. histolytica* in samples obtained after purging.[65]

Adequately trained laboratory personnel and proper laboratory techniques are critical for accurate diagnosis by microscopy. In their evaluation of parasitologic laboratories, Krogstad et al. found widespread methodologic shortcomings.[87] Improper sample storage, failure to use correct staining methods, and misidentification of leukocytes as cysts were common errors. Many laboratories did not measure cyst size with ocular micrometers and as a result confused *E. hartmanni* with *E. histolytica*. A recent laboratory-induced pseudo-outbreak of intestinal amebiasis demonstrates that these diagnostic inadequacies are still prevalent.[88]

Although first developed in 1925, the in vitro culture of stool for *E. histolytica* remains primarily an investigational technique. Numerous studies have shown this method to be more sensitive than the microscopic examination of stools for cysts and trophozoites. In surveys of amebiasis acquired by travelers or missionaries overseas, 10 percent of cases were diagnosed by culture only.[46] Among homosexuals in western Europe, 10 to 22 percent of patients have no detectable amebic organisms on microscopy but are culture-positive.[66,78]

Gastrointestinal endoscopy is a valuable diagnostic procedure in patients who are thought to have amebic infection but have nondiagnostic results on microscopy.[86] Inspection of the colonic mucosa may reveal punctate hemorrhages or characteristic ulcers. In addition, intestinal scrapings or biopsies may provide specimens that can be examined for *E. histolytica*.[76]

Treatment

Conventional therapy of amebiasis has targeted both infection limited to the bowel lumen and more extensive disease involving tissue invasion.[89,90] In trials performed in less developed countries, no single agent has proved effective for both stages of infection. If treated with a luminal drug alone, patients with intestinal disease frequently progressed to extraintestinal involvement. Conversely, therapy with systemic antimicrobials often failed to eradicate intestinal disease. For these reasons most patients are treated with both a luminal and a systemic agent. However, combination therapy has proved less than ideal owing to problems with cost, adverse reactions, and patient compliance.

Few studies have examined the benefits or efficacy of antimicrobials for treatment of amebiasis in homosexual men. As discussed previously, clinical studies, serologic surveys, and zymodeme analyses all indicate that the natural history of amebic infection is very different in this population when compared with disease in less developed nations. In particular, intestinal disease tends to be mild, and invasive amebiasis is exceedingly rare. These data suggest that for patients with sexually acquired infection, single-drug therapy with a luminal agent may be as effective as combination therapy. To date, this possibility has been addressed by only one study,[80] which is discussed below in the section on paromomycin.

Owing to the paucity of information available, recommendations for the therapy of amebiasis in homosexual men must be extrapolated from trials performed in less developed countries. In the discussion that follows only agents of potential value for the homosexual population will be examined (Table 10-2).

Nitroimidazoles

Metronidazole, first available in 1959, has been employed extensively for treatment of protozoan infections. The drug is directly amebicidal and is thought to act by inhibiting electron transport. When taken orally, it is well absorbed in the small intestine.[91] The recommended dosage is 750 mg three times daily for 10 days. While highly effective at extraintestinal sites of infec-

Table 10-2. Treatment of Intestinal Amebiasis in Adults

Antimicrobial Agent	Dosage	Microbiologic Cure Rate, %	Adverse Reactions
Paromomycin	25–35 mg/kg/day in three daily doses × 7 days;	70–92	Gastrointestinal disturbance
Metronidazole + iodoquinol	750 mg tid × 5–10 days + 650 mg tid × 20 days	90–95	Nausea, headache, metallic taste, disulfiram-like reaction + Rash, diarrhea, iodine allergy
Diloxanide[a] Furoate	500 mg tid × 10 days	80	Gastrointestinal disturbance
Tinidazole[b]	600 mg bid × 5–10 days or 2 g qid × 2–3 days	80–87 85–98	Identical to metronidazole

[a] Available in the United States only from the Centers for Disease Control.
[b] Not available in the United States.

tion (90 to 98 percent cure rate in hepatic abscesses),[92,93] the drug is less successful in eradicating intestinal disease; results vary somewhat with dose, frequency of administration, and duration of therapy, but in general rates of cure do not exceed 85 percent, and may be as low as 50 percent.[10,94] These poor results are attributed to low drug concentrations within the colon.[95] As a consequence, 10 days of metronidazole therapy is often coupled with the luminal agent iodoquinol (650 mg given orally three times daily for 20 days). Although combination therapy has a 90 to 95 percent rate of cure,[96] the long duration of drug administration is an obvious disadvantage.

In addition, metronidazole therapy is associated with adverse reactions in 15 to 35 percent of patients.[92,94,97,98] Frequent gastrointestinal disturbances include nausea, vomiting, abdominal pain, and diarrhea; headache, paresthesias, and dizziness are also common, and a disulfiram-like reaction occurs if alcohol is ingested during therapy. One long-standing theoretical concern has been possible carcinogenesis. Although metronidazole is mutagenic for some bacteria[99,100] and can produce tumors in animals,[101] no increased incidence of malignancies has been demonstrated in humans despite its widespread use.[102]

While not available in the United States, tinidazole has been used extensively in Europe and Asia. This agent is highly effective in the therapy of extraintestinal disease and in contrast to metronidazole, may also be successful in treatment of luminal infection. Joshi and Shah reported a 92 to 97 percent rate of microbiologic cure with 600 mg of tinidazole administered orally twice daily for 5 to 10 days, as compared with an 80 percent cure rate for metronidazole.[103] When tinidazole is given as single daily 2-g dose, 2 or 3 days of treatment have resulted in cure rates of 85 to 98 percent.[92,97,104] Adverse reactions identical to those seen with metronidazole have been reported but with lower frequency. These encouraging data indicate several advantages of tinidazole when compared with metronidazole therapy. However, most studies have been open-label trials with small numbers of patients. Less successful results have been reported, including one double-blind study in which tinidazole was no more effective than a placebo.[105] Until these conflicting data are resolved by large, well-controlled trials, single-agent therapy with tinidazole can only be recommended with caution.

Paromomycin

Paromomycin is an aminoglycoside that is amebicidal against both the cyst and trophozoite forms of *E. histolytica*. The drug is minimally absorbed systemically when taken orally.[106] Limited clinical trials performed in less developed countries have demonstrated that paromomycin cures 70 to 92 percent of patients with intestinal disease.[107–111]

A group of investigators in San Francisco recently assessed the efficacy of paromomycin therapy in 114 homosexual men with proven *E. histolytica* infection.[80] The drug was given for 7 days, 25 to 35 mg/kg daily, in three divided oral doses. When evaluated 4 to 6 weeks after therapy, 92 percent of the patients were cured, as determined by stool microscopy. Of the 80 patients with symptoms at the onset of treatment, 80 percent were asymptomatic at follow-up. The most frequent adverse reaction was mild diarrhea, which was reported in 67 percent of patients. More severe diarrhea (more than five loose stools per day) was less common (16 percent). Nausea, constipation, and vertigo were unusual side effects. No patient discontinued therapy because of drug toxicity. Thus, paromomycin proved to be a very effective treatment for amebiasis in homosexual men, with a rate of cure comparable with that of metronidazole-iodoquinol combination therapy. In addition, it eliminated symptoms in most individuals, a further benefit of treatment. Aside from minor adverse effects, the only disadvantage of this agent is cost; 1 week of paromomycin treatment is as expensive as 20 to 30 days of therapy with metronidazole and iodoquinol.

Iodoquinol (Diodohydroxyquin)

Of the many 8-hydroxyquinoline amebicides developed, iodoquinol is the only member of this group available in the United States. While highly effective when administered with metronidazole, iodoquinol alone has variable efficacy in intestinal amebiasis. Cure rates of 52 to 75 percent have been reported both in mild intestinal disease and in patients with dysentery.[112–114] Adverse reactions include transient abdominal discomfort, chills, fever, generalized furunculosis (iodine toxicoderma), diarrhea, and headache. Iodoquinol is contraindicated in patients allergic to iodine or with hepatic disease. Thyroid enlargement is seen on occasion. A rare toxic reaction ascribed to prolonged high doses of iodoquinol is subacute optic neuropathy.

Diloxanide Furoate

Diloxanide is regarded by some authors as the drug of first choice for asymptomatic amebiasis. In two series of patients with mild to moderate disease an 80 percent rate of cure has been described.[110,115] However, Wilmot et al. reported a 60 percent failure rate in 10 patients with dysentery.[116] The efficacy of this drug in homosexual men with amebic infection is unknown.

Only minor adverse effects occur with diloxanide therapy. Increased flatulence is a nearly universal complaint (87 percent); nausea, vomiting, and diarrhea are also reported. In the United States diloxanide can be obtained only from the Centers for Disease Control.

Other Agents

Tetracycline has been evaluated extensively in therapeutic trials in less developed countries. Although therapy with 1 g/day of tetracycline for 15 days produces a microbiologic cure in 90 to 97 percent of patients, 15 to 45 percent will relapse within 3 to 12 months after treatment.[112,117] Better results are seen when tetracycline is combined with another agent. In one series, for example, tetracycline and diloxanide cured 89 percent of patients with dysentery without a significant rate of relapse.[118] Tetracycline is well tolerated, mild gastrointestinal disturbances and photosensitivity being the only common complaints in adults.

Quinfamide is a newly developed luminal amebicide that appears to have the desirable properties of high efficacy, low toxicity, and short duration of therapy.[119] One day of treatment with 300 mg (given orally in three divided doses) results in a microbiologic cure in 75 to 100 percent of patients.[120–122] Side effects, which are generally mild, include flatulence, nausea, abdominal cramps, and dizziness. Further trials are needed to confirms these promising results. Although it has been approved for marketing in several countries, commercial production of quinfamide has not been initiated.

In summary, an ideal regimen for the treatment of amebiasis would be highly effective and inexpensive, require few days of administration, and have little toxicity. It is apparent that no regimen currently available meets all these criteria, so physicians must choose between two equally efficacious but dissimilar regimens. Therapy with paromomycin is highly effective, is well tolerated, and requires only 7 days of administration. Such a regimen is especially valuable in members of occupation groups (e.g., food handlers) who are prohibited from returning to work until they are free of parasites. The major drawbacks of paromomycin therapy are expense and frequent minor complaints. Combination therapy with metronidazole and iodoquinol has comparable efficacy. However, the associated expense, the long duration of treatment, and the high incidence of side effects are significant disadvantages.

Beyond these two regimens, the physician is faced with inconvenience and incertitude. Diloxanide may be a very effective agent, but further studies are needed to confirm this. Moreover, its restricted availability renders its use cumbersome. Several theoretically effective regimens include tetracycline combined with iodoquinol, short-course therapy with metronidazole and a luminal agent, and single-drug therapy with diloxanide, tinidazole, or quinfamide. However, until further data are available, these regimens must be regarded as experimental.

It should be recognized that the need to treat amebiasis in homosexuals has been questioned[79] because some studies have failed to correlate infection with symptoms. As has been discussed above, however, therapy produces a high rate of microbiologic cure and symptomatic improvement.[80] Moreover, avirulent strains may become more invasive on repeated passage.[8] For these reasons most investigators still recommend treatment in this population.[123]

GIARDIASIS

Microbiology and Life Cycle

Giardia lamblia (see also Ch. 9), a member of the order Diplomonadia and the family Hexamitidae, is a flagellate protozoan with both a trophozoite and a cyst form. Trophozoites are 10 to 12 μm in length, 5 to 7 μm in width, and have a characteristic pear shape. Two distinct nuclei are located in the anterior third of the organism. The nuclear karyosome is usually located centrally and varies in density. Four pairs of flagella are distributed across the convex dorsal surface of the trophozoite. The ventral surface is concave, and contains a prominent disc anteriorly, which is thought to mediate adherence.[124] On electron microscopy the adhesive disc has a striated appearance due to microtubules within its cytoskeleton. Giardia cysts are oval in shape and measure 8 to 12 μm in length by 7 to 10 μm in width. On light microscopy, the cyst wall is highly refractile and usually appears separated from the finely distributed cytoplasm.[126] Newly formed cysts have two nuclei while mature cysts contain four. The compact nuclear karyosome may be either central or eccentric in distribution.

The life cycle of *G. lamblia* is relatively simple. Infection begins with ingestion of cysts from a fecally contaminated source. Only a small inoculum is required to establish disease; studies in human volunteers have demonstrated that ingestion of as few as 10 cysts will produce infection.[127] Excystation occurs in the stomach and duodenum, where low pH may serve as a stimulus for trophozoite release.[128] The highly motile trophozoites migrate into the distal duodenum and proximal jejunum, where they attach to the endothelial surface by means of their adhesive discs.[129]

The mechanisms for adherence are not fully known. However, attachment of trophozoites to plastic surfaces requires calcium and is inhibited by iodoacetic acid, which indicates a dependence on glycolysis.[130] In addition, adherence is blocked by cytochalasin B, which suggests a role for microfilaments, as does the presence of actin and myosin within trophozoite discs.[125]

Intestinal mucus may further enhance trophozoite binding. Zenian and Gillin found that the adherence of trophozoites to glass is increased by mucus isolated from the small intestine.[131] In contrast, colonic mucus has no effect. Fractionation of the small bowel mucus revealed that adherence is augmented by a protein-rich, high-density (1.38 g/ml) nonmucin component, which on polyacrylamide gel chromatography was resolved into four major and four minor protein bands of unspecified molecular weight. It has not been determined if these proteins mediate trophozoite binding to endothelial cells.

The *Giardia* life cycle is completed by encystment of trophozoites in the small bowel or colon, followed by excretion into the external environment. Both cysts and trophozoites may be shed by infected individuals. However, trophozoites survive poorly outside the host, whereas cysts, in contrast, may remain viable for weeks under moist conditions. Thus, cysts are the usual infective form.

Pathogenesis and Host Response

Infection with *G. lamblia* results in several abnormalities of intestinal structure and function.[132] Jejunal biopsies frequently show morphologic changes in the intestinal villi, varying from mild blunting to complete atrophy.

Variable degrees of lymphocyte and PMN infiltration have been described,[133] and increased mitoses among crypt cells have been noted.[134] Numerous derangements of intestinal physiology accompany these morphologic changes. Abnormalities of vitamin B_{12}, folate, D-xylose, and fat absorption may be detected in 60 to 75 percent of patients with acquired hypogammaglobulinemia and *Giardia* infection.[135,136] In otherwise healthy adults with giardiasis and diarrhea, Wright et al. found that only 11 of 40 patients had normal small bowel function as measured by the above parameters of absorption.[137] The degree of malabsorption correlated directly with the severity of mucosal abnormalities detected by small bowel biopsy. For most patients both intestinal morphology and function reverted to normal after treatment with antimicrobial therapy specific for *G. lamblia*.

Although several pathogenetic mechanisms have been proposed, it is unclear how infection with *G. lamblia* results in these derangements of intestinal structure and physiology. While enterotoxin production has been hypothesized, studies employing several different biologic and immunologic assays have failed to demonstrate enterotoxin activity, either in trophozoites or in filtrates of their culture media.[138] A second purported pathogenetic mechanism, mucosal invasion by trophozoites, has been observed only rarely and therefore is not critical for disease production.

Kinetic studies in mice infected with *Giardia muris* have shown an increase in endothelial cell production and enterocyte migration from crypt to villous tip.[134] This increase in enterocyte turnover could result in a less differentiated intestinal cell population, which may be physiologically less competent and thereby produce malabsorption. However, in subsequent experiments defects in disaccharidase function antedated changes in intestinal morphology.[139] Thus, loss of enterocyte maturity is not likely to be a primary pathogenetic event in giardiasis.

The host inflammatory response may contribute to mucosal abnormalities. In nude (hypothymic) mice with persistent *G. muris* infection restoration of T-cell function by thymus transplantation produces clearing of infection[140] but exacerbates abnormalities of small bowel histology. The mechanisms by which T-cell response produces these changes in intestinal morphology are ill-defined, and their relative contributions to malabsorption are poorly delineated.

Several epidemiologic observations indicate that acquired host immunity may prevent or modulate the course of infection with *Giardia*. Studies in regions where giardiasis is endemic, such as Bangladesh or Aspen, Colorado, demonstrate that the prevalence of infection is greatest in children 4 to 14 years of age and declines thereafter.[43,51] In one outbreak long-term residents of an endemic region were four times less likely to develop symptomatic disease than recent arrivals, which further suggests that immunity to infection is acquired with repeated exposure.[141] Protection against reinfection has been demonstrated both in animal models[142] and in limited studies with human volunteers.[142]

The importance of humoral immunity was first indicated by the association of giardiasis with the common varied immunodeficiency syndrome, in which levels of circulating and secretory immunoglobulins are diminished.[135,136,144] Numerous studies have since demonstrated that infection with *G. lamblia* leads to the production of circulating immunoglobulin G that is specific for *Giardia*.[145–147] Experiments in vitro have shown that specific IgG enhances PMN and macrophage adherence, phagocytosis, and killing of trophozoites.[148] This opsonization of trophozoites by IgG does not require complement. In addition, IgG binding to *G. muris* trophozoites is correlated with their clearance from the intestine of infected mice.[149]

A role for IgA in immunity was suggested by Zinneman and Kaplan, who reported decreased concentrations of intestinal secretory IgA in 10 patients with giardiasis, 2 of whom had diminished serum levels as well.[150] These deficiencies persisted after eradication of infection with antimicrobials, which indicated a primary defect in host immunity. However, subsequent studies of patients with giardiasis have not detected any diminution in intestinal or serum IgA concentrations,[151] and many investigators have questioned the techniques employed in assaying intestinal immunoglobulins.[152] More recently, Loftness et al. have shown that infection of rats with *G. lamblia* leads to the appearance in bile of secretory IgA that is specific for trophozoites, as shown by IgA binding to the surface of trophozoites recovered from infected animals.[144] In addition, IgA binding to trophozoites in vivo is correlated with the spontaneous elimination of organisms from the bowel.[149]

Numerous studies indicate a role for cellular immunity in limiting infection with *Giardia*. Murine peritoneal macrophages are spontaneously cytotoxic to trophozoites in vitro, and their cytotoxicity is enhanced by antibodies specific for *Giardia*.[153,154] Moreover, macrophages located within Peyer's patches have been shown to ingest *G. muris*.[155] Although without spontaneous cytotoxicity, human PMNs in the presence of immune serum are lethal to trophozoites.[153,154]

Lymphocytes are another important component of cellular immunity in giardiasis. In contrast to most strains of immunocompetent mice, which promptly eliminate *G. muris* from the gut, athymic mice develop persistent infection.[140] Reconstitution of T-cell function produces a rapid clearing of organisms. However, the precise function of lymphocytes in giardiasis remains unclear. Lymphocytes are not directly cytotoxic to trophozoites even in the presence of immune serum.[154] Heyworth noted that lymphocytes isolated from infected mice were not adherent to trophozoites, which further argues against direct killing by lymphocytes.[149] Histologic studies indicate that lymphocytes may be involved in the processing of antigens within Peyer's patches.[129]

Epidemiology

Giardia lamblia is distributed throughout the world in a variety of climates. Ingestion of contaminated water is the most common mode of acquisition, although foodborne outbreaks have been reported. The prevalence of infection in less developed countries ranges from 4 percent in asymptomatic persons at one Bombay hospital[156] to 42% among southeast Asian refugees.[44]

As mentioned, children are more likely than adults to carry *Giardia;* in one study, for example, 28 percent of Columbian children 5 to 14 years of age were infected as compared with 12 percent of adults.[157] In some regions exposure to *Giardia* is nearly universal. Islam et al. evaluated the incidence of giardiasis in a cohort of mothers and infants in Bangladesh, who underwent monthly examination for the presence in their stools of *G. lamblia.*[158] Over the course of 1 year 82 percent of mothers and 42 percent of infants were at least transiently infected during the period of evaluation. Serologic surveys have also demonstrated high levels of endemicity in certain populations. In a survey of Mexican mothers 77 percent had circulating IgG to *Giardia,* indicative of a high prevalence of past infection.[159]

In the United States a prevalence of 5 to 10 percent was noted in older studies of housing project residents and in rural populations.[35,48,49] More recent data indicate a lower prevalence, 1 to 2 percent, among urban inhabitants.[70,160] Until 1977 outbreaks of infection were uncommon among adults except in municipalities with inadequate water purification systems. However, several communities have recently reported an increase in giardiasis[2,161,162] in association with homosexual activity. In San Francisco, for example, the number of reported cases has risen from less than 200 in 1982 to more than 500 in 1985. Risk of infection is associated with oral-anal contact and is correlated directly with the number of sexual partners.[64,69,71]

As has been discussed for amebiasis, the prevalence of giardiasis among homosexuals is difficult to calculate, owing to problems with sampling groups that may not be representative of the population as a whole. Estimates of prevalence in homosexual men attending sexually transmitted disease clinics vary from 3 to 18 percent (Table 10-1). Surveys that attempt to sample the homosexual population more broadly indicate a 4 to 9 percent rate of infection, as compared with 0 to 2 percent in heterosexual controls.[64,65,68,70]

Clinical Manifestations

The clinical features of *Giardia* infection in homosexual men are very similar to those in heterosexuals. Although patients with AIDS have a diminished monocyte chemotactic response to *G. lamblia* antigens in vitro,[163] this group has not been shown to have either a higher frequency of giardiasis or unusual complications. Infected persons are frequently asymptomatic, or they may have a variety of gastrointestinal complaints. The most common manifestation is diarrhea, which can be acute and self-limited or chronic and intermittent.[64,65] Stools often contain visible mucus, but hematochezia is rare. Other symptoms include nausea, lassitude, anorexia, a weight loss of 5 to 10 pounds, epigastric cramps, and flatulence. Proctitis is a frequent presenting manifestation. Although some symptoms, such as lactose intolerance, may be suggestive of giardiasis, most complaints are common to infection by numerous other pathogens.

Frequently giardiasis cannot be distinguished clinically from infection with

E. histolytica. In patients with proctitis, infection due to herpes simplex virus, *Neisseria gonorrhoeae,* or chlamydia must be considered. Thus, the clinical diagnosis of *Giardia* infection requires confirmation by microbiologic techniques.

Diagnosis

The most commonly employed method for the diagnosis of *G. lamblia* infection is microscopic examination of stools for cysts and trophozoites.[164] As with suspected amebiasis, both fresh and preserved samples should be examined to maximize the diagnostic yield. Trichrome staining of fresh specimens is especially valuable for detecting trophozoites. Formalin concentration of specimens enhances the diagnostic sensitivity of microscopy by 20 percent.[160] Since shedding of organisms is often intermittent, multiple samples should be collected on separate occasions.

In 15 to 50 percent of cases no cysts or trophozoites will be detected on microscopic examination of fecal specimens. For such patients a diagnosis of *G. lamblia* infection can be confirmed by sampling the contents of the small bowel, either by duodenal intubation and drainage or by the Enterotest.[165] The latter is performed by having the patient swallow the distal end of a weighted, encapsulated string, which is retrieved approximately 4 hours later. The adherent intestinal secretions are collected and examined by microscopy. Both duodenal drainage and the Enterotest have sensitivities of 82 to 84 percent.[166,167] For those few infected patients in whom duodenal sampling does not demonstrate *Giardia,* small bowel endoscopy coupled with mucosal brushing or biopsy will usually provide a diagnosis.[168]

Several investigators have demonstrated circulating IgG antibodies to *G. lamblia,* both by indirect immunofluorescence[145,146] and by enzyme-linked immunosorbent assay (ELISA).[147,169] The value of serologic testing in diagnosing acute infection has not been assessed. However, this technique has been useful to epidemiologists, both for estimating the prevalence of past exposure and for evaluating outbreaks retrospectively.

A newly developed diagnostic method is the immunologic assay of feces for giardial antigens. By means of counterimmunoelectrophoresis Craft and Nelson were able to detect coproantigens in 65 of 66 patients with giardiasis.[171] Both Unger et al. and Green et al. have recently described ELISA methods that are 92 to 99 percent sensitive and 98 to 100 percent specific as compared with light microscopy.[172,173] The latter group's test appears particularly sensitive; it reportedly can detect 25 ng of cyst protein and 40 ng of trophozoite protein per milliliter of stool. Although these assays are still undergoing development, they offer many advantages over microscopy. Results are obtained within a few hours and can be interpreted by technicians with minimal training. In addition, the assay of Green et al. does not require special equipment for interpretation but is read by direct visual inspection.

In vitro culture of *Giardia* has been used primarily for nondiagnostic investigational purposes such as the preparation of trophozoite antigens.[174] Many researchers have encountered difficulties in successfully propagating organisms in vitro.[175] Moreover, the conditions necessary for growth are ill-defined. Notwithstanding these obstacles, Gordts et al. have developed a cultivation technique that may be applicable to the diagnostic laboratory.[176] In their study cultures of duodenal aspirates were positive in 10 of 10 patients with proven giardiasis. Growth was detected within 2 or 3 days of inoculating the culture medium in nine cases. While these data can only be viewed as preliminary, cultivation of stool or duodenal samples may prove to be a worthwhile addition to existing diagnostic methods.

Treatment

Since giardiasis in homosexual men is not associated with unique complications or therapeutic problems, the treatment of infection in this population is identical to that of heterosexual adults. Several antimicrobial agents have demonstrated high levels of efficacy in numerous clinical trials.[177,178] Although no study has rigorously examined their value in the homosexual population, it appears that these drugs have comparable efficacy in this group.

Quinacrine

Quinacrine, initially developed as an antimalarial drug, was the first agent to demonstrate activity in vivo against *G. lamblia*. The dosage in adults is 100 mg orally, three times daily, for 5 days. Rates of microbiologic cure as low as 63 percent have been noted,[137] but most studies report a success rate greater than 90 percent.[179,180] In one large prospective trial, quinacrine eradicated infection in 94 percent of patients as compared with a cure rate of 100 percent for metronidazole.[181] When reevaluated 5 months after therapy, 87 percent of patients in both treatment groups were free of infection. Several other studies have confirmed that quinacrine is as effective as metronidazole.[178]

Adverse reactions to quinacrine are reported with varying frequency. Headache, dizziness, and gastrointestinal complaints are often noted, and (as would be expected of an acridine dye derivative) yellow discoloration of the skin may occur during therapy but resolves within a few weeks after treatment. Toxic psychosis, exfoliative dermatitis, and hemolysis in glucose-6-phosphate dehydrogenase (G6PD)–deficient patients are rare complications.

Nitroimidazoles

Both metronidazole and tinidazole have been employed successfully in eradicating giardiasis. Metronidazole therapy for 5 to 10 days (250 mg orally three times daily) cures 60 to 100 percent of patients, with most studies reporting cure rates of greater than 90 percent.[178,182,183] Single dose therapy with 2.4 g of metronidazole is less effective (50 to 60 percent rate of cure), and is associated with frequent relapses, occurring up to 1 month after treatment. Short courses of therapy (2.4 g as a single daily dose, for 2 or 3 days) may be more effective.[184,185] Adverse reactions to metronidazole therapy for giardiasis are identical to those described for the treatment of amebiasis. The lower dosage employed for giardiasis has a lower incidence of side effects (0 to 23 percent). Although widely available, metronidazole has not been approved by the Food and Drug Administration for the treatment of *Giardia* infection.

In comparison with metronidazole, tinidazole has greater activity in vitro against *G. lamblia* trophozoites and clinically is at least as effective.[99,186–188] Cure rates of 74 to 100 percent have been noted with multidose tinidazole therapy (150 mg twice daily for 7 days).[184,189–191] When given as a single 2-g dose, the drug will eliminate infection in more that 90 percent of patients.[187,189,190,192] In most studies this regimen has been associated with minor, transient adverse reactions (dizziness, lassitude, etc.) in about 15 percent of treated individuals.

Furazolidone

Furazolidone is a synthetic nitrofuran, which has been used successfully in treating pediatric giardiasis. In several comparative trials, however, furazolidone was less effective in adults than either quinacrine or metronidazole.[178,179] Most studies report cure rates of 72 to 85 percent with furazolidone.[157,193] The recommended dosage is 100 mg, orally four times daily for 7 to 10 days.

Adverse reactions have been observed in 18 to 23 percent of patients treated with furazolidone, with nausea and vomiting being frequent complaints. When taken with alcohol the drug can produce a disulfiram-like reaction. Hemolytic anemia may occur in patients with G6PD deficiency. Although not shown to be carcinogenic in humans, furazolidone has produced adenocarcinomas in mice and rats.

Summary of Therapeutic Modalities for Giardiasis

In summary, several therapeutic options are available in treating giardiasis in homosexual men (Table 10-3). In the United States quinacrine is probably the treatment of choice since it is highly effective and far less expensive than metronidazole. In countries where tinidazole is available, single-dose therapy with this agent offers greater convenience with comparable rates of cure. Regimens employing any of these three drugs should produce rates of microbiologic cure of 90 percent or more. Patients whose symptoms persist after therapy should undergo reevaluation for continued infection with *G. lamblia*. Since concurrent infection with other organisms is common, these individuals should also be assessed for enteric infection by pathogenic protozoa and bacteria.

Table 10-3. Treatment of Giardiasis in Adults

Antimicrobial Agent	Dosage (PO)	Microbiologic Cure Rate, %	Adverse Reactions
Quinacrine	100 mg tid × 5 days	≥90	Gastrointestinal disturbance, dizziness, yellow staining of skin
Furazolidone	100 mg qid × 7–10 days	72–85	Gastrointestinal disturbance, disulfuram-like reaction
Metronidazole[a]	250 mg tid × 5–10 days	≥90	Nausea, headache, metallic taste, disulfiram-like reaction
Tinidazole[b]	150 mg bid ×7 days or 2-g single dose	75–100 ≥90	Identical to metronidazole

[a] Not approved by the FDA for this use.
[b] Not available in the United States.

REFERENCES

1. Krogstad DJ, Spencer HC Jr, Healy GR: Amebiasis. N Engl J Med 298:263, 1978
2. Dritz SK, Goldsmith RS: Sexually transmissible protozoal, bacterial, and viral enteric pathogens. Compr Ther 56:315, 1980
3. Ravdin JI, Guerrant RL: Current problems in diagnosis and treatment of amebic infections. In Remington JS, Swartz MN (eds): Current Clinical Topics in Infectious Diseases. Vol 7. McGraw-Hill, New York, 1986
4. Sepulveda B. Progress in amebiasis. Scand J Gastroenterol [B] 77:153, 1982
5. Ravdin JI: Pathogenesis of disease caused by *Entamoeba histolytica:* studies of adherence, secreted toxins, and contact-dependent cytolysis. Rev Infect Dis 8:261, 1986
6. Sargeaunt PG, Williams JE: Electrophoretic isoenzyme patterns of *Entamoeba histolytica* and *Entamoeba coli.* Trans R Soc Trop Med Hyg 72:164, 1978
7. Sargeaunt PG, Williams JE: Electrophoretic isoenzyme patterns of the pathogenic and nonpathogenic intestinal amoebae of man. Trans R Soc Trop Med Hyg 73:225, 1979
8. Mirelman D, Bracha R, Chayen A: *Entamoeba histolytica:* effect of growth conditions and bacterial associates on isoenzyme patterns and virulence. Exp Parasitol 62:142, 1986
9. Sargeaunt PG, Williams JE: The epidemiology of *Entamoeba histolytica* in Mexico City. A pilot survey. I. Trans R Soc Trop Med Hyg 74:653, 1980
10. Sargeaunt PG, Williams JE, Bhojnani R, et al: The epidemiology of *Entamoeba histolytica* in a rural and an urban area of Mexico. A pilot survey. II. Trans R Soc Trop Med Hyg 76:208, 1982
11. Sargeaunt PG, Jackson TFHG, Simjee A: Biochemical homogeneity of *Entamoeba histolytica* isolates, especially those from liver abcess. Lancet 1:1386, 1982
12. Jackson TFHG, Gathiram V: Seroepidemiological study of antibody response to the zymodemes of *Entamoeba histolytica*. Lancet 1:716, 1985
13. Gathiram V, Jackson TFHG: Frequency distribution of *Entamoeba histolytica* zymodemes in a rural South African population. Lancet 1:719, 1985
14. Chadee K, Smith JM, Meerovitch E: *Entamoeba histolytica:* electrophoretic

isoenzyme patterns of strains and their virulence in the cecum of gerbils (*Meriones unquiculatus*). Am J Trop Med Hyg 34:870, 1985
15. Jarumilinta R, Maegraith BG: Enzymes of *Entamoeba histolytica*. Bull WHO 41:269, 1969
16. Gadasi H, Kessler E: Correlation of virulence and collagenolytic activity in *Entamoeba histolytica*. Infect Immun 39:528, 1983
17. McGowan K, Deneke CF, Thorne GM, Gorbach SL: *Entamoeba histolytica* cytotoxin: purification, characterization, strain virulence, and protease activity. J Infect Dis 146:616, 1982
18. Lushbaugh WB, Kairalla AB, Cantey JR, et al: Isolation of a cytotoxin-enterotoxin from *Entamoeba histolytica*. J Infect Dis 139:9, 1979
19. Feingold C, Bracha R, Wexler A, Mirelman D: Isolation, purification, and partial characterization of an enterotoxin from extracts of *Entamoeba histolytica* trophozoites. Infect Immun 48:211, 1985
20. Ravdin JI, John JE, Johnston LI, et al: Adherence of *Entamoeba histolytica* trophozoites to rat and human colonic mucosa. Infect Immun 48:292, 1985
21. Ravdin JI, Murphy CF, Salata RA, et al: *N*-acetyl-D-galactosamine-inhibitable adherence lectin of *Entamoeba histolytica*. I. Partial purification and relation to amoebic virulence in vitro. J Infect Dis 151:804, 1985
22. Ravdin JI, Croft BY, Guerrant RL: Cytopathogenic mechanisms of *Entamoeba histolytica*. J Exp Med 152:377, 1980
23. Ravdin JI, Guerrant RL: Role of adherence in cytopathogenic mechanisms of *Entamoeba histolytica*. J Clin Invest 68:1305, 1981
24. Ravdin JI, Sperelakis N, Guerrant RL: Effect of ion channel inhibitors on the cytopathogenicity of *Entamoeba histolytica*. J Infect Dis 146:335, 1982
25. Long-Krug SA, Fisher KJ, Hysmith RM, Ravdin JI: Phospholipase A enzymes of the *Entamoeba histolytica:* description and subcellular localization. J Infect Dis 152:536, 1985
26. Ravdin JI, Murphy CF, Guerrant RL, Long-Krug SA: Effects of antagonists of calcium and phospholipase A on the cytopathogenicity of *Entamoeba histolytica*. J Infect Dis 152:542, 1985
27. Ghadirian E, Meerovitch E: Effect of immunosuppression on the size and metastasis of amoebic liver abscesses in hamsters. Parasite Immunol 3:329, 1982
28. Guerrant RL, Bush J, Ravdin JI, et al: Interaction between *Entamoeba histolytica* and human polymorphonuclear neutrophils. J Infect Dis 143:83, 1981
29. Ortiz-Ortiz L, Capin R, Capin NR, et al: Activation of the alternative pathway of complement by *Entamoeba histolytica*. Clin Exp Immunol 34:10, 1978
30. Davies P, Allison AC, Schorlemmer HU: Interactions between *Entamoeba histolytica* and complement. Nature 277:214, 1979
31. Reed SL, Sargeaunt PG, Braude AI: Resistance to lysis by human serum of pathogenic *Entamoeba histolytica*. Trans R Soc Trop Med Hyg 77:248, 1983
32. Leitch GJ, Dickey AD, Udezulu IA, Bailey GB: *Entamoeba histolytica* trophozoites in the lumen and mucus blanket of rat colons studied in vitro. Infect Immun 47:68, 1985
33. Ross GW, Knight R: Dietary factors affecting the pathogenicity of *Entamoeba histolytica* in rats. Trans R Soc Trop Med Hyg 67:560, 1973
34. Roa VG, Pedma MC: Effect of host's nutrition on immune response to amoebic antigen on susceptibility to infection with *Entamoeba histolytica*. Indian J Exp Biol 13:176, 1975

35. Murray MJ, Murray A, Murray CJ: The salutary effect of milk on amoebiasis and its reversal by iron. Br Med J 280:1351, 1980
36. Jones FE, Smith CS, Eyles DE: Epidemiologic study of *Entamoeba histolytica* and other parasites in the New Hope community of Tennessee. Am J Trop Med Hyg 3:266, 1954
37. Krupp IM: Antibody response in intestinal and extraintestinal amebiasis. Am J Trop Med Hyg 19:57, 1970
38. Ghadirian E, Meerovitch E, Kingshavn PAL: Role of macrophages in host defense against hepatic amoebiasis in hamsters. Infect Immun 42:1017, 1983
39. Ghadirian E, Meerovitch E, Hartmann D-P: Protection against amebic liver abcess in hamsters by means of immunization with amebic antigen and some of its fractions. Am J Trop Med Hyg 29:779, 1980
40. Ghadirian E, Meevrovitch E: In vitro amoebicidal activity of immune cells. Infect Immun 36:243, 1982
41. Salata RA, Martinez-Palomo A, Murray HW et al: Patients treated for amebic liver abcess develop cell-mediated immune responses effective in vitro against *Entamoeba histolytica*. J Immunol 133:2633, 1986
42. Walsh JA: Problems in recognition and diagnosis of amebiasis: estimation of global magnitude of morbidity and mortality. Rev Infect Dis 8:228, 1986
43. Hossain MM, Ljungstrom I, Glass RI, et al: Amoebiasis and giardiasis in Bangladesh: parasitological and serological studies. Trans R Soc Trop Med Hyg 77:552, 1983
44. Borchardt KA, Ortega H, Mahood JD, et al: Intestinal parasites in Southeast Asian refugees. West J Med 135:93, 1981
45. Grossman W: Amebiasis in Peace Corps volunteers. Am J Gastroenterol 51:418, 1969
46. McQuay R: Parasitologic studies in a group of furloughed missionaries. Am J Trop Med Hyg 16:154, 1967
47. Burrows KB: Prevalence of amebiasis in the United States and Canada. J Trop Med Hyg 10:172, 1961
48. Brooke MM: Epidemiology of amebiasis in the US. JAMA 188:147, 1964
49. Eyle DE, Jones FE: The prevalence of *Entamoeba histolytica* and other intestinal parasites in a selected urban population. Am J Trop Med Hyg 3:988, 1953
50. Brooke MM, Healy GR, Levy P, et al: A sample survey of selected areas in and near Little Rock, Arkansas, to access the prevalence of *Entamoeba histolytica*. Bull WHO 29:813, 1963
51. Gleason N: A stool survey for enteric organisms in Aspen, Colorado. Am J Trop Med Hyg 19:480, 1976
52. Markell EK, Kuritsubo RA: Intestinal protozoal infections: prevalence in the Bay area. West J Med 135:188, 1981
53. Sargeaunt PG, Oates JK, MacLennan I, et al: *Entamoeba histolytica* in male homosexuals. Br J Vener Dis 59:193, 1983
54. Juniper K Jr: Amebiasis in the United States. Bull NY Acad Med 47:448, 1971
55. Knobloch J, Bialek R, Hagemann J: Intestinaler Protozoenbefall durch Berufsbedingten. Dtsch Med Wochenschr 108:57, 1983
56. Marr JS: Amebiasis in New York City: a changing pattern of transmission. Bull NY Acad Med 57:188, 1981
57. Schmerin MJ, Gelston A, Jones TC: Amebiasis. An increasing problem among homosexuals in New York City. JAMA 238:1386, 1977

58. Kean BH, William DC, Luninais SK: Epidemic of amoebiasis and giardiasis in a biased population. Br J Vener Dis 55:375, 1979
59. Burnham WR, Reeve RS, Finch RG: *Entamoeba histolyica* infection in male homosexuals. Gut 21:1097, 1980
60. Pomerantz BM, Marr JS, Goldman WD: Ambiasis in New York City 1958–1978: identification of the male homosexual high risk population. Bull NY Acad Med 56:232, 1980
61. Dritz SK, Ainsworth TE, Garrard WF, et al: Patterns of sexually transmitted enteric disease in a city. Lancet 2:3, 1977
62. Medical Staff Conference: Veneral aspects of gastroenterology. West J Med 130:236, 1979
63. McKusick L, Horstman W, Coates TJ: AIDS and sexual behavior reported by gay men in San Francisco. Am J Public Health 75:493, 1985
64. William DC, Shookoff HB, Felman YM, De Ramos S: High rates of enteric protozoal infections in selected homosexual men attending a venereal disease clinic. Sex Transm Dis 5:155, 1978
65. Phillips SC, Mildvan D, Williams DC, et al: Sexual transmission of enteric protozoa and helminths in a venereal-disease-clinic population. N Engl J Med 305:603, 1981
66. Junod C: Résultats comparés des examens coprologiques effectués en vue du dépistage des amebes et flagellés intestinaux chez 200 homosexuels masculins. Bull Soc Pathol Exot Filiales 76:805, 1983
67. Ortega HB, Borchardt KA, Hamilton R, et al: Enteric pathogenic protozoa in homosexual men from San Francisco. Sex Transm Dis 11:59, 1984
68. Keystone JS, Keystone DL, Proctor EM: Intestinal parasitic infections in homosexual men: prevalence, symptoms, and factors in transmission. Can Med Assoc J 123:512, 1980
69. Bienzle U, Coester CH, Knobloch J, Guggenmoos-Holzmann I: Protozoal enteric infections in homosexual men. Klin Wochenschr 62:323, 1984
70. Markell EK, Havens RF, Kuritsubo RA: Intestinal parasitic infections in homosexual men at a San Francisco health fair. West J Med 139:177, 1983
71. Markell EK, Havens RF, Kuritsubo, RA, Wingerd J: Intestinal protozoa in homosexual men of the San Francisco bay area: prevalence and correlates of infection. Am J Trop Med Hyg 33:239, 1984
72. Judson FN, Penley KA, Robinson ME, Smith JK: Comparative prevalence rates of sexually transmitted diseases in heterosexual and homosexual men. Am J Epidemiol 122:836, 1980
73. Thin RN, Smith DM: Some characteristics of homosexual men. Br J Vener Dis 52:161, 1976
74. Goldmeier D, Sargeaunt PG, Price AB, et al: Is *Entamoeba histolytica* in homosexual men a pathogen? Lancet 1:641, 1986
75. Ostrow DG, Altman NL: Sexually transmitted diseases and homosexuality. Sex Transm Dis 10:208, 1983
76. Quinn TC, Corey L, Chaffee R, et al: The etiology of anorectal infections in homosexual men. Am J Med 71:395, 1981
77. Adams EB, MacLeod IN: Invasive amebiasis. I. Amebic dysentery and its complications. Medicine (Baltimore) 56:315, 1977
78. McMillan A, Gilmour HM, McNeillage G, Scott GR: Amoebiasis in homosexual men. Gut 25:356, 1984

79. Allason-Jones E, Mindel A, Sargeaunt P, Williams P: *Entamoeba histolytica* as a commensal intestinal parasite in homosexual men. N Engl J Med 315:353, 1986
80. Sullam PM, Slutkin G, Gottlieb AB, Mills J: Paromomycin therapy of endemic amebiasis in homosexual men. Sex Transm Dis 13:151, 1986
81. Ylvisaker JT, McDonald GB: Sexually acquired amebic colitis and liver abcess. West J Med 132:153, 1980
82. Thompson JE Jr, Freischlag J, Thomas DS: Amebic liver abcess in a homosexual man. Sex Transm Dis 10:153, 1983
83. Finch R, Burnham WR, Reeve RS: Amoebic liver abcess. Br Med J 283:1545, 1981
84. Mathew HM, Moss DM, Healy GR, Mildvan D: Isoenzyme analysis of *Entamoeba histolytica* isolated from homosexual men. J Infect Dis 153:793, 1986
85. Healy GR: Laboratory diagnosis of amebiasis. Bull NY Acad Med 47:478, 1971
86. Pehrson PO: Amoebiasis in a non-endemic country. Scand J Infect Dis 15:207, 1983
87. Krogstad DJ, Spencer HC Jr, Healy GR, et al: Amebiasis: epidemiologic studies in the United States 1971–74. Ann Intern Med 88:89, 1978
88. Garcia L, Sovillo F, Epstein M, et al: Pseudo outbreak of intestinal amebiasis—California. MMWR 34:125, 1985
89. Botero D: Intestinal parasitic infections. Antibiot Chemother 30:1, 1981
90. Biagi F: Amebiasis. Antibiot Chemother 30:20, 1981
91. Andersson KE: Pharmacokinetics of nitroimidazoles. Spectrum of adverse reactions. Scand J Infect Dis 26:60, 1981
92. Islam N, Hasan K: Tinidazole and metronidazole in hepatic amebiasis. Drugs 15: suppl. 1, 26, 1978
93. Cohen HG, Reynolds TB: Comparison of metronidazole and chloroquin for the treatment of amoebic liver abcess. Gastroenterology 69:35, 1975
94. Kanani SR, Knight R: Experiences with the use of metronidazole in the treatment of nondysenteric intestinal amoebiasis. Trans R Soc Trop Med Hyg 66:244, 1972
95. Powell SJ, Elsdon-Dew R: Some new nitroimidazole derivatives. Clinical trials in amebic liver abcess. Am J Trop Med Hyg 21:518, 1972
96. Adams EB, MacLeod IN: Invasive amebiasis. II. Amebic liver abcess and its complications. Medicine (Baltimore) 56:325, 1977
97. Misra NP: A comparative study of tinidazole and metronidazole as a single daily dose three times daily in symptomatic intestinal amebiasis. Drugs 15: suppl. 1, 19, 1978
98. Bakshi JS, Ghiara JM, Nanivadeker AS: How does tinidazole compare with metronidazole? Drugs 15: suppl. 1, 33, 1978
99. Speck WT, Stein AB, Rosenkranz HS: Mutagenicity of metronidazole: presence of several active metabolites in human urine. JNCI 56:283, 1976
100. Connor TH, Stoeckel M, Evrard J, Legator MS: The contribution of metronidazole and two metabolites to the mutagenic activity detected in urine of treated humans. Cancer Res 37:629, 1977
101. Rustia M, Shubik P: Induction of lung tumors and malignant lymophomas in mice by metronidazole. JNCI 48:721, 1972
102. Beard CM, Noller KL, O'Fallon WM, et al: Lack of evidence for cancer due to the use of metronidazole. N Engl J Med 301:519, 1979
103. Joshi HD, Shah BM: A comparative study of tinidazole and metronidazole in treatment of amoebiasis. Indian Practitioner 28:295, 1975
104. Welch JS, Rowsell BJ, Freeman C: Treatment of intestinal amoebiasis and giar-

diasis. Efficacy of metronidazole and tinidazole compared. Med J Aust 1:469, 1978
105. Spillmann R, Ayala SC, Elena de Sanchez C: Double blind test of metronidazole and tinidazole in the treatment of asymptomatic *Entamoeba histolytica* and *Entamoeba hartmanni* carriers. Am J Trop Med Hyg 26:549, 1976
106. Knight R: The chemotherapy of amoebiasis. J Antimicrob Chemother 6:577, 1980
107. Bianchini C, Sanguigni S, Cifarelli F, Paparo BS: Osservazioni sul trattamento di amebiasi intestinale. Clin Ter 91:351, 1979
108. Carter CH: Paromomycin (Humatin) in the treatment of intestinal amebiasis: a preliminary dose-range study. Antibiot Med Clin Ther 6:585, 1959
109. Courtney KO, Thompson PE, Hodgkinson R, Fitzsimmons JR: Paromomycin as a therapeutic substance for intestinal amebiasis and bacterial enteritis. Antibiot Annu 7:304, 1959–60
110. Forsyth DM: The treatment of amoebiasis: a field study of various methods. Trans R Soc Trop Med Hyg 56:400, 1962
111. Wilmot AJ, Powell SJ, Macleod I, Elsdon-Dew R: Paromomycin in acute amoebic dysentery. Ann Trop Med Parasitol 56:383, 1962
112. Armstrong TG, Wilmot AJ, Elsdon-Dew R: The treatment of amoebic dysentery in the Bantu African. Trans R Soc Trop Med Hyg 42:597, 1949
113. Elsdon-Dew R, Wilmot AJ, Powell SJ: The tetracyclines in amebiasis. Antibiot Annu 7:829, 1959-1960
114. Powell SJ, Wilmot AJ, Elsdon-Dew R: Potentiating effect of quinolines on the action of tetracycline in amoebic dysentery. Lancet 1:76, 1960
115. Wolfe MS: Nondysenteric intestinal amebiasis. Treatment with diloxanide furoate. JAMA 224:1601, 1973
116. Wilmot AJ, Powell SJ, McLeod I, Elsdon-Dew R: Some new amoebicides in acute amebic dysentery. Trans R Soc Trop Med Hyg 56:85, 1962
117. Killough JH, Magill GB: A comparative study of fumagillin and oxytetracycline in amebiasis. Am J Trop Med Hyg 3:999, 1954
118. Botero D: Treatment of intestinal amebiasis with diloxanide furoate, tetracycline, and chloroquine. Trans R Soc Trop Med Hyg 61:769, 1976
119. Slighter RG, Yarinsky A, Drobeck HP, Bailey DM: Activity of quinfamide against natural infections of *Entamoba criceti* in hamsters: a new potent agent for intestinal amoebiasis. Parasitology 81:157, 1980
120. Guevara L: Evaluacion de la tolerancia y eficacia en humanos de quinfamide, un nuevo amebicida intraluminal (tratamiento de un día). Estudio doble-ciego. Rev Gastroenterol Mex 45:93, 1980
121. Huggins D: Ensaio clinico duplo-cego com o Win 40014 no tratamento de amebiase intestinal cronica. Folha Med 85:869, 1982
122. Rojas FA, Ledezman MD, Martinez CV, Garza RG: Treatment of chronic amebiasis in pediatric patients with a suspension of quinfamide. Clin Ther 6:47, 1983
123. Krogstad DJ: Isoenzyme patterns and pathogenicity in amebic infection. N Engl J Med 315:390, 1986
124. Smith JW, Wolfe MS: Giardiasis. Ann Rev Med 31:373, 1980
125. Feely DE, Schollmeyer JV, Erlandsen SL: *Giardia* spp: distribution of contractile proteins in the attachment organelle. Exp Parasitol 53:145, 1982
126. Burke JA: The clinical and laboratory diagnosis of giardiasis. CRC Crit Rev Lab Sci 7:373, 1977
127. Rendtorff RC: The experimental transmission of human intestinal protozoan parasites. II. *Giardia lamblia* cysts given in capsules. Am J Hyg 59:209, 1954

128. Bingham AK, Meyer EA: *Giardia* excystation can be induced in vitro in acid solutions. Nature 277:301, 1979
129. Owen RL, Nemanic PC, Stevens DP: Ultrastructural observations on giardiasis in a murine model. I. Intestinal distribution, attachment, and relationship to the immune system of *G. muris*. Gastroenterology 76:757, 1979
130. Feely DE, Erlandsen SL: Effect of cytochalasin-B, low Ca^{++} concentration, iodoacetic acid, and quinacrine-HCl on the attachment of *Giardia* trophozoites in vitro. J Parasitol 68:869, 1982
131. Zenian A, Gillin FD: Interactions of *Giardia lamblia* with human intestinal mucus: enhancement of trophozoite attachment to glass. J Protozool 32:664:1985
132. Duncombe VM, Bolin TD, Davis AE, et al: Histopathology in giardiasis: a correlation with diarrheoea. Aust NZ J Med 8:392, 1978
133. Hoskins LC, Winawer SJ, Broitman SA, et al: Clinical giardiasis and intestinal malabsorption. Gastroenterology 53:265, 1967
134. Yardley JH, Takano J, Hendrix TR: Epithelial and other mucosal lesions of the jejunum in giardiasis. Jejunal biopsy studies. Bull Johns Hopkins Hosp 115:389, 1964
135. Ament MF, Rubin CE: Relation of giardiasis to abnormal intestinal structure and function in gastrointestinal immunodeficiency syndromes. Gastroenterology 62:216, 1972
136. Hartong WA, Gourley WK, Arvanitakis C: Giardiasis: clinical spectrum and functional-structural abnormalities of the small intestine. Gastroenterology 77:61, 1979
137. Wright SG, Tonkins AM, Ridley DS: Giardiasis: clinical and therapuetic aspects. Gut 18:343, 1977
138. Smith PD, Gillin FD, Spira WM, Nash TE: Chronic giardiasis: studies on drug sensitivity, toxin production, and host immune response. Gastroenterology 83:797, 1982
139. Gillon J, Thamery DA, Ferguson A: Features of small intestinal pathology (epithelial cell kinetics, intraepithelial lymphocytes, disaccharidases) in primary *Giardia muris* infection. Gut 23:498, 1982
140. Roberts-Thomson IC, Mitchell GF: Giardiasis in mice. I. Prolonged infections in certian mouse strains and hypothymic (nude) mice. Gastroenterology 75:42, 1978
141. Istre GR, Dunlop TS, Gaspard GB, Hopkins RS: Waterborne giardiasis at a mountain resort: evidence for acquired immunity. Am J Public Health 74:602, 1984
142. Roberts-Thompson IC, Stevens DP, Mahmoud AAF, Warren KS: Acquired resistance to infection in an animal model of giardiasis. J Immunol 117:2036, 1976
143. Rendtorff RC, Holt CJ: The experimental transmission of human intestinal protozoan parasites. IV. Attempts to transmit *Entamoeba coli* and *Giardia lamblia* by water. Am J Hyg 60:327, 1954
144. Loftness TJ, Erlandsen SL, Wilson ID, Meyer EA: Occurrence of specific secretory immunoglobulin A in bile after inoculation of *Giardia lamblia* trophozoites in rat duodenum. Gastroenterology 87:1022, 1984
145. Ridley MJ, Ridley DS: Serum antibodies and jejunal histology in giardiasis associated with malabsorption. J Clin Pathol 29:30, 1976
146. Moody AH, Ridley DS, Tomkins AM, Wright SG: The specificity of serum antibodies to *Giardia lamblia* and to enterobacteria in gastrointestinal disease. Trans R Soc Trop Med Hyg 76:630, 1982
147. Smith PD, Gillin FD, Brown WR, Nash TE: IgG antibody to *Giardia lamblia* detected by enzyme-linked immunsorbent assay. Gastroenterology 80:1476, 1981

148. Radulescu S, Meyer EA: Opsonization in vitro of *Giardia lamblia* trophozoites. Infect Immun 32:852, 1981
149. Heyworth MF: Antibody response to *Giardia muris* trophozoites in mouse intestine. Infect Immun 52:568, 1986
150. Zimmerman HH, Kaplan AP: The association of giardiasis with reduced intestinal secretory immunoglobin A. Am J Dig Dis 17:793, 1972
151. Jones EG, Brown WR: Serum and intestinal immunoglobulins in patients with giardiasis. Am J Dig Dis 19:791, 1974
152. McClelland DBC, Warwick RRG, Shearman DJC: IgA concentration. Am J Dig Dis 18:347, 1973
153. Smith PD, Elson CO, Deister DB: Human host response to *Giardia lamblia*. I. Spontaneous killing by mononuclear leukocytes in vitro. J Immunol 128:1372, 1982
154. Smith PD, Keister DB, Elson CO: Human host response to *Giardia lamblia*. II. Antibody dependent killing in vitro. Cell Immunol 82:308, 1983
155. Owen RL, Allen CL, Stevens DP: Phagocytosis of *Giardia muris* by macrophages in Peyer's patch epithelium in mice. Infect Immun 33:591, 1981
156. Antia FP, Desai HG, Jeejeebhoy KN, et al: Giardiasis in adults. Incidence, symptomatology, and absorption studies. Indian J Med Sci 20:471, 1966
157. Botero DR, Cano M, Perez GMA, Hurtado MI: Furazolidone en giardiasis intestinal. Rev Int Salud Publica 33:127, 1973
158. Islam A, Stoll BJ, Ljungstrom I, et al: *Giardia lamblia* infections in a cohort of Bangladeshi mothers and infants followed for one year. J Pediatr 103:996, 1983
159. Miotti PG, Gilman RH, Pickering LK, et al: Prevalence of serum and milk antibodies in *Giardia lamblia* in different populations of lactating women. J Infect Dis 152:1025, 1985
160. Petersen H: Giardiasis (lambliasis). Scand J Gastroenterol [Suppl] 7:1, 1972
161. Meyers JD, Kuharic HA, Holmes KK: *Giardia lamblia* infection in homosexual men. Br J Vener Dis 53:54, 1977
162. Schmerin MJ, Jones TC, Klein H: Giardiasis: association with homosexuality. Ann Intern Med 88:801, 1978
163. Smith PD, Ohura K, Masur H, et al: Monocyte function in the acquired immune deficiency syndrome. Defective chemotaxis. J Clin Invest 74:2121, 1984
164. Thornton SA, West AH, Dupont HL, Pickering LK: Comparison of methods for identification of *Giardia lamblia*. Am J Clin Pathol 80:858, 1983
165. Kamath KR, Murugasu R: A comparative study of four methods for detecting *Giardia lamblia* in children with diarrheal disease and malabsorption. Gastroenterology 66:16, 1974
166. Rosenthal P, Liebman WM: Comparison of stool examination, duodenal aspiration, and pediatric entero-test for giardiasis in children. J Pediatr 96:278, 1980
167. Bezjak B: Evaluation of a new technique for sampling duodenal contents in parasitologic diagnosis. Am J Dig Dis 17:848, 1972
168. Marshall JB, Kelly DH, Vogele KA: Giardiasis: diagnosis by endoscopic brush cytology of the duodenum. Am J Gastroenterol 79:517, 1984
169. Visvesvara GS, Smith PD, Healy GR, Brown WR: An immunofluorescence test to detect serum antibodies to *Giardia lamblia*. Ann Intern Med 93:802, 1980
170. Voight RL, Little AA, Spitalny KC: Investigation of a waterborne outbreak of giardiasis, using serologic testing by IFA. Am J Public Health 74:272, 1984
171. Craft JC, Nelson JD: Diagnosis of giardiasis by counterimmunoelectrophoresis of feces. J Infect Dis 145:499, 1982
172. Green EL, Miles MA, Warhurst DC: Immunodiagnostic detection of *Giardia* anti-

gen in faeces by rapid visual enzyme-linked immunosorbent assay. Lancet 2:691, 1985
173. Ungar BLP, Yolken RH, Nash TE, Quinn TC: Enzyme-linked immunosorbent assay for the detection of *Giardia lamblia* in fecal specimens. J Infect Dis 149:90, 1984
174. Wieder SC, Deister DB, Reiner DS: Mass cultivation of *Giardia lamblia* in a serum-free medium. J Parasitol 69:1181, 1983
175. Meyer EA: Culture of *Giardia lamblia*. Lancet 2:527, 1984
176. Gordts B, Retore P, Cadranel S, et al: Routine cultures of *Giardia lamblia* trophozoites from human duodenal aspirates. Lancet 2:137, 1984
177. Davidson RA: Issues in parasitology: the treatment of giardiasis. Am J Gastroenterol 79:256, 1984
178. Levi GC, De Avila CA, Neto VA: Efficacy of various drugs for treatment of giardiasis. A comparative study. Am J Trop Med Hyg 26:564, 1977
179. Craft JC, Murphy T, Nelson JD: Furazolidone and quinacrine. Comparative study of therapy for giardiasis in children. Am J Dis Child 135:164, 1981
180. Bassily S, Rarid Z, Mikhail JW, et al: The treatment of *Giardia lamblia* infection with mepacrine, metronidazole, and furazolidone. J Trop Med Hyg 73:15, 1970
181. Kavousi S: Giardiasis in infancy and childhood: a prospective study of 160 cases with comparison of quinacrine (Atabrine) and metronidazole (Flagyl). Am J Trop Med Hyg 28:19, 1979
182. Palomino H, Perez C, Donckaster R, et al: Ensayo terapeutico con cinco medicamentos en lambliasis. Bol Chil Parasitol 25:52, 1970
183. Garg BK: Furazolidone and metronidazole in the treatment of giardiasis. Indian J Pediatr 39:264, 1972
184. Jokipii L, Jokipii AMM: Comparison of four dosage schedules in the treatment of giardiasis with metronidazole. Infection 6:92, 1978
185. Khambatta RB: Metronidazole in giardiasis. Ann Trop Med Parasitol 65:487, 1971
186. Boreham PFL, Phillips RE, Sheperd RW: The sensitivity of *Giardia intestinalis* to drugs in vitro. J Antimicrob Chemother 14:449, 1984
187. Jokipii L, Jokipii AMM: Single dose metronidazole and tinidazole as therapy for giardiasis: success rates, side effects, and drug absorption and elimination. J Infect Dis 141:317, 1980
188. Kyronseppa H, Pettersson T: Treatment of giardiasis: relative efficacy of metronidazole as compared with tinidazole. Scand J Infect Dis 13:311, 1981
189. Sterner G, Lantorp K: Outbreak of *Giardia lamblia* infection in a tourist group: treatment with tinidazole. Infection 1:33, 1973
190. Salih SY, Abdalla RE: Symptomatic giardiasis in Sudanese adults and its treatment with tinidazole. J Trop Med Hyg 80:11, 1977
191. Andersson T, Forssell J, Sterner G: Outbreak of giardiasis: effect of a new antiflagellate drug, tinidazole. Br Med J 2:449, 1972
192. Apte VV, Packard RS: Tinidazole in the treatment of trichomoniasis, giardiasis, and amoebiasis. Drugs 15: suppl. 1, 43, 1978
193. Murphy TV, Nelson JD: Five v. ten days' therapy with furazolidone for giardiasis. Am J Dis Child 137:267, 1983

11 Advances in the Biology and Immunology of *Pneumocystis carinii*

Joseph A. Kovacs
Henry Masur

Pneumocystis carinii is an organism whose importance has increased dramatically in recent years, primarily because of the advent of the acquired immunodeficiency syndrome (AIDS) but also because of the increased use of immunosuppressive regimens for treatment of patients with malignant neoplasms, organ transplants, and immunologically mediated diseases such as vasculitis.[1] According to estimates by the U. S. Public Health Service, more than 200,000 cases of *P. carinii* pneumonia will occur between 1986 and 1991 in the United States alone.[2]

Despite this dramatic increase in the clinical importance of *P. carinii* there has not been a commensurate increase in understanding its epidemiology, biology, antigenic structure, host-organism interaction, and taxonomy. Two major problems are responsible for this lack of progress, namely the difficulties encountered in culturing *P. carinii* and those encountered in purifying the organism as obtained from infected lungs. Thus, inability to prepare large quantities of viable purified *P. carinii* remains a major obstacle to the rapid expansion of knowledge regarding it. In spite of these difficulties some significant advances have been made in the past few years.

Much of the understanding of the biology of *P. carinii*, as well as the development of effective therapy for *P. carinii* pneumonia, has been based on studies of an animal model of *P. carinii* pneumonia.[3–5] Administration of steroids to rats will result in spontaneous development of *P. carinii* pneumonia in the majority of rats by 6 to 10 weeks. Tetracycline is administered simultaneously to prevent bacterial superinfection, and a low-protein diet may be substituted for regular rat chow to increase the severity of disease. By using this model, for example, transmission of the organism from animal to animal by the respiratory route and not by contaminated food, water, or bedding has been documented.[3] The efficacy of trimethoprim-sulfamethoxazole and more recently trimethoprim-dapsone, was initially demonstrated in this model, which has also been used to assess prophylactic regimens.[4,5]

However, there are limitations to the usefulness of the model in studying human disease. Animals often fail to survive therapeutic trials because of pathologic processes other than pneumocystis (e.g., aspergillosis). Drug pharmacokinetics are often dramatically different in rodents and in humans; for example, trimethoprim has a half-life of about 1 hour in rats, compared with about 10 hours in humans. Immunologic function in rats is clearly different from that in humans—especially important is the recent observation that *P. carinii* in rodents may not be antigenically identical to the organism found in humans.[6,7] It is thus clear that although the rat model can provide a basis for investigating *P. carinii,* sole reliance on this model can lead to conclusions that may not apply to *P. carinii*–related disease in humans.

This chapter will review some of the recent advances in the biology and immunology of *P. carinii* and will cover morphologic studies that have led to a better understanding of the histopathology and life cycle of the organism as well as biochemical studies of its metabolic pathways. Finally, recent studies investigating the antigenic structure of *P. carinii* through immunoblot techniques and monoclonal antibodies will be summarized. Earlier studies not covered in this chapter have been recently reviewed by Young and others.[8]

BIOLOGY OF *P. CARINII*

P. carinii, presumed to be a protozoan, has been detected in a large number of animals, including rabbits, dogs, mice, and horses. The identity of a natural reservoir is unknown, and how long it can exist outside a host is also unknown. Transmission of the organism, at least in the rat, appears to occur by the respiratory route.[3] The stage of the organism that is infectious is unknown.

Morphology, Histopathology, and Life Cycle

P. carinii has traditionally been described on the basis of morphologic studies as having three separate stages: trophozoite, precyst, and cyst[9–11] (Fig. 11-1). The trophozoite is irregularly shaped, is 2 to 8 μm in size, and is surrounded by a thin outer wall, or pellicle. The cyst is a round structure 6 to 8 μm in diameter, with a thickened outer wall, and contains up to eight internal sporozoites. The precyst is more regular in shape than the trophozoite but does not contain clearly defined or completed sporozoites. Internal structures that have been identified in the organism include nuclei, mitochondria, ribosomes, and glycogen deposits.

The standard method for detecting *P. carinii* in fixed tissue has been to use stains that demonstrate the cyst wall, such as toluidine blue O, Gram-Weigert, or methamine silver. The trophozoite can be detected by Giemsa, Diff-quik, or related stains on lung imprints and in pulmonary specimens such as sputum or bronchoalveolar lavage specimens but not in standard paraffin sections. Recently a technique was developed for visualizing trophozoites as well as internal sporozoites in histologic sections by prolonged Giemsa staining of 1-μm sections of glutaraldehyde-fixed tissue embedded in plastic.[12,13] Use of this technique indicated that trophozoites apparently far outnumber cysts in infected lung, which confirms the impression obtained from lung imprints and observations made by phase contrast microscopy of infected lung homogenates.[13,14] These studies further suggested that the intra-alveolar, apparently

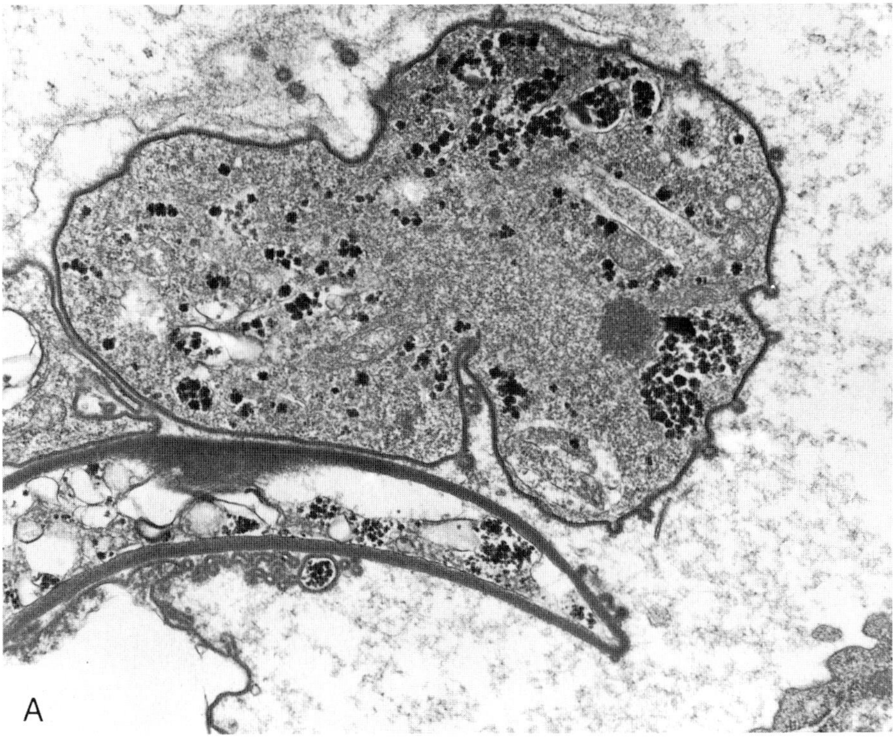

Fig. 11-1. Stages of *P. carinii* as identified by transmission electron microscopy. (**A**) Trophozoite (original 15,000 X) (*Figure continues.*)

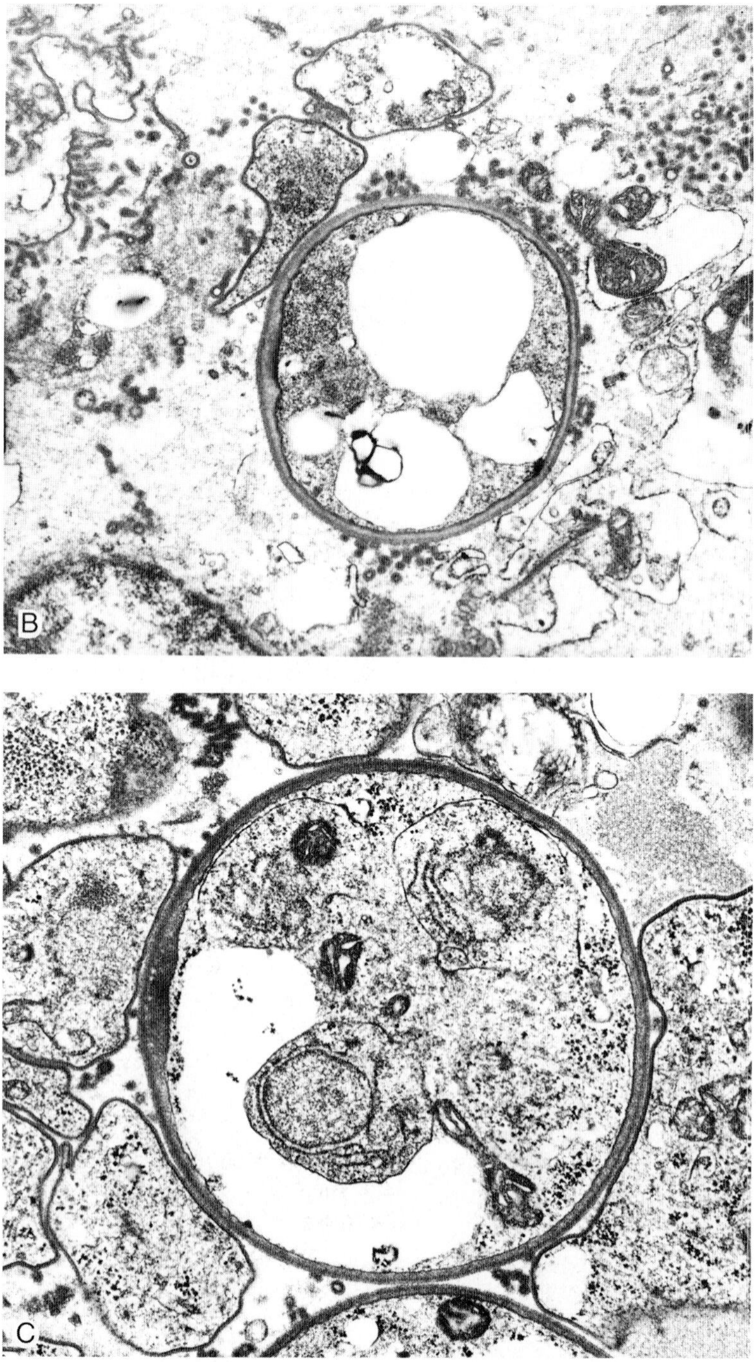

Fig. 11-1 (*Continued*). (**B** and **C**), Precyst forms (original 10,000 X and 15,000 X). (*Figure continues*.)

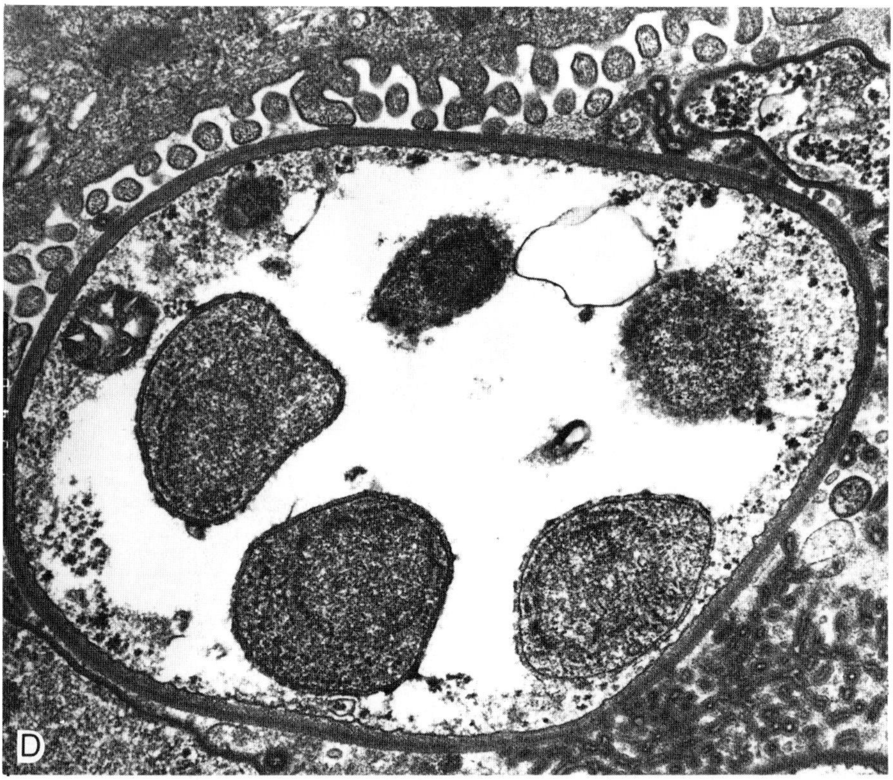

Fig. 11.1 (*Continued*). (**D**) Cyst with internal sporozoites (original 20,000 X).

acellular eosinophilic exudate that is characteristic of *P. carinii* pneumonia is largely composed of *P. carinii* organisms[13] (Fig. 11-2).

The life cycle of *P. carinii* and the relationship of the morphologically defined stages of the organism to each other are unknown. Purely on the basis of morphologic observations made by electron microscopy, a variety of life cycles have been proposed.[9,15] The generally accepted schema suggests progression from a trophozoite to a precyst to a fully matured cyst, with subsequent rupture of the cyst and release of the sporozoites to form new trophozoites (Fig. 11-3). Variations proposed for this basic cycle have included intracellular replication and a separate cycle of binary fission involving the trophozoite. There is very little evidence to support an intracellular phase in the life cycle of *P. carinii*.

In a recent electron microscopy study, evidence for a sexual phase in the organism, based on the presence of synaptonemal complexes and meiotic nuclear divisions in the precyst,[16] was obtained. A revised life cycle based on these observations was proposed. Ultimately, improved culture techniques will be needed to describe the life cycle more definitively by direct observation.

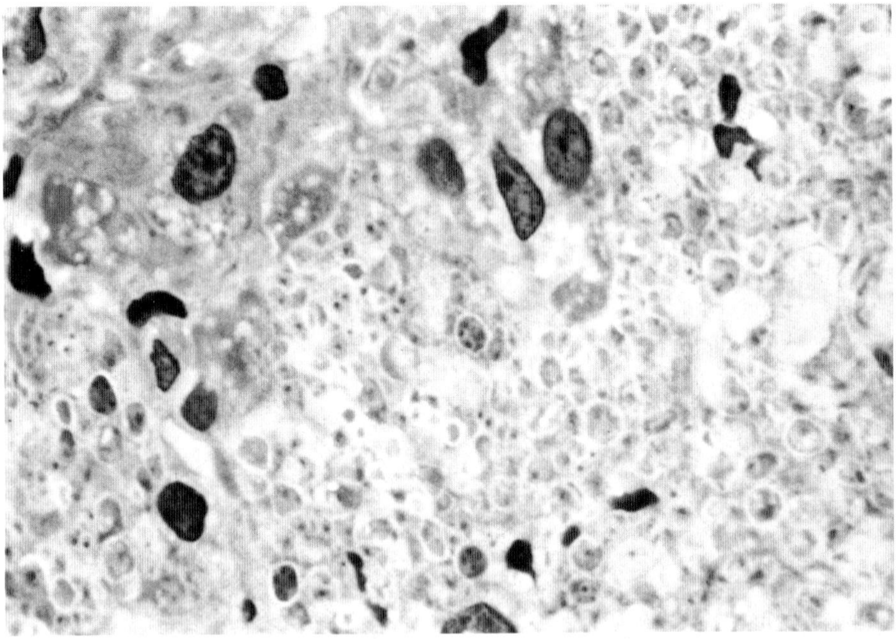

Fig. 11-2. Histopathologic section of a rat lung with steroid-induced *P. carinii* pneumonia. Lung was imbedded in plastic, and 1 μm sections were stained for 24 hours by the Giemsa technique. Alveolar spaces are filled with *P. carinii* organisms, primarily trophozoites (original 1,000 X).

P. carinii obtained from rat has been cultured in several laboratories by using a variety of feeder cells to support growth.[17–19] These cells have included WI-38 (a human embryonic lung fibroblast cell line), A549 (an alveolar type 2 cell line derived from human carcinoma), and primary rat lung cultures. Trophozoites appear to be the major stage that replicates in vitro. Difficulties in utilizing culture systems have been related to problems associated with sparse (two- to fourfold) replication of organisms, with documenting replication of organisms by reproducible techniques, with reproducing results from one laboratory to another, with variation from culture to culture, and with a very limited ability to effect serial passage of the organism. To date the utility of cultures has been limited to assays for drug susceptibility, although these results are subject to variable interpretation because of the problems noted above. Such in vitro studies have suggested that pentamidine and chloroquine are lethal to *P. carinii;* suramin, trimethoprim alone, and sulfamethoxazole alone are not; and, in a different system, trimethoprim-sulfamethoxazole and pentamidine can inhibit growth of *P. carinii* but α-difluoromethylornithine can do so only after erythrocytes are removed.[20,21] The reliability of such findings needs to be confirmed by other methods.

Development of a reliable, reproducible culture system that results in pro-

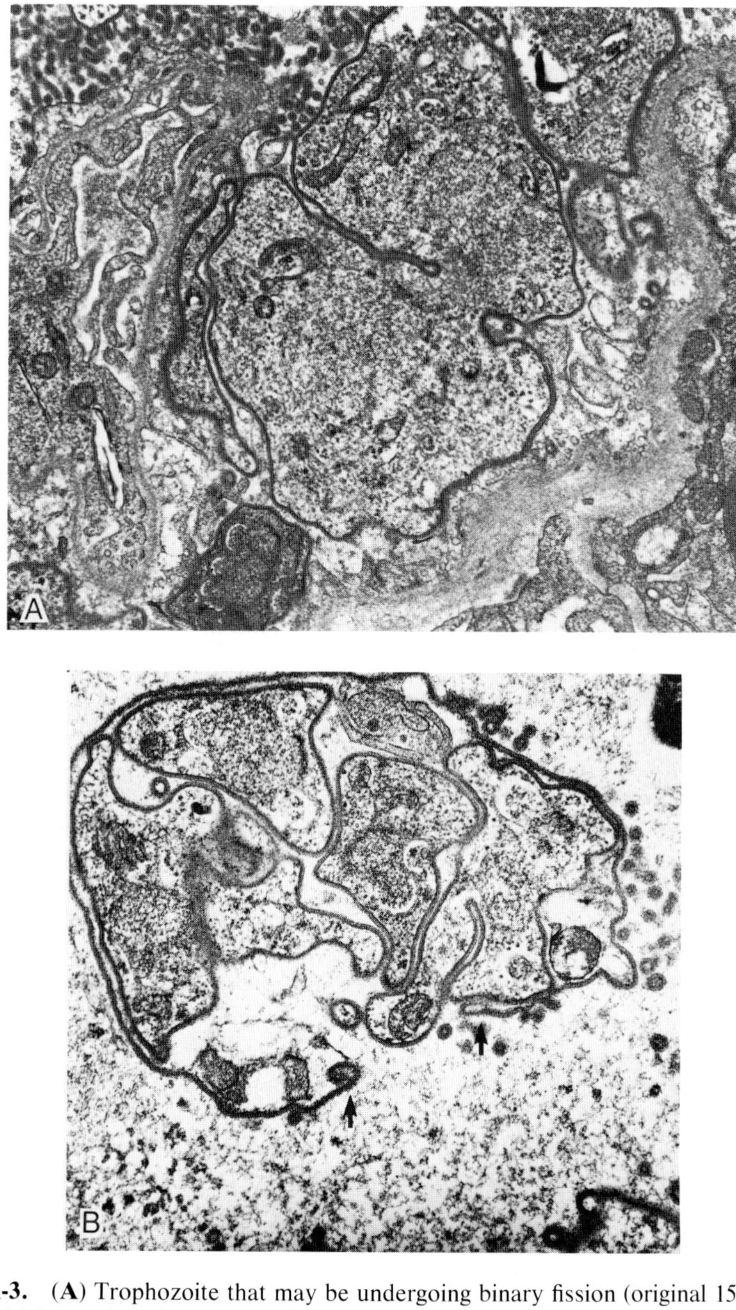

Fig. 11-3. (**A**) Trophozoite that may be undergoing binary fission (original 15,000 X). (**B**) Multiple trophozoites surrounded by a thin wall that contains an opening through which trophozoites could escape (arrows) (original 20,000 X).

duction of large quantities of purified organisms will provide a major advance in the understanding of *P. carinii*. Not only would such a system allow a more systematic evaluation of the *P. carinii* life cycle, but the availability of large quantities of organism would permit more definitive immunologic and epidemiologic studies as well as facilitate molecular investigation of the organism. Unfortunately, despite numerous attempts by a variety of laboratories, such a system has not yet been developed.

Biochemical Studies

Studies evaluating the metabolic pathways of *P. carinii* have been very limited in scope. Interpretation of results must be tempered by the realization that contamination with host cells, subcellular organelles, or contaminating organisms may be contributing to metabolic activity and that unknown proteolytic enzymes in crude extracts may be destroying activity. One series of investigations using such a crude extract suggested that *P. carinii* did not possess the antioxidant enzymes glutathione peroxidase and catalase but did possess significant amounts of superoxide dismutase.[22]

To circumvent the problem of potential contamination by host cells, our laboratory recently undertook a series of studies to evaluate metabolic pathways in *P. carinii* cysts by histoenzymology, a technique through which metabolic activity can be localized microscopically to *P. carinii*.[23] Immunofluorescence was used to document that reacting organisms were in fact *P. carinii*. By such techniques *P. carinii* cysts were determined to possess succinate dehydrogenase, lactate dehydrogenase, and glutamate dehydrogenase, while glucose-6-phosphate activity was minimal (Fig. 11-4). These results suggest that *P. carinii* cysts have the capacity for both aerobic and anaerobic metabolism, as suggested by the presence of enzymes important in glycolysis and the tricarboxylic acid cycle. They also possess a key enzyme of intermediary protein metabolism but may lack an enzyme important in shifting metabolism from glycolysis to the pentose shunt.

Dihydrofolate reductase (DHFR) is another enzyme being studied by our laboratory in conjunction with investigators from the National Cancer Institute. DHFR is important in the de novo synthesis of thymidylate and is involved in other metabolic pathways as well. It reduces dihydrofolate to tetrahydrofolate, which may subsequently act as a cofactor in thymidylate and purine nucleotide synthesis and amino acid metabolism. Previously, circumstantial evidence had strongly suggested that *P. carinii* possesses DHFR. Trimethoprim and pyrimethamine, both potent inhibitors of DHFR of bacteria and of other protozoa, have, when combined with sulfonamides, been found to be active against *P. carinii* both in the rat model and in human patients, and the target of these drugs has been presumed to be *P. carinii* DHFR.

Studies to characterize the DHFR of *P. carinii* were undertaken for two major reasons. First, since inhibitors of DHFR demonstrated marked variation

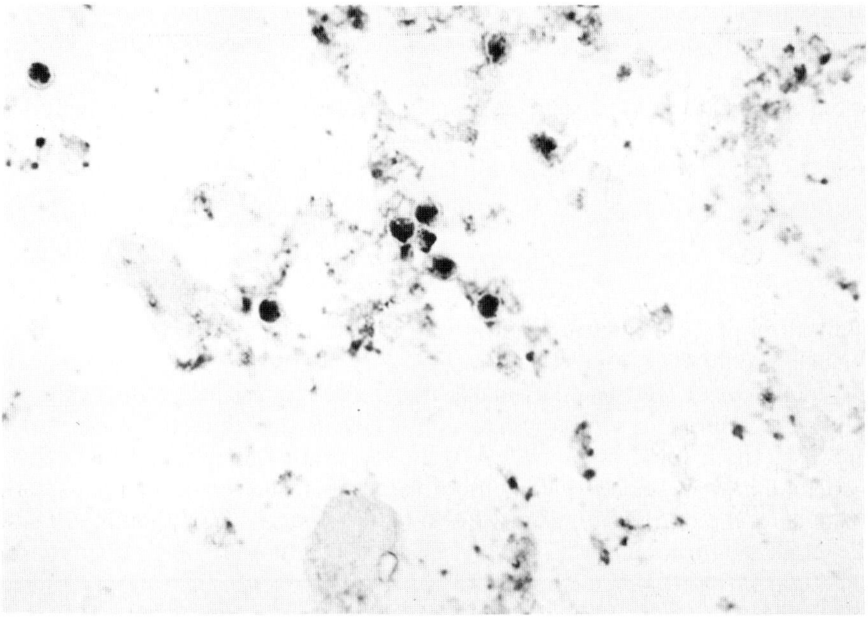

Fig. 11-4. Histoenzymologic documentation of the presence of succinate dehydrogenase in *P. carinii* cysts. In the presence of sodium succinate, formazan dye has been precipitated inside cysts that were identified by immunofluorescence (arrows) (original 1,000 X).

in their ability to inhibit enzymes from different organisms, characterization of *P. carinii* DHFR would allow rapid screening of other DHFR inhibitors and potentially allow the development of drugs more effective against the organism than currently available agents. Second, characterization of the enzyme would contribute to the understanding of the biology of the organism. It has been recently shown that all protozoa in which DHFR could be identified, including malarial and leishmanial species, possess a bifunctional enzyme that combines DHFR activity with thymidylate synthetase activity and that this bifunctional enzyme has a high molecular weight, usually over 100,000, as compared with 20,000 to 30,000 for the DHFR of bacteria, fungi, and mammals.[24]

It thus appeared that separation of *P. carinii* DHFR from potentially contaminating rat DHFR could be achieved by gel filtration and that such characterization would contribute to correct taxonomic classification of the organism. For comparison, parallel studies were conducted with *Toxoplasma gondii,* another protozoan that can cause disease in immunocompromised patients and that is also treated with pyrimethamine plus a sulfonamide.

In studies using a partially purified preparation of *P. carinii* isolated from rats, DHFR activity could only be found at a molecular weight of about 20,000, similar to that of rat.[25] No activity was found at a higher molecular weight.

Michaelis constants for the *P. carinii* DHFR as well as its interactions with a variety of inhibitors, especially trimethoprim and trimetrexate, differed markedly, however, from those for rat DHFR, which indicates that the identified enzyme came from *P. carinii.* As was expected from on the relatively low molecular weight, this enzyme did not possess thymidylate synthetase activity, unlike other protozoa. Studies with *T. gondii* documented that this protozoan did possess a high (110,000)-molecular-weight enzyme, which also exhibited thymidylate synthetase activity.[25]

Evaluation of Therapeutic Agents

Inhibitors of DHFR are available that could potentially be more effective than trimethoprim in inhibiting *P. carinii* DHFR and thus could potentially represent therapeutic advances. A series of studies undertaken to evaluate such inhibitors revealed that methotrexate and trimetrexate (a lipid-soluble analogue of methotrexate), were 1,000-fold more effective in inhibiting *P. carinii* DHFR than trimethoprim.[26] Pyrimethamine was 10-fold more effective than trimethoprim; however methotrexate, which requires an active transport process to be taken up by mammalian cells, could not be taken up by intact *P. carinii,* presumably because *P. carinii,* like most other protozoa, does not possess the active transport mechanism needed for this uptake. It could therefore be predicted that methotrexate would be ineffective for the treatment of *P. carinii* pneumonia, an expectation supported by clinical anecdotes. In contrast, trimetrexate, which enters cells by passive diffusion, was taken up by *P. carinii.* Of equal importance, folinic acid, or calcium leucovorin, a reduced folate that can bypass the blockade of DHFR, also requires an active transport mechanism for uptake, and thus also was not taken up by *P. carinii.* Leucovorin could, in contrast, be taken up by mammalian cells.

These studies provide a sound theoretical basis for treating *P. carinii* pneumonia with trimetrexate, with or without a sulfonamide, and simultaneously administering leucovorin to prevent toxicity due to inhibition of host DHFR. Studies using the rat model of *P. carinii* pneumonia have shown that trimetrexate plus sulfamethoxazole is at least as effective as trimethoprim in treating the infection. Preliminary studies in AIDS patients at the National Institutes of Health have shown that trimetrexate alone or trimetrexate combined with a sulfonamide can be effective in clearing *P. carinii* pneumonia. Simultaneous administration of leucovorin has minimized potential adverse reactions, apparently without interfering with antiprotozoal efficacy.[27] Analogous studies with *T. gondii* have demonstrated that trimetrexate appears superior to pyrimethamine, the drug usually used to treat toxoplasmosis, in inhibiting *T. gondii* DHFR as well as in inhibiting *T. gondii* replication in an infected in vitro macrophage system. Extension of these studies should lead to an improved understanding of the metabolism of these organisms and may allow development of more effective and less toxic drugs for treatment of *P. carinii* pneumonia and *T. gondii* encephalitis in immunocompromised patients.

IMMUNOLOGIC STUDIES OF *P. CARINII*

Immunologic evaluation of *P. carinii*–host interaction has been limited in scope because of difficulties in isolating or culturing the organism. The occurrence of *P. carinii* pneumonia in patients with isolated B-cell and T-cell deficiencies, as well as in patients with mixed deficiencies, suggests that both humoral and cell-mediated immunity play a role in protecting against development of clinical disease.[28] In vitro studies examining the interaction of *P. carinii* with host cells have been limited. Its interaction with rat alveolar macrophages has been investigated by two groups, both of whom reported that macrophages could phagocytize and destroy *P. carinii,* although in one study hyperimmune rabbit serum was required for phagocytosis when freshly cultivated alveolar macrophages were used.[29,30] In another study T-cell proliferative response in humans to crude rat *P. carinii* extracts was found to be present in most patients and controls; confirmation of these blastogenesis studies awaits investigations using more defined antigens of *P. carinii.*[31]

Immunofluorescence and ELISA Studies

The majority of studies of anti–*P. carinii* antibodies have used immunofluorescence techniques, with varying results. Factors responsible for the variation have included the techniques used by individual laboratories, the use of rat or human *P. carinii,* the use of fixed tissue sections or lung homogenates, or the use of partially purified organisms that have been separated from lung tissue by a variety of methods. In such studies anti-*P. carinii* antibodies have been found in 1.4 to 75 percent of normal controls and in up to 100 percent of patients with documented or suspected *P. carinii* pneumonia.[32,33] Rats have also been evaluated for the presence of antibodies to *P. carinii,* and such antibodies have been detected in about 50 percent of animals, with rate of positivity varying according to the age and drug therapy of animals.[34]

In the past few years other methods have been used to detect antibodies to *P. carinii.* For example, enzyme-linked immunosorbent assays (ELISA) using extracts of partially purified *P. carinii,* usually from rats, have been developed. In such studies antibodies against rat *P. carinii* have been found in most humans tested, including both normal controls and infected individuals.[35,36] However, antigens used in such assays have not been characterized or shown to be derived exclusively from *P. carinii* as opposed to contaminating host tissue. Nonspecific interactions may also play a role in positive results. Therefore the true significance of these ELISA findings is unknown.

A major problem in evaluating assays that detect antibodies to *P. carinii* is the absence of a "gold standard" with which to compare results. An additional complication is the inability to diagnose acute *P. carinii* infection by methods other than identification of the organism in pulmonary specimens. Based on studies using immunofluorescence to detect anti-*P. carinii* antibodies, the current concept of *P. carinii* infection assumes that most individuals are exposed to *P. carinii* as children, at which time they develop a nonspecific respiratory infection or an asymptomatic infection.[37] Following control of the infection by the normal host immune system, the organism becomes latent and does not cause further disease unless the immune system, primarily cell-mediated immunity, becomes suppressed. Studies supporting this hypothesis must be interpreted with caution, given the difficulties in conducting them outlined above (see Ch. 12). To document that this scenario does in fact occur, the initial acute infection needs to be identified by unequivocal serologic or culture techniques, and long-term studies following infection need to be undertaken.

Immunoblot Results

Immunoblot studies offer an approach to identifying antigens and antibodies that are specific for *P. carinii*. Using partially purified cysts, our laboratory had identified antigens with molecular weights of 40,000 to 100,000 that appear to be specific for rat *P. carinii* and antigens with molecular weights of 22,000 to 90,000 that are specific for human *P. carinii*.[38] Although cross-reactivity appears to exist between rat and human *P. carinii*, the antigenic pattern was different for the two isolates. Immunofluorescence studies using polyclonal sera had previously suggested that rat and human *P. carinii* differ antigenically, but such studies involve a subjective interpretation of fluorescence intensity and cannot characterize the specific nature of these differences.[6]

Antigens identified by immunoblot can be utilized in further immunoblot studies to identify antibodies specific for rat or human *P. carinii*. By such techniques antibodies apparently specific for human *P. carinii* have been detected in nearly all human sera tested.[38] Sera from 32 of 33 individuals, including normal controls and both AIDS and non-AIDS patients with *P. carinii* pneumonia, were found to contain antibodies against human *P. carinii*. Of note, only about half of the positive sera contained antibodies against rat *P. carinii*. Although further work is needed, this study supports the concept that most humans have been exposed to *P. carinii* by the time they are adults and that disease occurs following activation of a latent infection. Since all patients with *P. carinii* pneumonia had antibodies to the organism, this study also suggests that a B-cell response alone is inadequate to protect against disease.

Application of Monoclonal Antibodies

More specific identification of *P. carinii* antigens can be achieved by use of monoclonal antibodies, which offer a specificity that cannot be achieved by polyclonal sera. In 1986 three groups described the development of monoclonal antibodies directed against rat *P. carinii*.[39–41] All 12 antibodies developed by one group identified an antigen of about 110,000 molecular weight. In addition, minor antigens with molecular weights of 35,000 to 116,000 were also identified by each antibody. A second group prepared a single monoclonal antibody that reacted with antigens of 35,000, 65,000, and 110,000 molecular weight. A third group identified a major antigen of about 90,000 molecular weight using unreduced conditions.

Our laboratory has also been developing monoclonal antibodies directed against *P. carinii.*[7] Initially anti-rat *P. carinii* antibodies were developed and identified by immunofluorescence (Fig. 11-5). Only one of nine antibodies from the initial fusion reacted consistently with human *P. carinii,* and thus a second set of antibodies was developed against human *P. carinii.* None of six anti-human *P. carinii* antibodies was found to react with rat *P. carinii,* which supports the previously described finding that rat and human *P. carinii* are antigenically different.

Immunoblot studies with these monoclonal antibodies have identified antigens specific for rat and for human *P. carinii*[7]; the former antigens have molecular weights ranging from 40,000 to 100,000 and the latter have molecular weights of 22,000 to 100,000, as identified by these antibodies. Immunoblot studies have also documents that the method of processing can have an important effect on the antigens identified. For example, pretreatment of *P. carinii* with collagenase and hyaluronidase prior to partial purification leads to antigen degradation, as demonstarted by the presence of multiple bands, whereas only a single band was seen without such pretreatment.

Monoclonal antibodies have a number of potential uses. Such antibodies can be used to purify specific antigens (e.g., use of affinity columns) and may

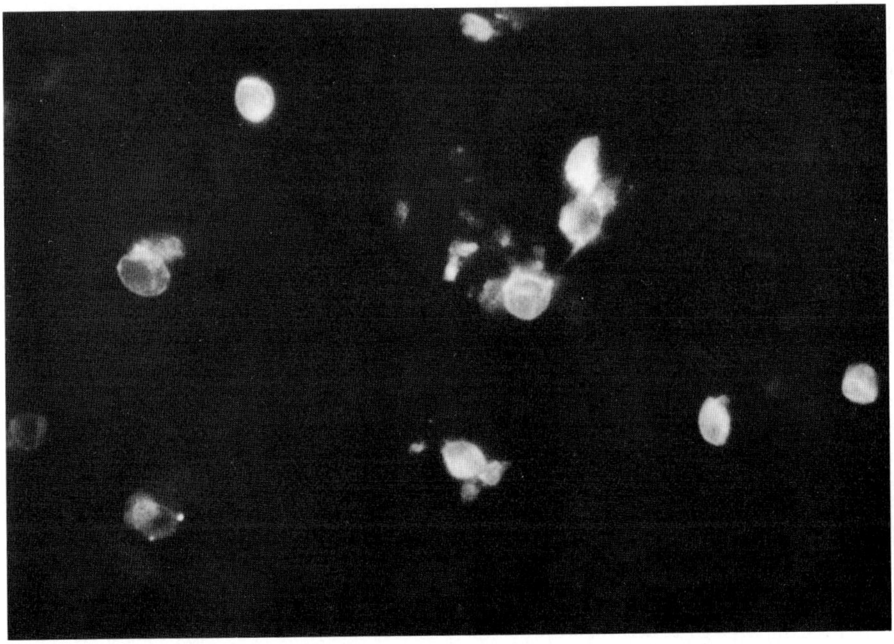

Fig. 11-5. Reactivity of a monoclonal antibody with partially purified rat *P. carinii* cysts, demonstrated by indirect immunofluorescence (original 1,000 X).

also be useful in the diagnosis of *P. carinii* pneumonia. One of the antibodies developed by our laboratory, antibody 2G2, exhibits brilliant fluorescence against human *P. carinii* although it does not react with rat *P. carinii* (Fig. 11-6). In a recent study 2G2 was evaluated prospectively for its ability to detect *P. carinii* in pulmonary specimens, primarily bronchoalveolar lavage specimens, and compared with the standard toluidine blue O stain.[42] *P. carinii* was correctly identified in 15 of 16 specimens that were positive by toluidine blue O; no false positives were seen. The advantages of immunofluorescence with this monoclonal antibody are that the procedure can be performed rapidly and that many microbiology laboratories, especially those in smaller hospitals, are more experienced in immunofluorescence techniques than in the specialized staining techniques needed to diagnose *P. carinii* pneumonia.

Other attempts to diagnose *P. carinii* pneumonia by immunologic techniques have centered on antigen detection by counterimmunoelectrophoresis. These studies have obtained the hyperimmune sera by utilizing uncharacterized rat *P. carinii* antigens to immunize rabbits. Although reports from one group have suggested that this technique may be useful in noninvasively diagnosing *P. carinii* pneumonia, attempts to confirm the results in other laboratories have been unsuccessful.[36,37,43] We have found that antigen detection, when performed by the former laboratory on frozen serum samples provided by our laboratory, does not correlate with clinical status or lung histopathology. At

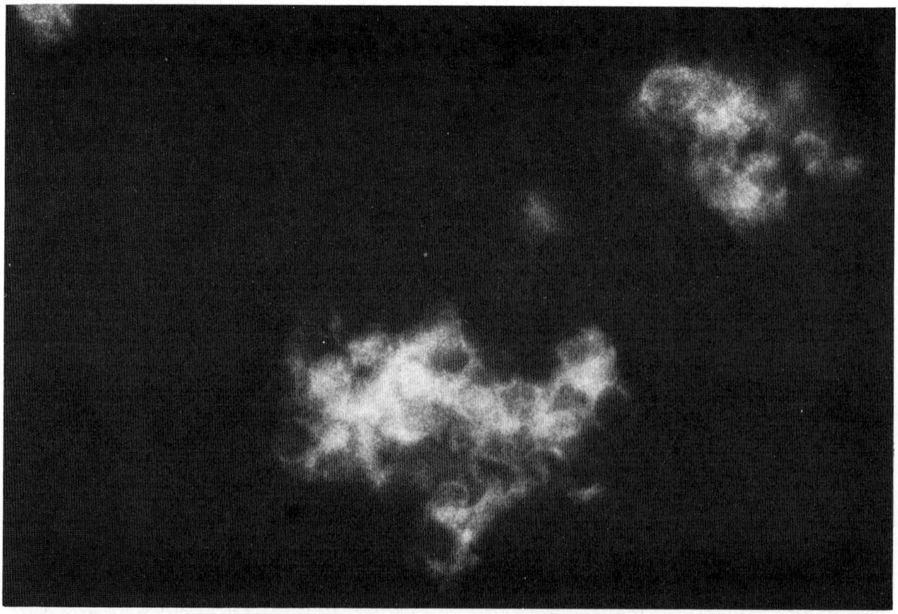

Fig. 11-6. Identification of *P. carinii* in a bronchoalveolar lavage specimen from a patient with AIDS and *P. carinii* pneumonia, using an antihuman *P. carinii* monoclonal antibody in an indirect immunofluorescent assay (original 1,000 X).

present antigen detection in serum has not been shown to be a reliable method of diagnosing *P. carinii* pneumonia in humans.

CONCLUSION

In summary, the dramatic increase in importance of *P. carinii*–related disease has not been accompanied by a concomitant increase in our understanding of the organism. Much needs to be done to better understand the epidemiology, life cycle, biology, and immunology of *P. carinii* and its interaction with hosts. Advances have been made through the development of culture techniques that allow limited replication of *P. carinii,* through enzyme studies that have allowed a rational approach to the identification of agents potentially active against *P. carinii,* through immunoblot studies of *P. carinii* antigens, and through the devlopment of monoclonal antibodies that are specific for both rat and human *P. carinii*. These studies should be initial steps to improving diagnostic, therapeutic, and preventive strategies. However, a great deal more remains to be done to better understand this enigmatic pathogen and hopefully to better control disease caused by it.

REFERENCES

1. Kovacs JA, Hiemenz JW, Macher AM, et al: *Pneumocystis carinii* pneumonia: a comparison between patients with the acquired immunodeficiency syndrome and patients with other immunodeficiencies. Ann Intern Med 100:663, 1984
2. Coolfont report: a PHS plan for prevention and control of AIDS and the AIDS virus. Public Health Rep 101:341, 1986
3. Hughes WT: Natural mode of acquisition for de novo infection with *Pneumocystis carinii*. J Infect Dis 145:842, 1982
4. Hughes WT, McNabb PC, Makres TD, et al: Efficacy of trimethoprim and sulfamethoxazole in the prevention and treatment of *Pneumocystis carinii* pneumonia. Antimicrob Agents Chemother 5:289, 1974
5. Hughes WT, Smith BL: Efficacy of diaminodiphenylsulfone and other drugs in murine *Pneumocystis carinii* pneumonitis. Antimicrob Agents Chemother 26:436, 1984
6. Walzer PD, Rutledge ME: Comparison of rat, mouse, and human *Pneumocystis carinii* by immunofluorescence. J Infect Dis 142:449, 1980
7. Kovacs JA, Swan JC, Gill V et al: Monoclonal antibodies against *Pneumocystis carinii:* utility for establishing diagnosis and species differences. Am Soc Microbiology, ICAAC, Washington, 1986 (Abstr. No. 688)
8. Young LS (ed): *Pneumocystis carinii* Pneumonia. Marcel Dekker, New York, 1984
9. Campbell WG: Ultrastructure of pneumocystis in human lung. Life cycle in human pneumocystis. Arch Pathol 93:312, 1972
10. Ham EK, Greenberg SD, Reynolds RC, Singer DB: Ultrastructure of *Pneumocystis carinii*. Exp Mol Pathol 14:362, 1971
11. Huneycutt HC, Anderson WR, Hendry WS: *Pneumocystis carinii* pneumonia. Case studies with electron microscopy. Am J Clin Pathol 41:411, 1964

12. Yoshida Y, Shiota T, Yamada M, Matsumoto Y: Further light microscopic studies on morphology and development of *Pneumocystis carinii.* Zentralbl Bakteriol [A] 250:213, 1981
13. Kovacs JA, Trische T, Swan J, et al: Persistence of pneumocystis trophozoites and sporozoites following anti-pneumocystis therapy. (Submitted for publication.)
14. Masur H: Interaction between *Pneumocystis carinii* and phagocytic cells. p. 77. In Young LS (ed): *Pneumocystis carinii* Pneumonia. Marcel Dekker, New York, 1984
15. Hasleton PS, Curry A, Rankin EM: *Pneumocystis carinii* pneumonia: a light microscopical and ultrastructural study. J Clin Pathol 34:1138, 1981
16. Matsumoto Y, Yoshida Y: Sporogeny in *Pneumocystis carinii:* synaptonemal complexes and meiotic nuclear divisions observed in precysts. J Protozool 31:420, 1984
17. Bartlett MS, Verbanac PA, Smith JW: Cultivation of *Pneumocystis carinii* with WI-38 cells. J Clin Microbiol 10:796, 1979
18. Cushion MT, Walzer PD: Growth and serial passage of *Pneumocystis carinii* in A549 cell line. Infect Immun 44:245, 1985
19. Pifer L, Hughes WT, Murphy MJ: Propogation of *Pneumocystis carinii* in vitro. Pediatr Res 11:305, 1977
20. Pesanti EL: In vitro effects of antiprotozoan drugs and immune serum on *Pneumocystis carinii.* J Infect Dis 141:775, 1980
21. Cushion MT, Stanforth D, Linke MJ, Walzer PD: A method of testing the sensitivity of *Pneumocystis carinii* to antimicrobial agents in vitro. Antimicrob Agents Chemother 28:796, 1985
22. Pesanti EL: *Pneumocystis carinii:* oxygen uptake, antioxidant enzymes, and susceptibility to oxygen mediated damage. Infect Immun 44:7, 1984
23. Mazer MA, Kovacs JA, Swan JC, et al: A histoenzymologic study of selected dehydrogenase enzymes in *Pneumocystis carinii.* Infect Immun 55:727, 1987
24. Garrett CE, Coderre JA, Meek TD, et al: A bifunctional thymidylate synthetase-dihydrofolate reductase in protozoa. Mol Biochem Parasitol 11:257, 1984
25. Kovacs JA, Allegra CJ, Swan JC, et al: Identification and characterization of dihydrofolate reductase from *Pneumocystis carinii* and *Toxoplasma gondii.* Clin Res 34:522A, 1986
26. Allegra CJ, Kovacs JA, Chabner BA, et al: Potent in vivo and in vitro activity of a lipid soluble antifolate, trimetrexate, against *Pneumocystis carinii.* Clin Res 34: 674A, 1986
27. Allegra CJ, Drake J, Swan J, et al: Preliminary results of a phase I-II trial for the treatment of *Pneumocystis carinii* pneumonia using a potent lipid soluble dihydrofolate reductase inhibitor, trimetrexate. Abstracts of the 1986 Soc Microbiology, ICAAC, Washington, 1986 (Abstr. No. 691)
28. Walzer PD, Krogstad DJ, Rawson PG, Schultz MG: *Pneumocystis carinii* pneumonia in the United States: epidemiologic, diagnostic, and clinical features. Ann Intern Med 80:83, 1974
29. Masur H, Jones TC: The interaction in vitro of *Pneumocystis carinii* with macrophages and L-cells. J Exp Med 147:157, 1978
30. Von Behren LA, Pesanti EL: Uptake and degradation of *Pneumocystis carinii* by macrophages in vitro. Am Rev Respir Dis 118:1051, 1978
31. Herrod HG, Valenski WR, Woods DR, Pifer LL: The in vitro response of human lymphocytes to *Pneumocystis carinii* antigen. J Immunol 126:59, 1981
32. Norman L, Kagan IA: Some observations on the serology of *Pneumocystis carinii* infections in the United States. Infect Immun 8:317, 1973

33. Meuwissen JHET, Tauber I, Leeuwenberg ADEM, et al: Parasitologic and serologic observations of infection with *Pneumocystis* in humans. J Infect Dis 136:43, 1977
34. Walzer PD, Rutledge ME: Humoral immunity in experimental *Pneumocystis carinii* infection. I. serum and bronchial lavage fluid antibody responses in rats. J Lab Clin Med 97:820, 1981
35. Maddison SE, Hayes GV, Slemenda SB, et al: Detection of specific antibody by enzyme-linked immunosorbent assay and antigenemia by counterimmunoelectrophoresis in humans infected with *Pneumocystis carinii.* J Clin Microbiol 15: 1036, 1982
36. Maddison SE, Walls KW, Haverkos HW, Juranek DD: Evaluation of serologic tests for *Pneumocystis carinii* antibody and antigenemia in patients with acquired immunodeficiency syndrome. Diagn Microbiol Infect Dis 2:69, 1984
37. Pifer LL, Hughes WT, Stagno S, Woods D: *Pneumocystis carinii* infection: evidence for high prevalence in normal and immunosuppressed children. Pediatrics 61:35, 1978
38. Kovacs JA, Halpern JL, Swan JC, et al: Identification of antigens and antibodies specific for *Pneumocystis carinii.* J Immunol 140:2023, 1988
39. Graves DC, McNabb SJN, Ivey MH, Worley MA: Development and characterization of monoclonal antibodies to *Pneumocystis carinii.* Infect Immun 51:125, 1986
40. Lee CH, Bolinger CD, Bartlett MS, et al: Production of monoclonal antibody against *Pneumocystis carinii* by using a hybrid of rat spleen and mouse myeloma cells. J Clin Microbiol 23:505, 1986
41. Gigliotti F, Stokes DC, Cheatham AB, et al: Development of murine monoclonal antibodies to *Pneumocystis carinii.* J Infect Dis 154:315, 1986
42. Kovacs JA, Gill V, Swan J, et al: Prospective evaluation of a monoclonal antibody in diagnosis of *Pneumocystis carinii* pneumonia. Lancet 2:1, 1986
43. Meyers JD, Pifer LL, Sale GE, Thomas ED: The value of *Pneumocystis carinii* antibody and antigen detection for diagnosis of *Pneumocystis carinii* pneumonia after marrow transplantation. Am Rev Respir Dis 120:1283, 1979

12 Diagnosis and Treatment of *Pneumocystis carinii* Pneumonia

Philip C. Hopewell

Pneumocystis carinii was first identified by Chagas in guinea pig lungs in 1909 and in human lung tissue in 1911. Although originally the organism was said to cause disease in humans, it was not until the early 1950s that the clinical illness produced by *P. carinii* was described. The first reports of *P. carinii* causing what was then known as "interstitial plasma cell pneumonia" originated in central Europe and involved premature or debilitated infants 6 weeks to 4 months of age. However, the parasitic etiology of the disease was not accepted initially by North American physicians.[1,2] Nearly all the early cases reported involved infants, but subsequently *P. carinii* pneumonia was diagnosed in older children and adults.[3] In each patient with the disease there was a recognized condition that impaired host responsiveness, leading to the classification of the organism as an opportunist.[1,4]

Presumably because the wartime conditions and postwar food shortages that led to malnutrition among infants in Europe abated by the late 1950s, the near epidemics in orphanges that characterized the epidemiology of *P. carinii* pneumonia disappeared. The pattern seen later was one of sporadic cases occurring in patients with congenital or acquired immunodeficiency states.[5] Between 1955 and 1967 a total of 130 cases were reported in the American literature.[6] With few exceptions, until 1981 *P. carinii* pneumonia continued to be a sporadic opportunistic infection involving mainly patients who had hematologic or lymphoreticular malignancies or who were receiving immunosuppressive therapy.[7,8] In fact, although there are no supporting data, it is likely that the frequency of *P. carinii* was decreasing because of the routine use of trimethoprim-sulfamethoxazole (TMP-SMX) to prevent the disease.[9]

Beginning in 1981 the epidemiology of *P. carinii* pneumonia changed drastically with the recognition of its frequency in patients with the acquired immunodeficiency syndrome (AIDS).[10,11] Consistently, since data describing the incidence of AIDS began to be collected and reported, *P. carinii* pneumonia has been the most common index diagnosis.[12] Of the reported cases of AIDS, 64 percent have *P. carinii* pneumonia either alone (56 percent) or in combination with Kaposi's sarcoma as the index diagnosis.[13] It is estimated that another 20 percent of AIDS patients develop the disease later in their course. Moreover, many patients have more than one episode of the illness. In the face of these data it is obviously of considerable importance for physicians to be aware of the clinical features of *P. carinii* pneumonia, to have an understanding of the diagnostic approaches that are most expeditious and efficient, and to be able to utilize the available therapies effectively.

PATHOGENESIS OF *P. carinii* PNEUMONIA

There is substantial albeit inferential evidence that *P. carinii* pneumonia results from recrudescence of infection that occurred earlier and had been easily suppressed by normal host defense mechanisms (see Ch.11). In animals, especially rats and mice, *P. carinii* pneumonia develops as a consequence of corticosteroid administration without obvious exposure to exogenous sources of infection.[14–17]

In humans evidence for early infection comes from serologic testing. Studies using several different antigen and antibody detection systems have suggested that most children have acquired *P. carinii* infection by 4 years of age. Meuwissen and associates[18] used an indirect fluorescent antibody (IFA) test with antigen prepared from *P. carinii* cyst walls and found immunoglobulin M (IgM) and IgG antibody titers greater than 1:40 in nearly 100 percent of children aged 2 to 4 years. Pifer et al.[19] used IFA tests to identify antibody and counterimmunoelectrophoresis to detect circulating antigen in normal children. Although antigenemia was not found in any of the normal children, 83 percent of those 3 to 4 years old had antibody titers of 1:16 or greater. In a separate group of 23 children studied longitudinally, acquisition of antibody (discounting maternal antibody) began at age 7 months and increased to a peak of 63 percent of the subjects by 4 years of age. Sheppard et al.[20] using similar techniques, found antibody to *P. carinii* in 53 percent of a group of normal subjects. Likewise, Hofmann et al.[21] found IgM antibodies to *P. carinii* in 72 percent, IgG in 38 percent, and IgA in 31 percent of healthy subjects.

Running somewhat counter to the hypothesis that *P. carinii* pneumonia is a recrudescence of a latent infection is the infrequency with which the organisms have been found in the autopsied lungs of persons dying of nonimmunosuppressive conditions.[18,22–24] These findings may, however, simply reflect the fact that a very small number of organisms has been sought with relatively insensitive techniques.

In spite of the evidence suggesting that latent infection is responsible for most clinical pneumonia caused by *P. carinii,* some reports of clustering of cases imply that horizontal transmission may also play a role.[4,7,8,25] While transmission from person to person could possibly be of importance in some instances, the lack of a consistent epidemiologic pattern seems to argue against a significant role for recent infection in causing the clinical illness.

The mode of acquisition of *P. carinii* seems to be the airborne route. Hughes[26] demonstrated that when germ-free, *P. carinii*–free rats were isolated and given sterile food and water but exposed to nonsterile air, they acquired the organism. When the air that they breathed was filtered they remained uninfected with *P. carinii.* This observation again suggests that horizontal airborne transmission from potential sources of infection to susceptible persons in the vicinity may occur.

The specific abnormalities of host defenses that set the stage for *P. carinii* pneumonia are not well understood. It appears, however, that defects in cellular immunity are the major factors involved. The most frequent clinical conditions with which *P. carinii* pneumonia has been associated are those that predominantly affect T lymphocytes and the expression of cell-mediated immunity.[4,27,28] However, humoral antibodies are probably important as well, as indicated by reports of *P. carinii* pneumonia in children with congenital agammaglobulinemia or hypogammaglobulinemia.[27] Given the important interrelationships between cell-mediated and humoral immunity, it is probably not of major clinical relevance to determine which system is the more important. Experimental studies using rat macrophages have suggested that both specific anti-*pneumocystis* antibody and intact macrophage function are necessary for ingestion and killing of *P. carinii.*[28,29]

DIAGNOSIS OF *P. carinii* PNEUMONIA

Clinical Presentation

As noted previously, patients who develop *P. carinii* pneumonia nearly always have clinically obvious immunosuppression. Often the patient's medical history is dominated by symptoms of the underlying disease process (e.g., leukemia or lymphoma). In such patients respiratory symptoms may be a consequence of the preexisting disease, its treatment, or a new process; thus, the differential diagnosis may contain a large number of processes, including an array of opportunistic infections. Although in patients with AIDS *P. carinii* pneumonia is the most frequent index diagnosis, these patients usually have had nonspecific symptoms such as fever, fatigue, and weight loss for weeks to months prior to developing respiratory symptoms and often have disorders that categorize them as having AIDS-related complex. Because of the prevalence of AIDS in some areas, a history in a person with an undiagnosed pulmonary disease must include information relating to whether or not the patient is from a recognized AIDS transmission category. It should be kept in mind, however, that 4 percent of AIDS patients reported in the United States and 18 percent of those reported in Europe do not fit into any of the recognized categories.

The most common presenting symptoms of *P. carinii* pneumonia are fever, cough, and, subsequently, shortness of breath. The shortness of breath usually progresses from being present only with exertion to being present at rest. Cough is generally nonproductive but may be associated with sputum in patients who smoke cigarettes or who have bacterial bronchitis or non-*pneumocystis* pneumonia, as well as *P. carinii* pneumonia.

The physical examination of patients with *P. carinii* pneumonia is not particularly helpful and again may be dominated by the underlying disease process. Patients with AIDS may appear somewhat wasted, and generally febrile, and those with more severe pulmonary involvement may be tachypneic. Diffuse lymphadenopathy is often noted, and a substantial percentage will have oral candidiasis or hairy leukoplakia. Perianal ulcers caused by herpes virus may also be present. Cutaneous lesion of Kaposi's sarcoma should be sought. Findings related to the lungs per se generally are not striking; dry rales may be heard, but findings indicative of consolidation are unusual.

Initial laboratory evaluation also is not especially helpful. Lymphopenia is common but not invariable. A variety of other hematologic abnormalities, including anemia, leukopenia, and thrombocytopenia, may also occur.

Radiographic Findings

In patients with respiratory symptoms the initial diagnostic study generally is a chest film, which provides information that is very useful in directing subsequent evaluations. The film may show abnormalities that are not likely to have an opportunistic cause such as hyperinflation from asthma or focal consolidation consistent with a pyogenic bacterial pneumonia (although this may be opportunistic). The radiographic patterns of the opportunistic processes are nonspecific, although some diagnoses may be more likely if certain radiographic changes are observed.[30,31]

P. carinii pneumonia most often causes diffuse interstitial infiltration involving all portions of the lungs rather evenly (Fig. 12-1).[30–32] Several variations of the basic pattern may be seen; the infiltration may be somewhat heterogenously distributed throughout the lung or it may be more miliary in appearance. Diffuse and focal air-space consolidation may also be caused by *P. carinii* pneumonia and usually occurs as the disorder becomes more severe (Fig. 12-2). Cystic changes or pneumatoceles (Fig. 12-3) have been noted, particularly during the healing process, and cavitation within a preexisting nodular lesion

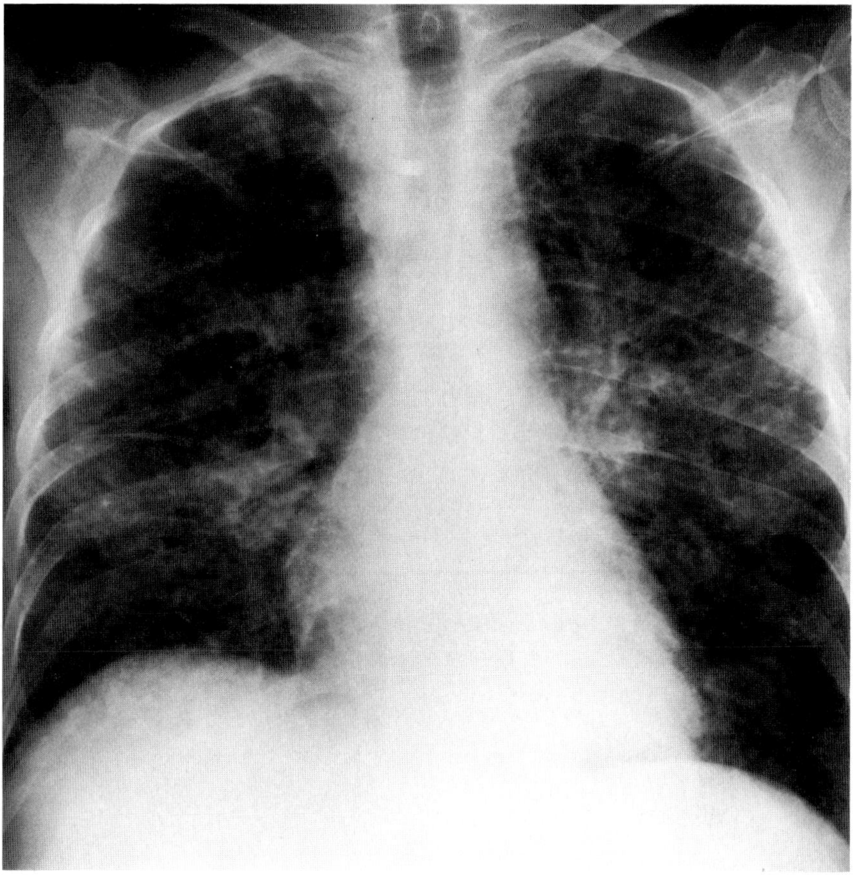

Fig. 12-1. Chest radiograph showing diffuse interstitial infiltration typical of *P. carinii* pneumonia.

may occur. Spontaneous pneumothorax may occur probably as an extension of the cystic or cavitary processes. Pleural effusions and intrathoracic adenopathy are very uncommon in patients with *P. carinii* pneumonia; adenopathy, if present, is probably due to another process and likewise when significant amounts of pleural fluid are present, other diagnoses should be considered.

A normal film may indicate that the respiratory symptoms reported by the patient are not being caused by lung disease or that the disease, if present, is not sufficiently advanced to cause radiographic findings. Approximately 5 to 10 percent of patients with AIDS who are proved to have *P. carinii* pneumonia have normal chest films.[30] Other pathogens, such as cytomegalovirus and *Mycobacterium avium* complex, may also be present without causing abnormal chest films. For this reason, if the symptoms are judged to be significant, further evaluation is warranted.

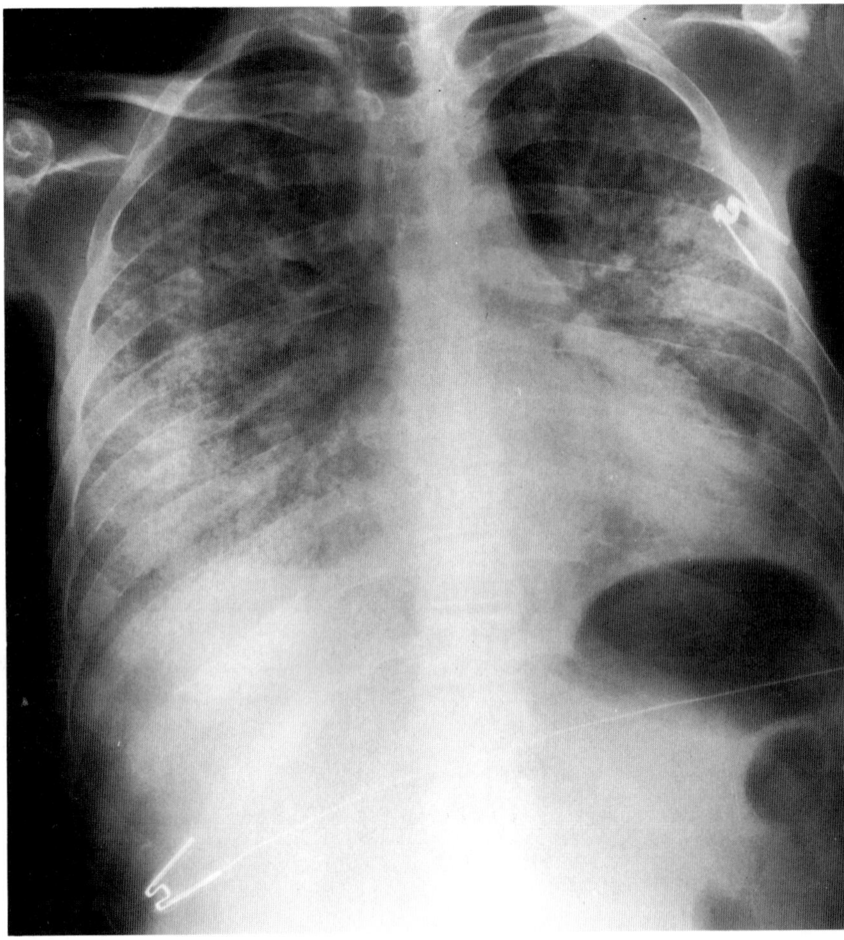

Fig. 12-2. Chest radiograph demonstrating diffuse air space consolidation in a patient with severe *P. carinii* pneumonia.

Pulmonary Function Tests

Abnormalities in lung function are found commonly in patients who have *P. carinii* pneumonia although, as with radiographic abnormalities, the changes cannot be viewed as specific. Typical findings include reductions in vital capacity (VC), total lung capacity (TLC), and single-breath diffusing capacity for carbon monoxide (DLco). Table 12-1 shows the values for VC, TLC, and DLco in 143 patients, of whom 91 were found to have *P. carinii* pneumonia and 52 had other diagnoses or no diagnosis.[33] There are statistically significant differences between the two groups with respect to VC, TLC, and DLco. Only seven patients with a normal DLco were shown to have *P. carinii* pneumonia. It should be noted that intravenous drug abuse, an AIDS risk factor, may cause

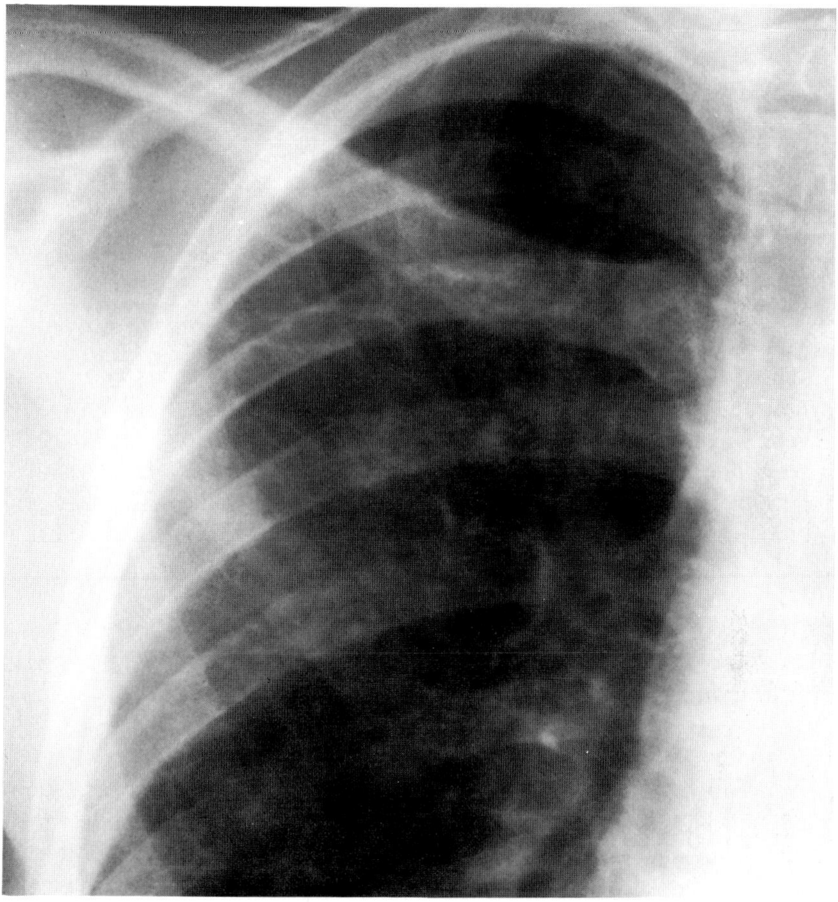

Fig. 12-3. Chest radiograph showing pneumatoceles caused by *P. carinii*

abnormalities on the chest film as well as a reduction in DLco and thus may confound the evaluation of patients in this risk group.

Arterial blood gas measurements are helpful in determining the severity of pulmonary involvement. Hypoxemia is frequent but not invariable, and hypocarbia may also be seen. An increase in the alveolar to arterial O_2 tension difference, especially with exercise, has also been reported to be common in patients with *P. carinii* pneumonia.[32]

Gallium Lung Scans

Gallium lung scanning has proved to be a very sensitive, although nonspecific, test for *P. carinii* pneumonia.[34] At San Francisco General Hospital only 4 of 65 patients shown to have *P. carinii* on lung biopsy had a normal gallium lung scan.[33]

Table 12-1. Mean values for pulmonary Function Tests in AIDS Patients with *carinii* Pneumonia

	VC (% pred)	TLC (% pred)	DLco (% pred)
PCP	59	72	63
No PCP	81	88	71
P	< 0.001	< 0.001	< 0.001

VC = vital capacity TLC = total lung capacity; DLco = diffusing capacity of carbon monoxide (single breath corrected for hemoglobin concentration); PCP = P. *carinii* pneumonia. (From Curtis, et al.,[33] with permission.)

Table 12-2 shows the overall diagnostic value of noninvasive tests for *P. carinii* pneumonia. As can be seen, both the DLco and the gallium lung scan are very sensitive to the presence of *P. carinii* but have a low specificity. None of the studies alone has a high enough positive or negative predictive value to be definitive. However, when grouped together, the noninvasive tests enable identification of persons who should undergo further diagnostic studies.

Means to Identify *P. carinii*

Sputum Examination

Although patients with *P. carinii* pneumonia often complain of cough, they rarely produce sputum that is suitable for examination. However, adequate specimens can be obtained by having patients inhale a mist of 3 percent saline produced by an ultrasonic nebulizer. Both Pitchenik and co-workers[35] and Bigby et al.[36] have documented that sputum examination provides diagnoses in a substantial number of patients with AIDS. In both studies *P. carinii* was found in 40 to 50 percent of the specimens examined, and the sensitivity was between 50 and 60 percent. In the group studied by Bigby et al.[36] there were no features that predicted which patients would have positive sputum, although those who were positive tended to have a lower arterial O_2 tension and DLco. Subsequent experience at San Francisco General Hospital has shown sputum examination to have a 79 percent sensitivity.

Table 12-2. Diagnostic Value of Noninvasive Tests for *P. carinii* Pneumonia

	VC	TLC	DLco	CXR	GALS
Sensitivity (%)	85.2	71.4	89.3	82.8	90.7
Specificity (%)	52.2	64.4	23.8	45.4	40.9
Positive predictive value (%)	75.8	77.5	67.7	68.8	75.0
Negative predictive value (%)	66.7	56.9	55.6	64.5	69.2

VC = vital capacity; TLC = total lung capacity; DLco = Single-breath diffusing capacity for carbon monoxide; CXR = Chest radiograph; GALS = gallium[67] citrate lung scan. (From Hopewell,[94] with permission.)

These studies demonstrate that sputum induction can provide a noninvasive and relatively inexpensive means of diagnosing *P. carinii* pneumonia in a significant proportion of patients with AIDS. Nevertheless, the sensitivity and negative predictive values are such that a negative result cannot be regarded as definitively excluding *P. carinii*. The diagnostic value of sputum examination in patients with other forms of immunosuppression has not been established. It should be noted that trophozoites of *P. carinii* are seen in sputum more commonly than in bronchoalveolar lavage or biopsy specimens. For this reason, Giemsa staining may be more sensitive than methenamine silver, which stains cyst walls only. A fluorescein-tagged anti-*pneumocystis* monoclonal antibody has also been used for staining of sputum smears (see Ch. 11). Preliminary data suggest that this method may be slightly more sensitive than Giemsa staining.

Bronchoalveolar Lavage and Transbronchial Lung Biopsy

Bronchoalveolar lavage and transbronchial lung biopsy have proved to be highly sensitive in identifying pulmonary infections in patients with AIDS.[37–41] These procedures, performed through a fiberoptic bronchoscope, are obviously much less invasive than open-lung biopsy, which was felt to be the procedure of choice to diagnose *P. carinii* pneumonia in patients without AIDS.[8] In an early series of AIDS patients, fiberoptic bronchoscopy with transbronchial biopsy and in some instances bronchoalveolar lavage and brush biopsy yielded 91 percent of the total diagnoses of infections.[38] The yield was higher when transbronchial biopsy and lavage were combined. An infecting agent was identified by open-lung biopsy after a nondiagnostic transbronchial biopsy in 10 of 24 patients. Five of seven patients whose initial bronchoscopic procedures were nondiagnostic had repeat transbronchial biopsies that identified infecting organisms. Open-lung biopsy was also performed in nine patients with bronchoscopically proven *P. carinii* pneumonia who were failing treatment. Only *P. carinii* was found in these patients.

Stover et al.[39] reported the results of bronchoscopic procedures in 72 patients with AIDS. Both transbronchial biopsy and bronchoalveolar lavage had high yields (88 and 85 percent, respectively); when these procedures were used together, the yield was 94 percent. The yield was especially high (94 percent) for *P. carinii*. Similar results were reported by Broaddus and coworkers,[41] who described the efficacy of bronchoalveolar lavage and transbronchial biopsy in detecting pulmonary pathogens in 276 fiberoptic bronchoscopic examinations performed on 171 patients with known or suspected AIDS. Of 173 pathogens identified during the initial evaluation or in the subsequent month, the initial bronchoscopy detected 166 (96 percent). Bronchoalveolar lavage and transbronchial biopsy had similar sensitivities of 86 percent (124 of 145) and 87 percent (133 of 153), respectively. For *P. carinii,* lavage had an 89 percent sensitivity, and transbronchial biopsy a 97 percent sensitivity. In patients who had both procedures performed, the sensitivity was 100 percent.

More recently bronchoalveolar lavage alone has been reported by Golden and co-workers[42] to have a sensitivity for *P. carinii* of 97 percent. At the San Francisco General Hospital we have reviewed our experience subsequent to the report by Broaddus et al.[41] and found that in no instance was *P. carinii* identified in transbronchial biopsy specimens when it was not seen in bronchoalveolar lavage fluid. Thus, as a matter of routine in patients with or suspected of having AIDS in whose sputum *P. carinii* is not found, we perform only bronchoalveolar lavage. If that procedure is not diagnostic, the lavage is repeated and a transbronchial biopsy is performed to look for other diagnoses.

The yields from bronchoscopic procedures in non-AIDS patients with *P. carinii* pneumonia are not as high as those described in AIDS patients.[43,44] The reasons for the lower yields are presumably related to the fact that there are fewer organisms in patients with lesser degrees of immunosuppression than is associated with AIDS. In addition, as a result of the AIDS epidemic physicians and laboratory technologists have become much more experienced and proficient in collecting, processing, and examining specimens for *P. carinii*.

Bronchoscopic Procedure. Fiberoptic bronchoscopy with bronchoalveolar lavage and transbronchial biopsy can be safely performed under local anesthesia via a transnasal or transoral approach without an endotracheal tube. Unless there is a focal abnormality on the chest film, the procedure can be done without fluoroscopic guidance, thereby saving time, cost, and discomfort to the patient.[45] The bronchoscopic procedure should involve inspection of the hypopharynx, vocal cords, and airways from the trachea to the subsegmental bronchi.

Bronchoalveolar Lavage. After inspection of the airways the bronchoscope is positioned in a peripheral airway, usually in the right middle lobe, and 80 to 100 ml of sterile, nonbacteriostatic saline is instilled in 20 ml aliquots. Suction is applied after each bolus. The aspirated return is usually 40 to 50 ml. Bronchoalveolar lavage can also be performed with a fiberoptic catheter or a double-lumen balloon-tipped catheter, neither of which requires bronchoscopy.[46]

Transbronchial Biopsy. If a transbronchial biopsy is to be performed, it should be done after the lavage. The bronchoscope is repositioned, generally in the right lower lobe. If the radiographic abnormality is localized, the biopsies should be taken in the area of greatest abnormality. Multiple specimens are generally obtained. At our institution the specimens for microbiologic evaluation are placed on a moistened gauze sponge and transported in a tightly capped specimen jar. Specimens for histologic study are placed in formalin. The use of touch imprints made from unfixed tissue specimens and smears of lavage sediment stained with Giemsa, Wright-Giemsa, or Gram-Weigert stains is a very sensitive means of detecting *P. carinii* and has the advantage of being rapid, as opposed to the slower methenamine-silver staining of fixed tissue sections.[40] Routine tissue histopathology with hematoxylin and eosin staining provides only inferential information concerning *P. carinii*. Typically, collections of eosinophilic material filling alveoli are seen. The amount of cellular infiltration is variable and *P. carinii* cannot be seen.

The complications of transbronchial biopsy consist mainly of hemorrhage and pneumothorax. In the series of transbronchial biopsies in patients with AIDS or suspected AIDS reported by Broaddus et al.,[41] pneumothorax occurred in 9 percent (23 of 253), with 15 (5.9 percent) requiring placement of a chest tube for reexpansion. Hemoptysis sufficient to cause respiratory compromise or to necessitate blood transfusion did not occur, and there were no deaths. The presence of an uncorrectable coagulopathy is an absolute contraindication to transbronchial biopsy, and respiratory failure sufficiently severe to require mechanical ventilation is usually viewed as a relative contraindication. However, bronchoalveolar lavage can be safely performed in these situations.

Open-Lung Biopsy

Open-lung biopsy in patients with AIDS should be reserved for several situations that are infrequently encountered: (1) patients with progressive pulmonary disease in whom sputum induction and a carefully performed fiberoptic bronchoscopy with bronchoalveolar lavage and transbronchial biopsy were nondiagnostic; (2) patients with an uncorrectable coagulopathy in whom lavage has been nondiagnostic; and (3) patients who require mechanical ventilation and in whom biopsy and or lavage has been nondiagnostic. Even in these situations a second bronchoscopic procedure may be indicated prior to open-lung biopsy. If possible, one should wait until the results of all microbiologic evaluations of the initial specimens have been returned before performing an open biopsy.

In immunosuppressed patients who do not have AIDS, open-lung biopsy may be indicated more frequently.[47] This seems to be true because of both the lower yields from bronchoscopic procedures and the often broader array of diagnostic possibilities in this group of patients.

Other Approaches to Diagnosis

Other means of establishing a diagnosis of *P. carinii* pneumonia include percutaneous cutting needle lung biopsy and needle aspiration.[48,49] Both these approaches have relatively high yields but are associated with a significant rate of complications and therefore are less useful than bronchoscopic techniques.

In some patients an empiric treatment trial may be used to infer a diagnosis. Generally, however, this is unsatisfactory—first, because another treatable process may be missed, and second, because such an approach exposes the patient to the risks of therapy, perhaps without benefit.

Antibody and antigen detection have not proved useful in establishing a diagnosis of *P. carinii* pneumonia. Meyers and co-workers[50] studied 424 patients who had had bone marrow transplants, of whom 33 later developed *P. carinii* pneumonia. Antibody was found in 13 of 25 tested prior to transplantation. Convalescent serum specimens demonstrated an increase in antibody in only 5 of 13 patients tested. Both the prevalence of antibody and the frequency of an increase in titer were the same as found in a group of transplant patients who had idiopathic interstitial pneumonia on lung biopsy. Circulating antigen was detected in 22 of 28 patients (79 percent) with *P. carinii* pneumonia. A similar frequency of antigenemia was found in 52 patients with cytomegalovirus or idiopathic pneumonia (35 of 52, or 67 percent). Antigen was also detected frequently in nonimmunocompromised patients with pneumonia (79 percent) and in transplant patients without pneumonia (44 percent) but not in healthy marrow donors (2 percent). These findings suggest that lung inflammation and perhaps immunosuppression without lung injury liberate *P. carinii* antigen and that antigenemia is a nonspecific finding.

Diagnostic Strategy

The results described above permit formulation of a logical diagnostic sequence by which patients suspected of having *P. carinii* pneumonia can be evaluated. This scheme is shown in Figure 12-4. Although several possible modifications could be envisioned, a logical, orderly approach of this sort should result in reaching a diagnosis more expeditiously and using resources most efficiently. Patient discomfort is also minimized by using more invasive studies only after less invasive approaches have failed. Obviously, clinical circumstances and institutional experience and resources will influence the determination of a diagnostic approach. It is important that institutions evaluate their results on an ongoing basis in order to determine the most effective diagnostic strategy based on prevailing local conditions.

TREATMENT

Evolution of Treatment

Although numerous agents have been used in attempts to treat *P. carinii* pneumonia, none were successful until 1958, when Ivady and Paldy[51] began trials of pentamidine. In 1967 pentamidine became available in the United States through the Parasitic Disease Drug Service of the National Communicable Disease Center (now Centers for Disease Control) and has since been used routinely in treating *P. carinii* pneumonia.

In 1971 Kirby et al.[52] reported successful pyrimethamine and sulfadiazine treatment of two of three patients with *P. carinii* pneumonia. None of four previous patients treated with these agents had survived.[53,54] Further experience with this combination has been very limited.

The combination of trimethoprim (TMP) and sulfamethoxazole (SMX) was first shown to be effective in treating and preventing *P. carinii* pneumonia in the rat model by Hughes and associates in 1974.[55] Subsequent clinical studies documented the usefulness of this combination in humans.[56–59]

Currently both TMP-SMX and pentamidine isethionate are approved for

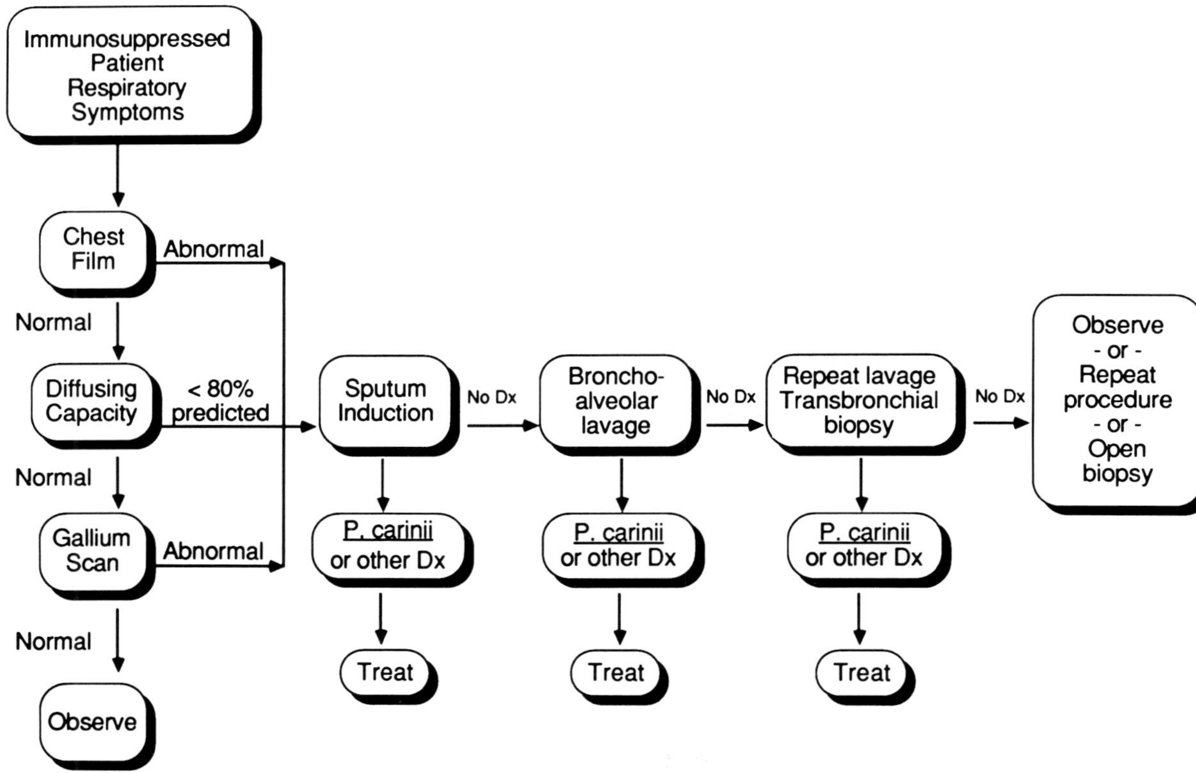

Fig. 12-4. Flow diagram of the sequence of diagnostic studies for evaluation of patients suspected of having *P. carinii* pneumonia or other opportunistic pulmonary infection.

treating *P. carinii* pneumonia. In analyses of non-AIDS patients with *P. carinii* pneumonia, TMP-SMX appeared to be more effective, with response rates in the range of 85 percent compared with approximately 65 percent for pentamidine when either drug was given for more than 9 days.[60] In addition, adverse effects were more frequent with pentamidine than with TMP-SMX. For these reasons, in the pre-AIDS era TMP-SMX was considered to be the drug of choice for *P. carinii* pneumonia. In patients with AIDS, however, TMP-SMX is not so clearly superior to pentamidine, as will be discussed subsequently.

Specific Anti-*Pneumocystis* Agents

Pentamidine

Pharmacology. Pentamidine is an aromatic diamidine that was first used in the 1940s to treat African trypanosomiasis and leishmaniasis. As noted previously, it was not used in treating *P. carinii* pneumonia until the late 1950s,[51] and the drug was not marketed in the United States until 1984. The spectrum of activity of pentamidine in nontoxic doses includes only *Trypanosoma rhodesiense, Trypanosoma gambiense, Leishmania donovani,* and *P. carinii*.[61]

The mechanism of action of pentamidine on *P. carinii* has not been firmly established. It inhibits dihydrofolate reductase (DHFR) in vitro, although it is not so potent in this regard as other folate antagonists.[62] In addition, it has been found to interfere with anaerobic glycolysis, to inhibit oxidative phosphorylation, and to limit nucleic acid and protein synthesis.[63]

Until recently the pharmacokinetics of pentamidine had not been well studied; however, the recent availability of a specific and sensitive assay has enabled more accurate studies to be conducted.[64] Conte and colleagues[65] measured plasma and urine concentrations of pentamidine in six patients who received the drug intravenously (IV) and in six given intramuscular (IM) doses; the dose in both groups was 4 mg/kg body weight. Mean peak concentrations occurred at 0.67 hours after administration in the IM patients and at 2 hours after initiation of a 2-hour infusion in the IV patients. There was a wide range of concentrations in each group, but the mean peak values were 209 ng/ml and 612 ng/ml in the IM and IV groups, respectively. The elimination half-life was 9.36 hours in the IM and 6.40 hours in the IV patients. The apparent volume of distribution was very large in both groups, indicating tissue sequestration. All patients had measurable concentrations 24 hours after administration. Urinary excretion in 24 hours was 2.5 to 4.1 percent of the total dose.

Previous studies in animals have shown high concentrations in kidneys and liver, with lower concentrations in lungs, after systemic administration of pentamidine.[66,67] Waldman and co-workers[67] also demonstrated selective sequestration of pentamidine in the lungs of rats given the drug by aerosol. Recently, Debs and associates have shown lung uptake with little or no systemic absorption when the drug was given as an aerosol[68] and have also reported that rats with *P. carinii* pneumonia could be treated successfully with aerosolized pentamidine.[69] Extending the observations on aerosol delivery of pentamidine to humans, Montgomery et al.[70] measured very high concentrations of the drug in bronchoalveolar lavage fluid with little or none in the plasma after aerosol administration in patients with *P. carinii* pneumonia. Both Golden et al.[71] and Montgomery et al.[72] have reported high rates of successful treatment with no systemic toxicity in pilot studies of aerosol pentamidine in AIDS patients with *P. carinii* pneumonia.

Dosage and Administration. The standard dose of pentamidine isethionate is 4 mg/kg body weight per day. For the methanesulfonate salt, the dose is 2.3 mg/kg/day. These doses are based loosely on animal studies and empiric observations. Because *P. carinii* cannot be maintained in culture, a minimum inhibitory concentration of pentamidine cannot be determined. Using a determination of dye uptake as an index of viability, Pesanti[73] showed that pentamidine concentrations of 5 and 10 μg/ml sharply decreased the uptake of neutral red after a lag of 6 hours. The 5-μg/ml concentration corresponds roughly to the plasma concentrations produced by IM or IV administration of 4 mg/kg of pentamidine isethionate.[65,66] Given the tissue tropism of the drug, it is likely that concentrations in the lung are substantially greater and that lower doses could perhaps be used.[67]

Because pentamidine is not absorbed from the gastrointestinal tract, parenteral administration is necessary. The approved route of administration is IM; however, because of the pain of the injection and the frequency of sterile abscesses, IV administration has come to be preferred.[74] Intravenous administration should be done only under circumstances such that the patient's blood pressure can be measured and the patient observed. The drug should be dissolved in 250 ml of 5 percent dextrose in water and administered at a constant infusion rate over 1 hour. The dosing interval of 24 hours should be increased for patients with impaired renal function for whom there is no suitable alternative agent.

The minimum duration of treatment with pentamidine has also not been established in a systematic fashion, but in most trials the drug was given for 14 to 21 days.[58,75,76,79] In addition, in patients with AIDS retropective analysis has suggested that 21 days of administration is superior to 14 days.[77]

Adverse Reactions. Western and co-workers[6] reported the first systematic compilation of adverse reactions to pentamidine. Of 164 patients given the drug 69 (42 percent) had untoward effects. Walzer et al.[78] extended these observations to include 404 patients, of whom 190 (47 percent) had adverse reactions. The most frequent reactions were azotemia, pain at the injection site, hypoglycemia, and sterile abscesses. A variety of other reactions, including hypotension, nausea and/or vomiting, skin rashes, and hypocalcemia, also were reported.

In patients with AIDS, adverse reactions to pentamidine occur with approximately the same frequency, but the array has broadened. In the study by Wharton et al.,[76] 14 of 32 patients (44 percent) given pentamidine for any period of time had a major adverse reaction which necessitated changing the drug, and all patients given the drug had minor adverse reactions. In this group the most frequent major adverse reaction was neutropenia (<1,000 polymorphonuclear leukocytes/μL) whereas hyponatremia, abnormal liver function, and azotemia were the most frequent minor reactions. Most reactions in these patients occurred between day 7 and day 14 of treatment.

Reported Effectiveness. The use of pentamidine clearly decreased mortality in the epidemic form of *P. carinii* pneumonia reported from Europe. Without treatment the estimated case fatality rate was 50 percent, whereas with pentamidine therapy mortality was reduced to 3.5 percent.[51]

In the United States data from Western et al. demonstrated a 76.7 percent rate of successful treatment for patients who received pentamidine for 9 or more days.[6] Overall, 36 of 75 patients (48 percent) recovered. Subsequently, Hughes and co-workers[58] prospectively evaluated 24 immunosuppressed children treated with pentamidine, 18 (75 percent) of whom recovered. In a similar study, Siegel et al.[75] reported recovery in 9 of 10 children treated with pentamidine. In a prospective study of *P. carinii* pneumonia in patients with AIDS, Wharton et al.[75] reported success in all but 1 of 20 patients randomized to receive pentamidine. Similar results in AIDS patients were reported by Klein et al.[79]

To summarize, treatment with pentamidine has resulted in cure rates ranging from 75 to 90 percent in both non-AIDS and AIDS patients. Adverse reactions that in many instances necessitate changing to an alternate agent occur in 40 to 50 percent of patients. Although the frequency of these reactions is approximately the same in non-AIDS patients, the spectrum is different. Especially notable is the frequency of neutropenia in patients with AIDS.

Trimethoprim-Sulfamethoxazole

Pharmacology. Sulfonamides were first synthesized in 1932 and used as anti-infective agents in 1935. Trimethoprim was synthesized in 1956 as a result of a systematic search for potential antimicrobial agents. The combination of TMP and SMX has a broad range of antimicrobial activity, including many gram-positive and aerobic gram-negative bacteria.[80]

These two agents act on separate sites to inhibit purine synthesis[80]: sulfonamides inhibit dihydrofolic synthetase, preventing the conversion of microbial para-aminobenzoic acid to dihydrofolic acid, and TMP acts on DHFR, thereby decreasing synthesis of tetrahydrofolic acid (see Ch. 6). In this effect TMP is at least 2,000 to 10,000 times more potent an inhibitor of microbial DHFR than of the human enzyme. Both drugs are well absorbed from the gastrointestinal tract. After an oral TMP dose of 240 mg, peak serum levels of 2 to 3 μg/ml are reached in 1 to 2 hours. The serum half-life of TMP is approximately 13 hours, with measurable concentrations present 24 hours after administration. Peak SMX concentrations of approximately 60 μg/ml are reached 2 hours after an oral dose of 1,200 mg. Its serum half-life is 9 to 12 hours, and measurable concentrations of the drug are present 24 hours after administration. Because the rates of absorption and the half-lives of the drugs are similar, they can be administered simultaneously. Their synergy in inhibiting purine synthesis is optimum at a TMP/SMX ratio of 1 : 20, this serum ratio being achieved by administration of a 1 : 5 dose ratio. For both drugs, both peak concentrations and serum half-lives increase linearly with increasing doses. Most of the administered dose of both drugs is excreted in the urine within 24 hours.

Concentrations of the drugs are generally higher in tissues than in serum. The TMP concentration in sputum is approximately twice the serum concentration, but the SMX concentration is only half that in serum.[81]

Dosage and Administration. As with pentamidine, minimal inhibitory concentrations of TMP and SMX for *P. carinii* have not been determined. In spite of the clinical efficacy of the combination no effect on neutral red dye uptake was noted by Pesanti[73]; thus, this assay provided no clues to the necessary serum concentrations.

In the studies of *P. carinii* pneumonia in the rat model that first documented the effectiveness of TMP-SMX, Hughes and co-workers[15] used a dose of 50 mg/kg/day for TMP and 250 mg/kg/day for SMX. Serum concentrations of the drugs were not measured. In the first report of treatment of patients with the combination, two doses were used, 4 to 7 mg/kg/day of TMP with 20 to 35 mg/kg/day of SMX and 20 and 100 mg/kg/day of TMP and SMX, respectively.[58] Peak serum concentrations of TMP were approximately 2 and 7 to 10 μg/ml for the lower and higher dose, respectively, and those of SMX were 50 to 60 and 80 to 120 μg/ml for the low and high doses, respectively. Two of six patients treated with low doses died, as did 2 of 14 who received high doses.

On the basis of this experience Hughes et al[58] conducted a prospective randomized study comparing TMP-SMX with pentamidine in immunosuppressed children with *P. carinii* pneumonia. They chose doses of 20 and 100 mg/kg/day for TMP and SMX, respectively. Serum levels of both agents were measured 2 and 6 hours after oral ingestion of one-fourth of the respective daily doses (5 and 25 mg/kg) on days 1, 3, 6, 9, and 12. The concentrations of both drugs tended to remain constant from the third day, although there was moderate variability from day to day. The 2- and 6-hour mean concentrations were not substantially different for either drug: for TMP the mean concentrations ranged from approximately 4 to 6.5 μg/ml and for SMX the range was approximately 115 to 175 μg/ml. All studies reported since the 1975 paper by Hughes et al.[56] have used these doses.[57–60,75,76,79,82] Whether or not lower doses would be effective has not been established.

Although the earlier reports used oral administration, concern about absorption prompted investigators to administer the drug intravenously.[60,76,79,82–84] Currently it is recommended that the daily dose be divided into four 6-hourly doses. If there is no suggestion that the drug will not be completely absorbed, it can be given orally, usually in the form of tablets containing TMP 160 mg and SMX 800 mg. In patients who require parenteral administration the drug should be diluted in 250 ml of 5 percent dextrose in water and given over a 30- to 60-minute period at 6-hour intervals. It is not clear whether the high dose of TMP-SMX should be continued for the full course of therapy or whether the dose can be reduced once a response is evident.[83] Likewise, the minimum duration of treatment necessary has not been established. In nearly all published reports, however, the drugs have been given for 14 to 21 days or occasionally longer depending on the clinical course.

Adverse Reactions. The major benefit offered by TMP-SMX over pentamidine in the early reports was a much lower frequency of adverse reactions.[56–60,74] In the prospective trial conducted by Hughes et al.,[58] the therapy of only one patient was changed because of an adverse reaction, an urticarial rash. Three patients had nausea and vomiting but were able to continue with the drug. Winston and co-workers[60] reported one patient with a skin rash and one with nausea and vomiting among 11 patients treated. Sattler and Remington[82] reported mild rash, phlebitis, and vomiting in 3 of 15 patients. Siegel et al.[75] noted skin rashes in 3 of 15 patients, but in only one was a change in therapy necessary. Also noted were mild elevations in serum transaminases and a 50 percent decrease in white blood cell count in two patients each.

Unfortunately, in treating patients with AIDS the frequency of significant adverse reactions has proved to be much higher. Gordin et al.[84] retrospectively reviewed adverse reactions among AIDS patients who were being treated with TMP-SMX and found that 19 of 35 patients treated for more than 2 days were not able to complete a full course of the agent because of adverse reactions. Severe skin rashes, often associated with fever, were the most common reactions; leukopenia and thrombocytopenia were the next most frequent reasons for discontinuing the drug; and hepatitis occurred in a small number of patients. These investigators noted that the adverse reactions nearly always occurred between days 6 and 14 of a planned 21-day course of treatment.

In the prospective study conducted by Wharton et al.,[76] adverse reactions to TMP-SMX were encountered frequently. Of 20 patients assigned to receive the drug, 10 had major adverse reactions, necessitating its discontinuation after a median of 11 days. As was noted by Gordin et al.,[84] nearly all adverse reactions occurred between days 6 and 14. Again, the most frequent major reactions were severe skin rash (20 percent) hepatitis (20 percent), neutropenia (15 percent), and thrombocytopenia (15 percent). Minor adverse reactions that did not necessitate discontinuation of the drug were seen in all patients. In addition to lesser degrees of the severe reactions, minor adverse effects included nausea and vomiting and hyponatremia.

Reported Effectiveness. In spite of the differences in adverse reactions between AIDS and non-AIDS patients with *P. carinii* pneumonia, rates of success in those who complete therapy are similar. In the two early papers by Hughes et al.,[56,58] survival rates in children were 75 and 77 percent. Early experience in adult patients was not as good as in children. Five (62 percent) of eight patients reported by Lau and Young[57] survived, as did 7 of 11 (64 percent) patients reported by Winston et al.[60] and 8 of 15 (53 percent) patients reported by Sattler and Remington.[82] In each of these groups the underlying disease processes and their treatments contributed to the mortality rates, thereby reducing the apparent rates of cure. For example, autopsied lung tissue from five of the seven patients who died in Sattler and Remington's series showed no *P. carinii,* indicating a "microbiologic cure."

Evaluating the success rates of TMP-SMX in patients with AIDS is difficult because of the frequency with which the drug must be discontinued owing to adverse reactions. In a retrospective review Haverkos[77] reported 91 percent (40 of 44 patients) survival in patients who were treated with a full course of the agent. On the other hand, survival was only 31 percent (11 of 35) in patients who were changed to pentamidine because of ineffectiveness of TMP-SMX and 69 percent in patients changed because of adverse reactions. Overall, 74 of 97 (76 percent) patients who were initially begun on TMP-SMX survived. Notably, this rate was not significantly different from survival rates in adults (65 percent) and children (70 percent) with other forms of immunosuppression.[77]

Among the patients reported in the National Heart, Lung, and Blood Institute workshop on the pulmonary complications of AIDS, 88 of 107 (82 percent) treated with TMP-SMX alone survived.[38] Of 37 patients who failed on TMP-SMX, only 4 (11 percent) survived, whereas 41 of 41 patients who were changed to pentamidine because of adverse reactions survived.

In the prospective studies by Wharton et al.[76] and Klein et al.,[79] survival rates for patients assigned to receive TMP-SMX were 75 percent (15 of 20) and 63 percent (22 of 35), respectively.

Dapsone (Diaminodiphenylsulfone)

Dapsone is a sulfone used nearly exclusively in the treatment of leprosy. In screening a number of agents for anti-*Pneumocystis* effects, Hughes and Smith[85] found that dapsone was effective in both preventing and treating *P. carinii* pneumonia in the cortisone-treated rat. A dose of 25 mg/kg/day had an effect similar to that of TMP-SMX (50 and 250 mg/kg/day), whereas 5 mg/kg/day had a lesser but still apparent effect.

On basis of these experimental results, Leoung and colleagues[86] conducted an open trial of the combination of dapsone 100 mg/day and TMP 20 mg/kg/day in treating mild to moderate *P. carinii* pneumonia in patients with AIDS. All of 15 patients recovered, and, although 14 of the 15 had minor adverse reactions, the drug had to be discontinued in only two patients, both because of rash. The most common minor reactions were nausea and vomiting. Subsequently these investigators have completed an open trial of dapsone 100 mg/kg/day without TMP and a prospective comparative trial of dapsone-TMP versus TMP-SMX.[87,88] Treatment with dapsone alone in a dose of 100 mg/day was associated with treatment failure or lack of improvement in 7 of 18 patients (39 percent).[87] There were no adverse effects that required stopping the drug. From this study it was concluded that dapsone alone was less effective than standard therapy for *P. carinii* pneumonia.

In the trial comparing dapsone-TMP with TMP-SMX, treatment failure occurred in 2 of 29 patients (7 percent) in each group.[88] Major toxicity occurred in 16 of 29 patients (55 percent) given TMP-SMX and 9 of 29 (31 percent) given TMP-dapsone. The adverse effects of TMP-dapsone included skin rash (three patients), nausea and vomiting (two patients), and leukopenia, thrombocytopenia, hepatitis, and methemoglobinemia (all one patient each). From this study it was concluded that dapsone-TMP was as effective as TMP-SMX and produced fewer adverse reactions.

α-Difluoromethylornithine

α-Difluoromethylornithine (DFMO) inhibits ornithine decarboxylase, thereby decreasing polyamine synthesis. It has been shown to be effective in treating African trypanosomiasis and has effects on other protozoa as well.[89] Although the drug was tested in the rat model of *P. carinii* pneumonia and had no effect,[85] clinical studies have shown some promise. Golden and co-workers[90] used the drug in six AIDS patients who had been treated with standard therapy and either had failed or were intolerant of the agents. The dose given was 6 g per square meter of body surface area daily divided into three doses given for 8 weeks. Each of the six patients had a successful outcome. Leukopenia and/or thrombocytopenia occurred in five of the six.

McLees et al.[91] have reported on the results of DFMO in 234 patients with *P. carinii* pneumonia who were said to have failed on standard treatment. The dose was 400 mg/kg/day given in four doses. The intended duration of IV administration was 14 days followed by 4 to 6 weeks of oral therapy with a dose of 75 mg/kg every 6 hours. These patients were severely ill, 45 percent being mechanically ventilated. Survival was 36 percent (84 of 234). Reversible thrombocytopenia occurred in 43 percent and leukopenia in 11 percent.

Although both clinical trials of DFMO suggest that the agent might be useful, a prospective comparative evaluation will be necessary to determine its true effectiveness.

Trimetrexate

Trimetrexate (TMX) is a potent inhibitor of DHFR that has antipneumocystis effects (see Ch. 11). Preliminary studies reported by Allegra and associates[92] showed complete responses in 9 of 13 previously untreated patients who received TMX, 30 mg/m^2 of body surface area daily, plus sulfadiazine, 1.0 g at 6-hour intervals and leucovorin. Of 14 previously untreated patients given TMX and leucovorin, 9 responded, as did 9 of 13 patients who had failed conventional therapy. All treatment was given for 21 days. Relapse rates within 1 month appeared to be rather high. Thrombocytopenia occurred in 8, granulocytopenia in 5, transaminasemia in 8, and skin rash in 1 of the 42 patients.

TREATMENT STRATEGIES

A synthesis of information available concerning the treatment of *P. carinii* pneumonia leads to both general and specific recommendations. As a general rule treatment should be based on a proven diagnosis. This is especially true in view of the frequency of adverse drug reactions. Moreover, given the rather large number of processes that comprise the differential diagnosis in immunocompromised patients with respiratory symptoms, establishing a precise diagnosis before undertaking treatment is sound practice.

In either AIDS or non-AIDS patients who can take oral medications without problems, treatment should be initiated with oral TMP, 20 mg/kg/day and SMX, 100 mg/kg/day. The total dose can be divided into two or four doses, although twice daily administration may not be tolerated because of gastrointestinal upset. If possible, either a TMP or an SMX serum concentration should be measured 2 hours after administration of the oral dose on day 2 or 3 of therapy. The concentration of TMP should be in the range of 4.5 to 6 μg/ml and that of SMX approximately 100 to 120 μg/ml.

For patients who are more severely ill or who cannot take oral drugs, TMP-SMX should be given IV in the same doses at 6-hour intervals. It should be kept in mind that administration of the total amount of drug requires infusion of approximately 1 L of 5 percent dextrose in water. Patients who require fluid restriction may not tolerate this volume. With IV administration serum concentrations of the drugs do not need to be checked.

Patients who have had adverse reactions to sulfa agents or specifically to TMP-SMX should be started on treatment with pentamidine, as should patients who cannot be given the fluid volume required to administer TMP-SMX. The dose of pentamidine isethionate is 4 mg/kg/day given IV or IM as a single daily administration. Especially with IV administration, patients should be monitored for hypotension during and shortly after the infusion.

The usual median time to respond to either agent is approximately 4 days, and some patients worsen before they begin to improve. Response should be judged by standard indexes, including degree of dyspnea, fever, respiratory rate, arterial O_2 tension, and chest film. Patients probably should not be considered as treatment failures with either drug until after 4 days of therapy. Continued worsening after 4 days or failure to improve after 7 to 10 days are indications to change therapy, generally from TMP-SMX to pentamidine.

All patients should be observed carefully for adverse reactions throughout the course of therapy. This is particularly true for patients with AIDS, especially in the second week of therapy. At the time treatment is initiated, baseline tests of hepatic and renal function and a complete blood count with differential and a platelet count should be obtained. Blood glucose should be measured in patients being given pentamidine. In AIDS patients these tests should be repeated at 3-day intervals at least through day 14 of treatment. For non-AIDS patients testing at 5- to 7-day intervals should be sufficient. Adverse reactions that necessitate changing treatment include: neutropenia ($<$750 polymorphonuclear leukocytes/μL); thrombocytopenia ($<$40,000 platelets/μL); elevation of serum creatinine to $>$3.0 mg/dl; increased aspartate or alanine aminotransferase to $>$5 times normal; and progressively worsening skin rash, especially if accompanied by mucositis or fever. Hypotension or hypoglycemia produced by pentamidine does not necessarily mean that the drug should be discontinued, but special care should be taken in its administration.

Both dapsone-TMP and aerosol pentamidine would appear to be suitable alternative forms of therapy for patients who fail treatment or are intolerant to the standard drugs. For patients being given dapsone-TMP, methemoglobin saturations should be measured at 3- to 5-day intervals. Aerosol pentamidine does not appear to be associated with systemic toxicity, but there is not sufficient experience to state this with certainty. At this point neither DFMO nor TMX can be said to have an established role.

The necessary duration of therapy is not well established. In non-AIDS patients 10 to 14 days seems to be sufficient, whereas in patients with AIDS 14 to 21 days is probably preferable. Assessment of response to therapy should be based on clinical and radiographic evaluation. Repeat examinations for *P. carinii* in patients with AIDS who have been successfully treated show *P. carinii* in over 60 percent, indicating that this is not a reliable means of determining cure.[93]

REFERENCES

1. Gajdusek DC: *Pneumocystis carinii*—etiologic agent of interstitial plasma cell pneumonia of premature and young infants. Pediatrics 19:543, 1957
2. Deamer WC, Zollinger HU: Interstitial "plasma cell" pneumonia of premature and young infants. Pediatrics 12:11, 1953
3. Hamperl H: *Pneumocystis* infection and cytomegaly of the lungs in the newborn and adult. Am J Pathol 32:1, 1956
4. Dutz W: *Pneumocystis carinii* pneumonia. Pathol Annu 5:309, 1970
5. LeClair RA: Descriptive epidemiology of interstitial pneumocystic pneumonia; an analysis of 107 cases from the United States, 1955–1967. Am Rev Respir Dis 99:542, 1969
6. Western KA, Perera DR, Schultz MG: Pentamidine isethionate in the treatment of *Pneumocystis carinii* pneumonia. Ann Intern Med 73:695, 1970
7. Singer C, Armstrong D, Rosen PP, Schottenfeld D: *Pneumocystis carinii* pneumonia: a cluster of eleven cases. Ann Intern Med 82:772, 1975
8. Young LS: Clinical aspects of pneumocystosis in man: epidemiology, clinical manifestations, diagnostic approaches and sequelae. p. 139. In Young LS (ed): *Pneumocystis carinii* Pneumonia. Marcel Dekker, New York, 1984
9. Hughes WT, Kuhn S, Chaudhary S, et al: Successful chemoprophylaxis for *Pneumocystis carinii* pneumonitis. N Eng J Med 297:1419, 1977
10. Gottlieb MS, Schroff R, Schanker HM, et al: *Pneumocystis carinii* pneumonia and mucosal candidiasis in previously healthy homosexual men. N Engl J Med 305:1425, 1981
11. Masur H, Michelis MA, Greene JB, et al: An outbreak of community acquired *Pneumocystis carinii* pneumonia. N Engl J Med 305:1431, 1981
12. Curran JW, Morgan WM, Hardy AM, et al: The epidemiology of AIDS: current status and future prospects. Science, 229:1352, 1985
13. Centers for Disease Control: Update: acquired immunodeficiency syndrome, MMWR 35:757, 1986
14. Frenkel JK, Good JT, Schultz JA: Latent *Pneumocystis* infection of rats, relapse and chemotherapy. Lab Invest 15:1559, 1966

15. Hughes WT, McNabb PC, Makres TD, Feldman S: Efficacy of trimethoprim and sulfamethoxazole in the prevention and treatment of *Pneumocystis carinii* pneumonitis. Antimicrob Agents Chemother 5:289, 1975
16. Walzer PD, Schnelle V, Armstrong D, Rosen PP: Nude mouse: a new experimental model for *Pneumocystis carinii* infection. Science 197:177, 1977
17. Walzer PD, Powell RD Jr, Yoneda K: Experimental *Pneumocystis carinii* pneumonia in different strains of cortisonized mice. Infect Immun 24:939, 1979
18. Meuwissen JHET, Tauber I, Leeuwenberg ADEM, et al: Parasitologic and serologic observations of infection with *Pneumocystis* in humans. J Infect Dis 136:43, 1977
19. Pifer LL, Hughes WT, Stagno S, Woods D: *Pneumocystis carinii* infection: evidence for high prevalence in normal and immunosuppressed children. Pediatrics 61:35, 1978
20. Sheppard V, Jameson B, Knowles GK: *Pneumocystis carinii* pneumonitis: a serological study. J Clin Pathol 32:773, 1979
21. Hofmann B, Odum H, Platz P, et al: Humoral responses to *Pneumocystis carinii* in patients with the acquired immunodeficiency syndrome and in immunocompromised homosexual men. J Infect Dis 152:838, 1985
22. Hamlin WB: *Pneumocystis carinii.* JAMA 204:173, 1968
23. Esterly JA: *Pneumocystis carinii* in lungs at autopsy. Am Rev Respir Dis 97:935, 1968
24. Coleman DL, Luce JM, Wilber JC, et al: Antibodies to the retrovirus associated with the acquired immunodeficiency syndrome (AIDS): presence in presumably healthy San Franciscans who died unexpectedly. Arch Intern Med 146:713, 1986
25. Watanabe JM, Chinchinian H, Weitz G, et al: *Pneumocystis carinii* pneumonia in a family. JAMA 193:685, 1965
26. Hughes, WT: Natural mode of acquisition for de novo infection with *Pneumocystis carinii.* J Infect Dis 145:842, 1982
27. Burke BA, Good RA: *Pneumocystis carinii.* Medicine (Baltimore) 52:23, 1973
28. Masur H, Jones TC: The interaction in vitro of *Pneumocystis carinii* with macrophages and L-cells. J Exp Med 147:157, 1978
29. VonBehren LA, Pesanti EL: Uptake and degradation of *Pneumocystis carinii* by macrophages in vitro. Am Rev Respir Dis 118:1051, 1978
30. Goodman PC, Broaddus VC, Hopewell PC: Chest radiographic patterns in the acquired immunodeficiency syndrome. Am Rev Respir Dis 129:A36, 1984
31. Cohen BA, Pomeranz S, Rabinowitz JG, et al: Pulmonary complications of AIDS: Radiologic features. AJR 143:115, 1984
32. Stover DE, White DA, Romano PA, et al: Spectrum of pulmonary disease associated with the acquired immune deficiency syndrome. Am J Med 78:429, 1985
33. Curtis J, Goodman P, Hopewell PC: Noninvasive tests in the diagnostic evaluation for *P. carinii* pneumonia in patients with or suspected of having AIDS. Am Rev Respir Dis 113:A182, 1986
34. Coleman DL, Hattner RS, Luce JM, et al: Gallium lung scanning in patients with suspected pneumonia and the acquired immunodeficiency syndrome. Am Rev Respir Dis 130:1166, 1984
35. Pitchenik AE, Ganjei P, Torres A, et al: Sputum examination for the diagnosis of *Pneumocystis carinii* in the acquired immunodeficiency syndrome. Am Rev Respir Dis 133:226, 1986
36. Bigby T, Margolskee D, Curtis J, et al: The usefulness of induced sputum in the diagnosis of *Pneumocystis carinii* pneumonia in patients with the acquired immunodeficiency syndrome. Am Rev Respir Dis 133:515, 1986

37. Coleman DL, Dodek PM, Luce JM, et al: Diagnostic utility of fiberoptic bronchoscopy in patients with *Pneumocystis carinii* pneumonia and the acquired immunodeficiency syndrome. Am Rev Respir Dis 128:795, 1983
38. Murray JF, Felton CP, Garay S, et al: Pulmonary complications of the acquired immunodeficiency syndrome: report of a National Heart, Lung, and Blood Institute workshop. N Engl J Med 310:1682, 1984
39. Stover DE, White DA, Romano PA, Gellene RA: Diagnosis of pulmonary disease in the acquired immune deficiency syndrome: roles of bronchoscopy and bronchoalveolar lavage. Am Rev Respir Dis 131:659, 1984
40. Blumenfeld W, Wagar E, Hadley WK: Use of the transbronchial biopsy for diagnosis of opportunistic pulmonary infections in the acquired immunodeficiency syndrome. Am J Clin Pathol 81:1, 1984
41. Broaddus VC, Dake MD, Stulbarg MS, et al: Bronchoalveolar lavage and transbronchial biopsy for the diagnosis of pulmonary infections in patients with the acquired immunodeficiency syndrome. Ann Intern Med 102:747, 1985
42. Golden JA, Hollander H, Stulbarg MS, Gamsu G: Bronchoaveolar lavage as the exclusive diagnostic modality of *Pneumocystis carinii* pneumonia. Chest 90:18, 1986
43. Feldman NT, Pennington JE, Ehrie MG: Transbronchial lung biopsy in the compromised host. JAMA 238:1377, 1977
44. Nishio JM, Lynch JP: Fiberoptic bronchoscopy in the immunocompromised host; the significance of a "nonspecific" transbronchial biopsy. Am Rev Respir Dis 121:307, 1980
45. Hopewell PC, Luce JM, Sheppard D, et al: Blind transbronchial biopsy in diffuse lung disease associated with known or suspected acquired immunodeficiency syndrome. Am Rev Respir Dis 129:A76, 1984
46. Wong H, Caughey G, Gamsu G, Golden J: Nonbronchoscopic catheter bronchoalveolar lavage in the diagnosis of *Pneumocystis carinii* pneumonia. Am Rev Respir Dis 131:A222, 1985
47. Springmeyer SL, Silvestri RC, Sale GE, et al: The role of transbronchial biopsy for the diagnosis of diffuse pneumonias in immunocompromised marrow transplant recipients. Am Rev Respir Dis 126:763, 1982
48. Zavala DC, Bedell GN: Percutaneous lung biopsy with a cutting needle. Am Rev Respir Dis 106:186, 1972
49. Wallace JM, Batra P, Gong H Jr, Ovenfors C-O: Percutaneous needle lung aspiration for diagnosing pneumonitis in the patient with acquired immunodeficiency syndrome (AIDS). Am Rev Respir Dis 131:389, 1985
50. Meyers JD, Pifer LL, Sale GE, Thomas ED: The value of *Pneumocystis carinii* antibody and antigen detection for diagnosis of *Pneumocystis carinii* pneumonia after marrow transplantation. Am Rev Respir Dis 120:1283, 1979
51. Ivady G, Paldy L, Koltay M, et al: *Pneumocystis carinii* pneumonia. Lancet 1:616, 1967
52. Kirby HB, Kenamore B, Guckian JL: *Pneumocystis carinii* treated with pyrimethamine and sulfadiazine. Ann Intern Med 75:505, 1971
53. Rifkind D, Faris TD, Hill RB Jr: *Pneumocystis carinii* pneumonia. Studies on the diagnosis and treatment. Ann Intern Med 65:943, 1966
54. Ruskin J, Remington JS: The compromised host and infection. I. *Pneumocystis carinii* pneumonia. JAMA 202:96, 1967
55. Hughes WT: Treatment of *Pneumocystis carinii* pneumonitis. N Engl J Med 295:726, 1976

56. Hughes WT, Feldman S, Sanyal SK: Treatment of *Pneumocystis carinii* pneumonitis with trimethoprim-sulfamethoxazole. Can Med Assoc J 112:475, 1975
57. Lau WK, Young LS: Trimethoprim-sulfamethoxazole treatment of *Pneumocystis carinii* pneumonia in adults. N Engl J Med 297:1419, 1976
58. Hughes WT, Feldman S, Chaudhary SC, et al: Comparison of pentamidine isethionate and trimethoprim-sulfamethoxazole in the treatment of *Pneumocystis carinii* pneumonia. J Pediatr 92:285, 1978
59. Larter WE, John JT, Sieber OF, et al: Trimethoprim-sulfamethoxazole treatment of *Pneumocystis carinii* pneumonitis. J Pediatr 92:826, 1978
60. Winston DJ, Lau WK, Gale RP, Young LS: Trimethoprim-sulfamethoxazole for the treatment of *Pneumocystis carinii* pneumonia. Ann Intern Med 92:762, 1980
61. Drake S, Lampasona V, Nicks HL, et al: Pentamidine isethionate in the treatment of *Pneumocystis carinii* pneumonia. Clin Pharm 4:507, 1985
62. Waalkes TP, Makulu DR: Pharmacologic aspects of pentamidine. Natl Cancer Inst Monogr 43:171, 1976
63. Bornstein RS, Yarbro JW: An evaluation of the mechanism of action of pentamidine isethionate. J Surg Oncol 2:393, 1970
64. Lin J, Shi RJ, Lin ET: High performance liquid chromatographic determination of pentamidine in plasma. J Liquid Chromatog 9:2035, 1986
65. Conte JE Jr, Upton RA, Phelps RT, et al: Use of a specific and sensitive assay to determine pentamidine pharmacokinetics in patients with AIDS. J Infect Dis 154:923, 1986
66. Waalkes TP, Denham C, DeVita VT: Pentamidine: clinical pharmacological correlations in man and mice. Clin Pharmacol Ther 11:505, 1970
67. Waldman RH, Pearce DE, Martin RA: Pentamidine isethionate levels in lungs, livers, and kidneys of rats after aerosol or intramuscular administration. Am Rev Respir Dis 108:1004, 1973
68. Debs RJ, Straubinger RM, Brunette E, et al: Selective enhancement of pentamidine uptake in the lung by aerosolization and delivery in liposomes. Am Rev Respir Dis 135:731, 1987
69. Debs RJ, Blumenfeld W, Brunette EM, et al: Successful treatment with aerosolized pentamidine of *Pneumocystis carinii* in rats. Antimicrob Agents Chemother 31:37, 1987
70. Montgomery AB, Debs RC, Luce JM, et al: Selective delivery of pentamidine by aerosol Am Rev Respir Dis 137:477, 1988
71. Golden JA, Hollander H, Conte JE Jr: Inhaled pentamidine or low-dose intravenous pentamidine as novel therapy for *Pneumocystis carinii* pneumonia in the acquired immunodeficiency syndrome (AIDS). Am Rev Respir Dis 135:A168, 1987
72. Montgomery AB, Debs RJ, Luce JM, et al: Aerosolized pentamidine as sole treatment for *Pneumocystis carinii* pneumonia in patients with the acquired immunodeficiency syndrome. Lancet 2:480, 1987
73. Pesanti EL: In vitro effects of antiprotozoan drugs and immune serum on *Pneumocystis carinii*. J Infect Dis 141:775, 1980
74. Navin TR, Fontaine RE: Intravenous versus intramuscular administration of pentamidine. N Engl J Med 311:1701, 1984
75. Siegel SE, Wolff LJ, Baehner RL, Hammond D: Treatment of *Pneumocystis carinii* pneumonitis. An J Dis Child 138:1051, 1984
76. Wharton JM, Coleman DL, Wofsy CB, et al: Trimethoprim-sulfamethoxazole or pentamidine for *Pneumocystis carinii* pneumonia in the acquired immunodeficiency syndrome. Ann Intern Med 105:37, 1985

77. Haverkos HW, PCP Therapy Project Group: Assessment of therapy for *Pneumocystis carinii* pneumonia. Am J Med 76:501, 1984
78. Walzer PD, Perl DP, Krogstad DJ, et al: *Pneumocystis carinii* pneumonia in the United States: epidemiologic, diagnostic and clinical features. In Robbins JB, DeVita VT Jr (eds): Symposium on *Pneumocystis carinii* infection. Natl Cancer Inst Monogr 43:930, 1976
79. Klein MC, Duncanson FP, Lennox TH, et al: Prospective randomized treatment for *Pneumocystis carinii* pneumonia (PCP) in AIDS patients. Proc 2nd Int Conf AIDS:52, 1986
80. Kucers A, Bennett NMcK: Trimethoprim and co-trimoxazole. p. 687. In The Use of Antibiotics. William Heinemann Medical Books Ltd., London 1979
81. Hughes D: Chemoprophylaxis in chronic bronchitis. J Antimicrob Chemother 2:320, 1976
82. Sattler FR, Remington JS: Intravenous trimethoprim-sulfamethoxazole therapy for *Pneumocystis carinii* pneumonia. Am J Med 70:1215, 1981
83. Young LS: Treatment and prevention of *Pneumocystis carinii* infection. p. 175. In Young LS (ed): Pneumocystis carinii Pneumonia. Marcel Dekker, New York, 1984
84. Gordin FM, Simon GL, Wofsy CR, Mills J: Adverse reactions to trimethoprim-sulfamethoxazole in patients with the acquired immunodeficiency syndrome. Ann Intern Med 100:495, 1984
85. Hughes WT, Smith BL: Efficacy of diaminodiphenylsulfone and other drugs in murine *Pneumocystis carinii* pneumonitis. Antimicrob Agents Chemother 26:436, 1984
86. Leoung GS, Mills J, Hopewell PC, et al: Dapsone-trimethoprim for *Pneumocystis carinii* pneumonia in the acquired immunodeficiency syndrome. Ann Intern Med 105:45, 1986
87. Mills J, Leoung G, Medina J, et al: Dapsone treatment of *Pneumocystis carinii* pneumonia in the acquired immunodeficiency syndrome. Antimicrob Agents Chemother
88. Medina I, Leoung G, Mills J, et al: Oral therapy for *Pneumocystis carinii* pneumonia in AIDS: a randomized double-blind trial of trimethoprim-sulfamethoxazole versus dapsone-trimethoprim for first episode *Pneumocystis carinii* pneumonia in AIDS. Proc 3rd Int Conf on AIDS:208, 1987
89. McCann PP, Bacchi CJ, Clarkson JR, et al: Further studies on difluoromethylornithine in African trypanosomes. Med Biol 59:434, 1981
90. Golden JA, Sjoerdsma A, Santi DV: *Pneumocystis carinii* pneumonia treated with α-difluoromethylornithine. West J Med 141:613, 1984
91. McLees BD, Barlow JLR, Kuzma RJ, et al: Successful eflornithine (DFMO) treatment in AIDS patients failing conventional therapy. Am Rev Respir Dis 135:A167, 1987
92. Allegra CJ, Chabner B, Tuazon C: Preliminary results of a phase I–II trial of trimetrexate therapy for pneumocystis pneumonia in AIDS. Proc 3rd Int Conf AIDS:155, 1987
93. Michael P, Brodie H, Wharton M, et al: Significance of persistence of *P. carinii* after completion of treatment. Proc 1st Int Conf AIDS:23, 1985
94. Hopewell PC, Luce JM: Pulmonary manifestations of the acquired immunodeficiency syndrome. Clin Immunol Allergy 6:489, 1986

13 Host Defense in Leishmaniasis

Joseph P. Sypek
David J. Wyler

In the last decade there has been a resurgence of research interest in leishmaniasis. Several factors have contributed to the increased attention to this infection, one believed to afflict several hundred thousands if not millions of people worldwide.[1] First, the World Health Organization, through its Special Programme for Research Training in Tropical Disease (TDR), cosponsored by the U.N. Development Programme and the World Bank has brought attention to the fact that leishmaniasis in many endemic regions is probably far more prevalent and represents a greater public health problem than has been previously appreciated.[2] Second, the limitations of conventional chemotherapeutic regimens for leishmaniasis have stimulated the search for new agents.[3] Third, the development of recombinant DNA technology has provided new tools for rapid diagnosis[4,5] and, in conjunction with hybridoma methodology, has raised optimism for eventual development of a subunit vaccine for prevention of leishmaniasis. And fourth (a fact most compelling for the basic immunologist), the obligate intracellular nature of leishmanial infection provides an excellent model for studying principles of cell-mediated host defense against organisms that reside in host macrophages (e.g., bacteria, mycobacteria, fungi, chlamydia, and protozoa).

Leishmania spp. are obligate intracellular parasites transmitted to vertebrate hosts by the bite of infected sandflies. In mammalian hosts the organisms reside virtually exclusively within mononuclear phagocytes (macrophages and monocytes). Control of leishmaniasis transmission is complicated by a number of aspects of its epidemiology. For example, since the disease is zoonotic in most areas, nonhuman reservoirs remain potential sources for transmission even if all human cases could be cured. Unfortunately, elimination of these reservoirs is generally impractical. Another difficulty is that the insect vectors in most areas with endemic leishmaniasis are not peridomestic dwellers, so that their elimination through residual insecticide spraying is also impossible. On the other hand, kala azar (visceral leishmaniasis) has been virtually eradicated in many parts of China, where the major vector (*Phlebotomus chinensis*) is peridomestic and could be controlled with residual insecticides. Elimination of the dog reservoirs in China was also important in disease control.[6] Unfortunately, population migration into previously uninhabited regions where leishmaniasis is enzootic has more recently contributed to increased disease prevalence in China, the Amazon basin, and elsewhere.

At present the primary chemotherapy available for leishmaniasis is pentavalent antimonial compounds (sodium stibogluconate and N-methylglucamine antimonate); amphotericin B and pentamidine have also been used successfully in patients resistant to antimonials. Adverse toxic side effects, in addition to limited efficacy of conventional therapies in some cases and other complications, have dictated the need to identify newer agents. Newer therapeutic regimens, including use of pyrazylopyrimidine compounds such as allopurinol ribonucleoside[7] and agents such as rifampicin,[8] formycin B,[9] and liposome-associated amphotericin B,[10] are being assessed or considered. Currently no chemoprophylaxis against leishmaniasis is available.

A striking feature of some *Leishmania* infections of the skin (Old World cutaneous leishmaniasis) is their propensity to be self-limiting. Spontaneous self-cure is followed by long-lasting immunity with apparent resistance to reinfection.[11] Furthermore, protective immunity also appears to develop in successfully treated kala azar patients.[12] These observations suggest that perhaps vaccination could be feasible in the control of leishmaniasis. Certainly, this approach to disease control would seem most desirable since it circumvents the limitations imposed on other control modalities by the ecologic and epidemiologic factors mentioned above. No vaccine against leishmaniasis currently exists, however. Protection against reinfection has been successfully achieved by intentional inoculation of *Leishmania*-infected tissue or attenuated cultured parasites (promastigotes), a practice used for centuries in the Middle East and the Soviet Union.[13] While this approach (called "leishmanization" and reminiscent of Jenner's approach to cowpox called "jennerization") has been successful, it is not widely accepted because of disease complications that have recurred in some patients. Nonetheless, the experience supports the notion that a leishmaniasis vaccine is a reasonable possibility. Knowledge about defense mechanisms in leishmaniasis can be expected to aid in establishing a strategy for vaccine development.

HOST DEFENSE

In view of the obligate intracellular nature of *Leishmania* in mammalian hosts and supporting experimental evidence, current paradigms of immunity to this intramacrophage microbe suggest that host defense in leishmaniasis is largely if not exclusively cell-mediated.[14] Evidence obtained in animal models of leishmaniasis indicates that cell-mediated immunity is essential for healing of cutaneous lesions and development of protective immunity to reinfection.[15] Such studies have indicated that spontaneous resolution of leishmaniasis is generally associated with acquisition of antigen-specific T-cell responsiveness.[16,17] Further compelling evidence for a prominent role of cell-mediated immunity is provided by the observation that adoptive transfer of T cells—but not serum—from immune donors can impart protection to naive recipients in experimental murine models.[18,19] In addition, mice rendered agammaglobulinemic by treatment with anti-μ antibody are able to spontaneously heal their *Leishmania tropica*–induced skin lesions,[20] which strengthens the evidence against a direct role of antibody in antileishmanial defense.

Prophylactic immunization with irradiated *Leishmania* of highly susceptible BALB/c mice (which otherwise normally experience progressive and lethally disseminating leishmanial infections) has also been shown to depend on the generation of antigen-specific T cells, which presumably directly mediate defense.[21–23] Immunity acquired by this intravenous immunization protocol was transferable to naive recipients by T cells. These immune effector cells were specifically shown to bear the Lyl^+2^- phenotype. In addition to providing support for the notion that T cell–mediated immunity is essential for defense, these studies also indicate that immunity can indeed be established in nonhealer animals through vaccination. On the other hand, in none of the in vivo studies have the mechanism(s) whereby T cells impart protection in leishmaniasis been elucidated.

Host defense to intracellular microorganisms could theoretically occur by one of the following mechanisms: (1) activation of macrophages by lymphocyte-derived soluble mediators (lymphokines), as occurs in *Listeria* infection[24]; (2) direct cell lysis of host cells by cytotoxic T lymphocytes, as occurs in certain viral infections[25]; and (3) macrophage activation by direct physical contact of effector T lymphocytes with target macrophages, independently of host cell damage and soluble mediators (see below). The first and third of these mechanisms appear to be instrumental in host defense in leishmaniasis. No compelling evidence for a role of cytotoxic T cells in this disease has been presented.

LYMPHOKINE-MEDIATED DEFENSE

Studies of *Listeria*-infected mice carried out in the 1960s[26] revealed that while T cells develop specific immune responses to the invading intracellular microorganism, macrophages are the cells that eliminate the pathogen. Furthermore, these studies indicated that macrophages recovered from infected animals could destroy microorganisms antigenically unrelated to *Listeria*.[27] The observation that soluble mediators released by specifically sensitized T cells nonspecifically confer enhanced antimicrobial properties to macrophages[28,29] focused subsequent research attention on the role of lymphokines in macrophage activation.[30] In the specific case of *Leishmania* infection, Mauel and colleagues first demonstrated that *Leishmania enriettii* (pathogenic only to guinea pigs) was destroyed in lymphokine-activated mouse macrophages.[31,32] Although these earlier studies were the first to establish the principle of lymphokine involvement in antileishmanial defense, the facts that *L. enriettii* is not pathogenic for mice and that these parasites grow poorly in untreated mouse macrophages in vitro raised concern that the findings might not be relevant to defense against pathogenic species. Accordingly, in collaboration with Dr. Carol Nacy, one of us (DJW) initiated studies to examine the role of lymphokines in defense against *Leishmania major* (naturally pathogenic to humans and also pathogenic to experimentally infected mice).

L. major amastigotes were obtained from infected footpads of BALB/c mice, and resident peritoneal macrophages of uninfected C3H/HeN mice were infected in vitro by methods we had previously developed for infecting human mononuclear phagocytes.[33] When cells were incubated in polypropylene culture tubes (but not when macrophages were allowed to adhere to a plastic surface), intracellular amastigotes replicated approximately three- to fourfold over 72 hours.[34,35] Crude (unfractionated) lymphokine-containing culture supernatants were prepared from spleen cells of mice previously sensitized to bacille Calmette Guérin (BCG) and incubated in vitro with purified protein derivative of tuberculin (PPD). These supernatants were not directly toxic to the *Leishmania,* but when added to the murine macrophage cultures they had distinct antileishmanial effects.[35] Three different effects were observed depending on when the lymphokine-containing preparations were added to macrophage cultures (Fig. 13-1). If macrophages were first incubated with the lymphokine preparation, washed, and then infected with amastigotes, the infection rate (percent infected macrophages and number of amastigotes per 100 macrophages) was substantially reduced (30 to 50 percent) compared with that observed for untreated macrophages.[35] We subsequently observed that the decrease in infection resulting from lymphokine treatment was due to a specific, reversible reduction in the ingestion of amastigotes but not apparently in the expression of macrophage receptors for amastigotes. Lymphokine-treated macrophages were briefly exposed to cytochalasin E, washed, and then cocultured with amastigotes. This treatment permits amastigotes to attach to macrophages normally but prevents their entry into the host cells.[36] Since lymphokine treatment did not reduce parasite binding to the cytochalasin-treated cells but did reduce infection of cells not treated with cytochalasin, it seems most likely that its effect on infection was to interfere with subsequent entry (Fig. 13-2). Furthermore, since nonspecific (latex bead) and receptor-mediated (immunoglobulin G–coated erythrocyte) particle uptake was not altered by our lymphokine treatment (unpublished data), the effect on parasite infection was not due to a detectable widespread alteration in macrophage phagocytic function. This lymphokine effect is reversible. When treated macrophages were washed and incubated for 6 hours or more prior to adding amastigotes, they regained their ability to ingest the parasites (Fig. 13-3). We have evidence that this lymphokine effect may occur in vivo. Peritoneal macrophages obtained from *L. major*–infected mice (at the onset of spontaneous resolution of their cutaneous infection) have a reversible defect in their ability to ingest amastigotes but not IgG-coated erythrocytes or latex beads.[37] Because these macrophages obtained from infected mice function similarly to ones treated in vitro with lymphokines, our observation may indicate that lymphokines actually function in antileishmanial defense in vivo.

Another effect of lymphokines in antileishmanial defense in vitro is to inhibit parasite replication and kill *Leishmania* within macrophages. In the presence of lymphokines, intracellular parasites can be destroyed. Even pretreatment of uninfected macrophages (followed by washing and continued incubation in medium alone) results in an antimicrobial effect on the intracellular amastigotes (Fig. 13-1B).[35]

Several additional features of lymphokine-mediated activation of macrophages for antileishmanial effects in vitro have been analyzed by Nacy and her colleagues as well as by other groups. For example, it has been shown that macrophages preincubated in vitro prior to lymphokine treatment become progressively refractory to subsequent activation of microbistatic and microbicidal effects by lymphokines.[35,38] In addition, only resident macrophages activated by lymphokines develop increased resistance to infection and acquire the capacity to kill intracellular *Leishmania;* elicited (inflammatory) peritoneal macrophages are relatively refractory.[35,39]

Precisely how parasites are killed within activated macrophages is presently unclear. Marcrophage activation by lymphokines results in an array of physiologic and metabolic changes in the host cell, some of which might theoretically contribute to the antileishmanial effects.[40] Evidence has been provided that the enhanced capacity of lymphokine-activated mononuclear phagocytes to exert antimicrobial effects correlates closely with the ability of these cells to secrete high levels of superoxide anion (O_2^-) and hydrogen peroxide (H_2O_2).[41] However, since mononuclear phagocytes that are defective in generating an oxidative burst are nonetheless capable of exerting antileishmanial effects in vitro,[42,43] toxic oxygen radicals are clearly not the sole intracellular mediators of antileishmanial defense.

Recent studies have shed light on the molecular nature of one of the lymphokines that can activate antileishmanial defense in macrophages. Recombinant γ-interferon (rIFNγ) can activate macrophages for this defense.[44] On the other hand, monoclonal anti-IFNγ antibody treatment of unfractionated lymphokines diminishes but does not abolish the activating capacity of the preparation.[45,46,55] It therefore seems that IFNγ is the primary but not sole lymphokine responsible for stimulating macrophage oxidative bursts and activating antileishmanial activity in vitro.[45,46] The other, noninterferon lymphokine factors are apparently immunochemically unrelated to this molecule but have not as yet been identified.

The implication of these in vitro observations for understanding host defense in vivo is that they suggest the *possibility* that macrophage activation by lymphokines is important in defense. Evidence for such lymphokines actually being operative in vivo has so far been sought in only a few studies. By using murine models of leishmaniasis a correlation was observed between the ability

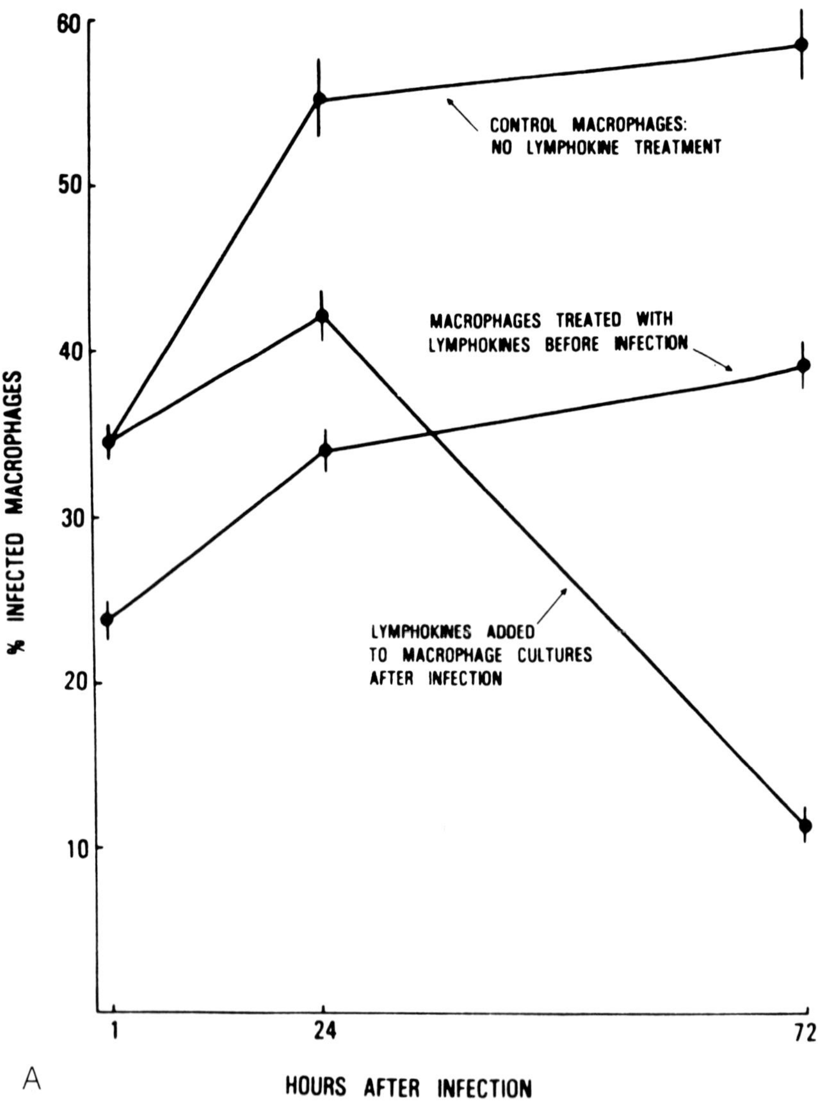

Fig. 13-1 Effects of lymphokines on infection and replication of *L. major* amastigotes in peritoneal macrophages. (**A**) Macrophages pretreated with lymphokines for 4 hours ingest fewer parasites on subsequent exposure to *L. major* amastigotes than do untreated macrophages. When lymphokines are added to infected macrophages, parasites are killed and digested over a subsequent 72-hour incubation (parasiticidal effect). When macrophages were treated with lymphokines only prior to infection (pretreatment), the percent of infected macrophages remained constant over 72 hours. (*Figure continues*).

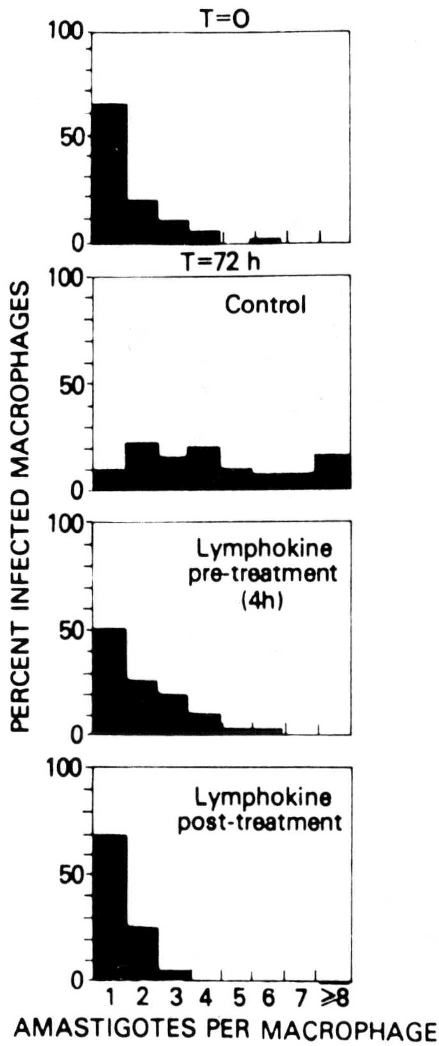

B

Fig. 13-1 (*Continued*). (**B**) By histogram analysis of the number of amastigotes per infected macrophage after a 1 hour infection (T = 0) or 72 hours later (T = 72), replication of parasites under different experimental conditions could be assessed. Untreated macrophages contained more amastigotes per infected cell at T = 72 than T = 0. Parasites did not replicate when macrophages were pretreated with lymphokines, which reflects a parasitistatic effect. (From Nacy CA, et al.,[35] with permission.)

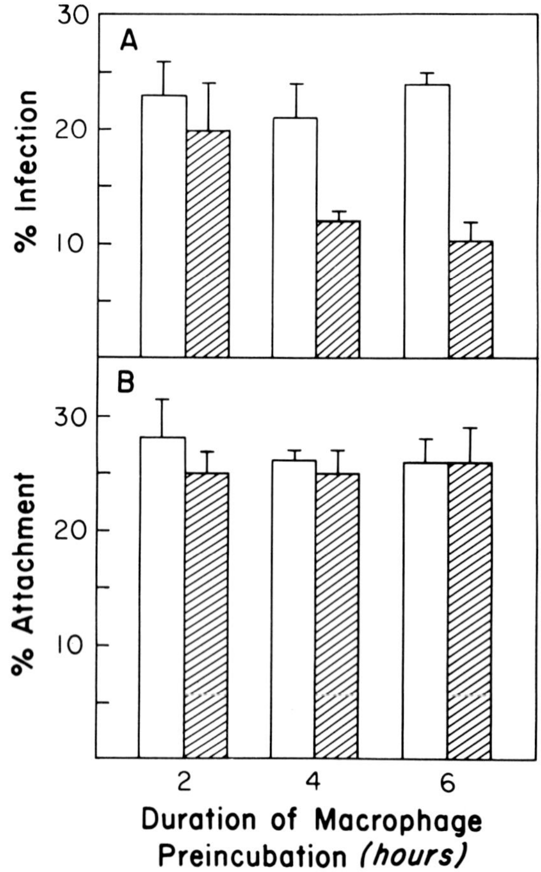

Fig. 13-2. Effect of lymphokine treatment of macrophages on (**A**) uptake or (**B**) attachment of *L. major* amastigotes in vitro. (**A**) Macrophages were preincubated either in the medium (open bars) or in a lymphokine preparation (striped bars) for 2, 4, or 6 hours prior to adding amastigotes (MOI = 0.5 : 1) for 2 hours. The magnitude of parasite ingestion (percent infected macrophages) was assessed by microscopic examination of cytocentrifuge preparations of macrophage-parasite cocultures. (**B**) Attachment (percent uninfected macrophages with $\geq$ 1 amastigote closely attached to the surface) was similarly assessed in preparations from cultures in which untreated and lymphokine-treated macrophages were exposed to cytochalasin E (1 μg/ml) for 30 minutes and washed prior to cocultivation with amastigotes for the duration shown. Cytochalasin treatment resulted in 0 to 2% infection. Mean ± standard error of triplicate cultures.

to spontaneously resolve infection with *L. major* (in C57BL/6 mice) and the capacity of lymph node lymphocytes from infected mice to generate IFNγ in vitro in response to leishmanial antigens.[47] In contrast, lymph node lymphocytes from mice (BALB/c) whose infections disseminated (and failed to self-cure) remained incapable of secreting IFNγ in response to leishmanial antigens irrespective of when in the course of infection they were obtained. However, when susceptible BALB/c mice were rendered capable of spontaneous self-cure (by sublethal irradiation), their lymph node lymphocytes developed the capacity to generate IFNγ upon in vitro leishmanial antigen stimulation. Our additional circumstantial evidence for lymphokine effects in vivo have been discussed above.[37] While it seems very likely that IFNγ and other macrophage-activating lymphokines play a role in antileishmanial defense in vivo, additional studies are needed to confirm this impression.

A general principle of lymphokine-mediated activation of macrophage antimicrobial defense is that antigen specificity resides in the interaction between antigen and specifically sensitized lymphocytes in triggering mediator secretion. Once secreted, activating lymphokines act in an antigen-nonspecific manner (i.e., regardless of the antigenic composition of the microbe residing with the macrophage). This principle is substantiated by our observation that supernatants of mycobacterial antigen-sensitized lymphocytes can effectively induce antileishmanial effects in infected macrophages.[35] The antigen-nonspecific nature of lymphokine-macrophage interaction limits the use of this in vitro assay in identifying parasite antigens that might serve as vaccine candidates. In contrast, conventional cytotoxic T cells interact with their targets in an antigen-specific manner, so that in vitro cytotoxicity assays might be useful in uncovering target antigens expressed on the surface of infected cells. This kind of strategy has been used on virus-infected cells, for example.[48] Unfortunately, preliminary in vitro studies that suggested the possible existence of T cells cytotoxic for *Leishmania*-infected macrophages[49] could not be confirmed. In vivo studies also provide evidence against a role of conventional cytotoxic T cells in antileishmanial defense. Adoptive transfer of protection to *Leishmania* in experimental murine models has been consistently achieved with T cells that lack the Ly 2 phenotypic marker characteristic of cytotoxic T cells.[18,23] Furthermore, resistance appears to depend on the induction of a Lyl^+2^- T cell subpopulation comprising cells presumably responsible for the activation of infected macrophages.[19,23]

CELL CONTACT-MEDIATED DEFENSE

We recently uncovered an antigen-specific mechanism of macrophage activation of antileishmanial defense by T cells that neither is cytotoxic to host cells nor involves secretion of soluble mediators but requires direct cell contact. We obtained draining popliteal lymph node lymphocytes from C57BL/6 mice with *L. major* footpad infections that had lasted for various numbers of days. These were added to suspension cultures of *L. major*–infected peritoneal macrophages obtained by starch elicitation from uninfected syngeneic mice. Control cultures consisted of infected macrophages without added lymphocytes or with equal numbers of draining popliteal lymph node lymphocytes from uninfected mice that had received an injection of complete Freund's adjuvant into their hind footpads. *Leishmania*-sensitized but not CFA-sensitized lymphocytes exerted antileishmanial effects on the *L. major*–infected

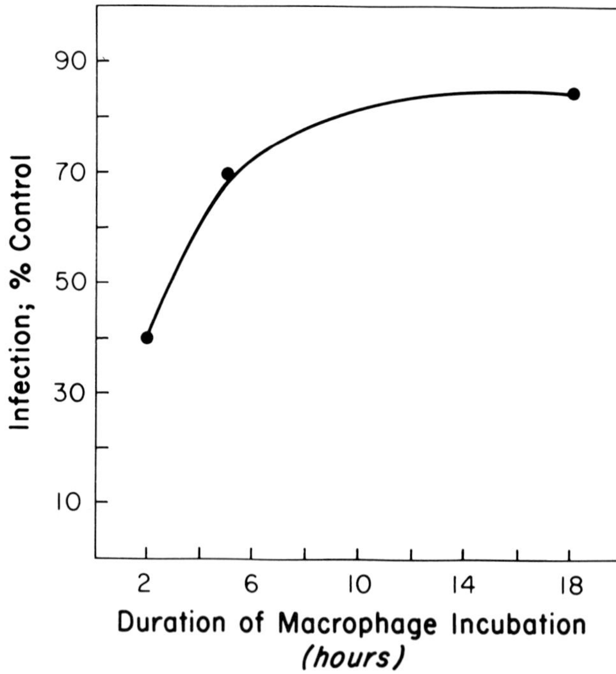

Fig. 13-3. Reversibility of lymphokine-induced inhibition of in vitro ingestion of *L. tropica* amastigotes. Macrophages were treated with medium or with lymphokine (1 : 4 dilution) for 4 hours, washed, resuspended in medium, and incubated for the duration indicated prior to the addition of amastigotes. The ingestion by lymphokine-treated macrophages of amastigotes during a subsequent 2-hour period of coculture is expressed as a percent of the magnitude of ingestion by macrophages cultured without lymphokine. For these calculations, the mean of triplicate determinations in parallel cultures at each time point was employed.

macrophages. Maximum effects were observed with lymph node cells of mice at 4 to 5 weeks of infection coinciding with the *onset* of spontaneous resolution of infection (Fig. 13-4). These effector lymphocytes were no longer detectable 3 to 4 weeks after the infection resolved.[50] Infected chromium 51–labeled macrophages did not release excess ^{51}Cr and retained their phagocytic function when cocultured with the lymph node T lymphocytes, indicating that they act without detectably damaging the host cells.[50] Furthermore, we established that the effector lymphocytes in our assay possess the $Lyl^{+}2^{-}$ phenotype.[51]

Evidence that the antileishmanial effect observed in our system is not strictly mediated by soluble factors includes the following observations: (1) Direct cell contact between T cells and *Leishmania*-infected macrophages is required; when lymphocytes are physically separated by a semipermeable membrane, minimal antileishmanial effects are observed, which are substantially less than when these cells are in direct contact.[50] (2) We could not detect macrophage-stimulating activity in supernatants collected from macrophage-

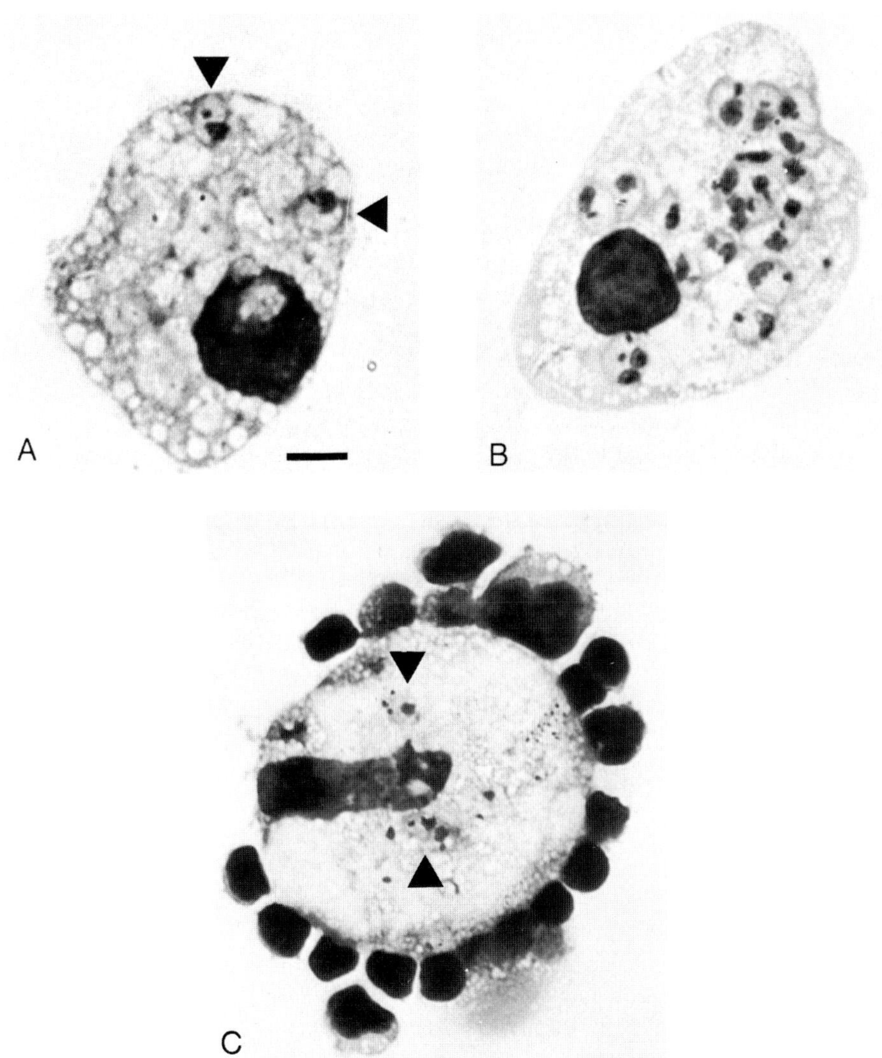

Fig. 13-4. Effect of popliteal lymph node lymphocytes from 5-week *L. major*–infected mice on in vitro intracellular growth of *L. major* in starch-elicited peritoneal macrophages. *L. major*–infected macrophages were infected for 24 hours (**A**) and cultured for an additional 48 hours (**B**) without or (**C**) with addition of effector lymphocytes. Note intracellular replication of amastigotes in (**B**) but not in (**C**). This observed antileishmanial activity is not lymphokine-mediated and requires cell-cell contact for maximum antileishmanial effect to occur. Arrows indicate amastigotes. Bar = 10μ. (From Panosian et al.,[50] with permission.)

lymphocyte cocultures.[50] (3) The mechanism is antigen-specific and genetically restricted to the I-A region of the major histocompatibility complex, which distinguishes it from antigen nonspecific, genetically unrestricted effects of macrophage-activating lymphokines.[52,53] (4) Starch-elicited (inflammatory) macrophages, although relatively refractory to lymphokine activation,[39] are fully susceptible to cell-contact–mediated activation.[50] (5) Lymphokine-mediated antileishmanial effects require macrophage incubation at 37°C and are substantially reduced at 34°C.[54] In contrast, contact-mediated effects are effective at both 34 and 37°C.[50] (6) Monoclonal antibody against murine γ-interferon does not abrogate contact-mediated effects but inhibits lymphokine-mediated macrophage activation for antileishmanial effect.[55] (7) When sensitized T cells are stimulated in vitro, they secrete lymphokines that can induce significant antileishmanial effects in infected macrophages.[35] When such cells are cultured in the presence of cyclosporin A, they fail to secrete lymphokines.[56–58] Although cyclosporin blocks all detectable lymphokines that activate antileishmanial effects, it does not inhibit the capacity of T cells to exert macrophage activation for antileishmanial effects even under the most stringent conditions.[55] We conclude therefore that there exists an apparently novel macrophage-activating mechanism for antileishmanial defense, which is independent of soluble lymphokine mediators and involves antigen-specific interactions between target macrophages and effector cells.

This lymphokine-independent macrophage activation mechanism appears to be antigen-specific in that the effector T cells must recognize appropriate antigens presumed to be displayed on the surface of infected macrophages in order for subsequent macrophage activation and parasite killing to occur. Specifically, we observed that draining lymph node lymphocytes from mice previously sensitized to other antigens—namely, mycobacterial or listerial antigens—induce only minimal antileishmanial effects in macrophages infected with *L. major* in vitro.[50,52] In contrast, when *L. major*–infected macrophages were primed with listerial antigens in vitro (by allowing the macrophages to ingest heat-killed *Listeria*), *Listeria*-sensitized lymphocytes could then induce antimicrobial effects against *Leishmania* in an apparently lymphokine-independent fashion, as described above (Fig. 13-5). These findings further suggested that antigen recognition in macrophage activation for antileishmanial effects was restricted to the initial interaction between appropriately sensitized T cells and infected macrophages.

Because of the antigen-specific nature of this interaction, it may be possible to identify parasite antigens expressed on the macrophage surface that participate in this contact-dependent effector mechanism, as well as to analyze immunoregulatory pathways in its expression. We have determined that genus-conserved antigens are among those recognized by the effector cells. Draining lymph node lymphocytes were obtained from *L. major*– or *L. mexicana*–infected mice and tested for their ability to induce antimicrobial effects in macrophages infected with the homologous or heterologous species (including *L. donovani*).[52] In all cases antimicrobial effects of lymphocytes against heterologous parasite species were comparable with those against the homologous

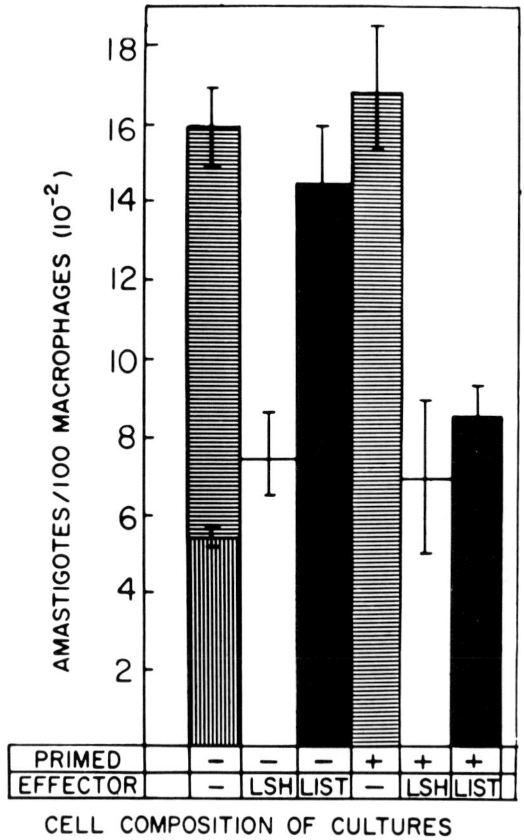

Fig. 13-5. Antigen specificity of contact-dependent antileishmanial effects in vitro. Macrophages were initially infected with *Leishmania major* amastigotes for 24 hours (magnitude of infection shown in vertical lined portion of bar) and cultured for an additional 48 hours (horizontal-striped, open or solid bars) with and without lymphocytes sensitized to *L. major* (LSH) or *Listeria monocytogenes* (LIST). Some of the macrophages infected with *L. major* were also primed with heat-killed *L. monocytogenes*. LIST-sensitized lymphocytes only exert antileishmanial effects in macrophages primed with listeral antigens. (Adapted from Sypek JP, et al.,[52] with permission.)

species. Indeed, cross-species protection has been previously noted in some mouse models of leishmaniasis,[21,22,59,60] which raises optimism that a vaccine might be developed that could protect against infection with different *Leishmania* species.

GENETICS OF SUSCEPTIBILITY

Identification of effector T cell populations responsible for antileishmanial defense may also permit a clearer understanding of how immunoregulatory pathways influence the clinical outcome. In addition to its intrinsic scientific interest, such knowledge might ultimately also influence strategies for immunoprophylaxis. Leishmaniasis, like leprosy, appears to be a spectral disease with distinct polar forms. At one pole (e.g., Old World cutaneous leishmaniasis) spontaneous resolution and resistance to reinfection are characteristic. In contrast, disseminated infections (cutaneous or visceral) define the other polar forms of the disease. Existing evidence supports the view that the clinically observed spectrum in both leprosy and leishmaniasis represents a subtle regulatory balance of T helper and T suppressor cells that determine the ultimate course of the disease.[15,61] The host and parasite factors that tip the balance toward one or the other pole have not been elucidated.

Models of leishmaniasis that employ different inbred strains of mice have been studied to assess factors that might affect disease outcome. Certain strains of inbred mice differ in their innate susceptibility to *Leishmania* as well as in their ability to control an established infection.[62,63] In the case of *Leishmania donovani* infection, the existence in mice of separate genetic determinants of innate resistance on the one hand and apparently acquired resistance on the other have been identified.[64] Innate susceptibility, apparently expressed by the relative resistance of macrophages to infection, is determined by a single regulatory locus, "Lsh," which resides on chromosome 1. The allele that imparts innate resistance to *L. donovani* also protects against two other obligate intracellular pathogens, *Salmonella typhimurium* and *Mycobacterium bovis*.[65,66] However, Lsh did not influence the outcome of other experimental leishmaniasis infections of mice. The acquisition of defense to *L. donovani* appears to be influenced by at least three regulatory genes, Rld-1 (an H-2–linked gene on chromosome 17[67]), an H-11–linked gene,[68] and an Ir-2–linked gene.[69]

The genetics of susceptibility to *L. major* in mice have not as yet been as well defined but are clearly not identical to those for *L. donovani*. Susceptibility to *L. major* appears to map to chromosome 8, and this gene has been provisionally designated "Scl."[70] As with *L. donovani,* an H-11–linked influence has also been found to determine resistance to *L. major* infections.[68] The implications from these studies is that genetic background, including non-MHC-linked loci, may play a role in determining clinical outcome. No comparable studies in human leishmaniasis have as yet been undertaken to assess whether genetic composition of the host determines susceptibility. There is evidence that in certain areas with endemic leishmaniasis some patients experience asymptomatic infections.[71] Possibly, this may reflect genetic polymorphism in susceptibility in the human population, although strain variation in the parasites transmitted in these areas has not been excluded as an alternative explanation.

IMMUNOREGULATION

The failure to control leishmanial infections appears to be influenced by definable immunoregulatory mechanisms. The most striking immunologic feature of disseminated leishmaniasis in humans is a depressed cell-mediated immune response characterized by a marked cutaneous anergy to leishmanial antigens.[72] The basis for immunologic dysfunction associated with disseminated leishmaniasis might be due to one or more of the following: (1) enhanced T-suppressor cell activity[73]; (2) the presence of adherent suppressor cells (macrophages)[74]; (3) the presence of circulating suppressor factors that might include immune complexes[75–79]; and (4) decreased lymphocyte-activating lymphokine production.[80]

Animal studies have begun to elucidate pathways toward immunosuppression in disseminated leishmaniasis. *Leishmania major* infection of the BALB/c mouse results in uncontrolled and ultimately fatal visceral disease. As in human kala azar, marked T-cell anergy to leishmanial antigens occurs in these mice. In marked contrast C57BL/6 mice spontaneously resolve *L. major* infections.[62,63] The impairment of cell-mediated immune responses in BALB/c mice has been shown to result from the activity of antigen-specific suppressor T cells of the Lyl^+2^- phenotype.[81,82] Interestingly, the generation of parasite-specific suppressor cells can be abrogated in BALB/c mice by sublethal irradiation before infection with *L. major*.[83] Furthermore, substantial protection can also be established by intravenously immunizing BALB/c mice with heavily irradiated *L. major* promastigotes (asexual stage present in the insect vector).[21,22] Paradoxically these immunized mice fail to display any cutaneous delayed-type hypersensitivity to leishmanial antigens, a feature previously thought to correlate with protective T cell responses. The adoptive transfer of a subpopulation of Lyl^+2^- cells but not Lyl^-2^+ cells from these treated donors to highly susceptible BALB/c mice protects the mice from subsequent challenge with *L. major* and with heterologous *Leishmania* spp.[19,21–23]

These findings do not define whether immunosuppression results from or is the cause of disseminated infection. Interestingly, BALB/c mice early in their infection with *L. major* develop many more *Leishmania* antigen–specific T-cell clones than strains of mice that subsequently progress to cure.[84] Preventing the overly exuberant expansion of T-cell clones with anti-L3T4 antibody or cyclosporin A treatment apparently renders the BALB/c mice capable of controlling the infection.[85–87] These findings suggest that an early hyperresponsiveness to leishmanial antigens might, in fact, underlie the subsequent immunosuppression.

IDENTIFICATION OF LEISHMANIAL ANTIGENS FOR VACCINE DEVELOPMENT

The application of knowledge concerning defense and immunoregulatory mechanisms in leishmaniasis with respect to vaccine development requires a greater understanding of relevant parasite antigens. Interest in identifying and characterizing leishmanial antigens—primarily through the use of monoclonal antibodies—has been motivated by the need for newer methods of taxonomic classification and serodiagnosis. Identification of potential antigenic targets for vaccine-induced protection has only very recently been established as an important goal. Monoclonal antibodies have identified classes of antigens that are

(1) stage-specific (i.e., present either only on promastigotes or only on amastigotes),[88–90] (2) species-specific,[91–94] and (3) common to many *Leishmania* species ("conserved" antigens).[89,90] The biologic role of the antigenic components of these parasites is defined in only a few cases, and for the most part their relevance to protection has yet to be determined. On the other hand, these antibodies have been valuable for species identification in clinical settings.

Given our present understanding of parasite biology and defense, two classes of antigens can be expected to serve as potential targets of defense in leishmaniasis: (1) those expressed on the parasite surface and involved in attachment to and entry into host macrophages, and (2) those expressed on the surface of infected macrophages that engage appropriate antigen receptors on specific T-cell clones, which subsequently activate antileishmanial defense in the infected cells. The expectation in the former case is that antibody directed at the parasite antigens will interfere with *Leishmania* entry into host cells. Although under natural circumstances antibody appears not to be important in defense,[18–20] it might be argued that vaccine-induced protection could, under certain circumstances, be antibody-mediated. On the other hand, antigens expressed on infected macrophage surfaces are likely to be essential in the triggering of specific T cell-mediated defenses.

The strategy used for identifying antigenic components that might be involved in parasite attachment to host cells has been to screen monoclonal antibodies for their ability to block promastigote-macrophage association in vitro. Results obtained by this approach indicate that at least two described components occurring on the promastigote plasmalemma appear to be involved in such parasite interactions. These include a 20,000- to 60,000-molecular-weight amphipathic glycolipid[95,96] and a 63,000-molecular-weight mannose-containing glycoprotein.[97] The monoclonal antibodies were employed to isolate these parasite surface antigens; the antigens could competitively interfere with promastigote association with host cells.[98,99] The combined observation that both the antigens and the monoclonal antibodies could interfere with parasite-host cell interaction makes it highly likely that one of the ligands involved in this association has been identified. Coincubation of certain antipromastigote monoclonal antibodies with promastigotes in vitro was also found to render them noninfectious when subsequently injected (along with the antibody) into susceptible mice.[100] Whether infusing mice with the monoclonal antibody would also be protective remains to be determined, however. On the other hand, a surface glycolipid was isolated from *L. major* promastigotes by affinity purification using monoclonal antibodies. When this antigen was injected with *Corynebacterium parvum* (as an adjuvant), either intravenously or intraperitoneally, it protected C3H and C57BL/6 mice from challenge with live *L. major* parasites.[101] High but not absolute levels of resistance (less than 90 percent) were also observed in the more susceptible BALB/c mice that were immunized.

Parasite antigens identified on the surface of infected macrophages (which may be important in antigen presentation) by which T cells may be stimulated for antileishmanial effects also appear promising as candidates for potential vaccine development. A number of workers have demonstrated parasite antigen(s) displayed on the surface of infected macrophages.[89,102–104] Furthermore, antigens that are expressed on the parasite surface and that can be shed have been identified. When released from inside the phagolysosome in which the parasites reside, these antigens may attach to the host cell membrane and be transported to the macrophage cell surface. Release of glycoconjugates from the surface of the *Leishmania* may involve the action of an endogenous phospholipase C.[95,96,104] The relationship between these antigens and those recognized by *Leishmania*-specific T cells mediating antileishmanial effects remains to be determined.[52]

These very early results are encouraging, and further development in this area may provide us with the necessary knowledge for designing vaccines for treatment of leishmaniasis. Since cell-mediated immunity appears to be critical in this disease, identification of appropriate adjuvants to promote these responses rather than antibody responses will be required, in addition to isolation of potential target antigens.

ACKNOWLEDGMENTS

Supported by U.S. Public Health Service grant AI 17151 (to DJW). The authors are grateful for the excellent secretarial and administrative assistance of Ms. Irene Doucette.

REFERENCES

1. Walsh JA, Warren KS; Selective primary health care. An interim strategy for disease control in developing countries. N Engl J Med 301:967, 1979
2. UN Development Programme/World Bank/WHO Special Programme for Research and Training in Tropical Diseases: The leishmaniases. Ch. 7. In Tropical Disease Research, 7th Programme Report. World Health Organization, Geneva, 1985
3. Berman JD: Experimental chemotherapy of leishmaniasis—a critical review. p. 111. In Chang K-P, Bray RS (eds): Human Parasitic Diseases. Vol. 1: Leishmaniasis. Elsevier Biomedical, New York, 1985
4. Wirth DF, McMahon-Pratt D: Rapid identification of *Leishmania* species by specific hybridization of kinetoplast DNA in cutaneous lesions. Proc Natl Acad Sci USA 79:6999, 1982
5. Lopes UG, Wirth DF: Identification of visceral *Leishmania* species with cloned sequences of kinetoplast DNA. Mol Biochem Parasitol 20:77, 1986
6. Wang C-T: Leishmaniasis in China: Epidemiology and control program. p. 469. In Chang K-P, Bray RS (eds): Human Parasitic Diseases. Vol. 1: Leishmaniasis. Elsevier Biomedical, New York, 1985
7. Berens RL, Marr JJ, Nelson DJ, LaFon SW: Antileishmanial effect of allopurinol and allopurinol ribonucleoside on intracellular forms of *Leishmania donovani*. Biochem Pharmacol 29:2397, 1980
8. Even-Paz Z, Weinrauch L, Livshin R, et al: Rifampicin treatment of cutaneous leishmaniasis. Int J Dermatol 21:110, 1982

9. Rainey P, Santi DV: Metabolism and mechanism of action of formycin B in *Leishmania*. Proc Natl Acad Sci USA 80:288, 1983
10. New RRC, Chance ML, Heath S: Antileishmanial activity of amphotericin and other antifungal agents entrapped in liposomes. J Antimicrob Chemother 8:371, 1981
11. Guirges SY: Natural and experimental reinfection of man with Oriental sore. Ann Trop Med Parasitol 65:197, 1971
12. Heyneman D: Immunology of leishmaniasis. Bull WHO 44:499, 1971
13. Greenblatt CL: The present and future of vaccination for cutaneous leishmaniasis. p. 259. In Mizrahi A (ed): New Developments with Human and Veterinary Vaccines. Alan R Liss, New York, 1980
14. Garnham PCC, Humphrey JH: Problems in leishmaniasis related to immunology. Curr Top Microbiol Immunol 48:29, 1969
15. Howard FRS, Liew FY: Mechanisms of acquired immunity in leishmaniasis. Philos Trans R Soc Lond [Biol] 307:87, 1984
16. Louis J, Moedder E, Behin R, Engers H: Recognition of protozoan parasite antigens by murine T lymphocytes. I. Induction of specific T lymphocyte-dependent proliferative response to *Leishmania tropica*. Eur J Immunol 9:841, 1979
17. Louis JA, Moedder E, MacDonald HR, Engers HD: Recognition of protozoan parasite antigens by murine T lymphocytes. II. Role of the H-2 gene complex in interactions between antigen-presenting macrophages and *Leishmania*-immune T lymphocytes. J Immunol 126:1661, 1981
18. Liew FY, Hale C, Howard JG: Immunologic regulation of experimental cutaneous leishmaniasis. V. Characterization of effector and specific suppressor T cells. J Immunol 128:1917, 1982
19. Mitchell GF: Murine cutaneous leishmaniasis: resistance in reconstituted nude mice and several F_1 hybrids infected with *Leishmania tropica major*. J Immunogenet 10:395, 1983
20. Sacks DL, Scott PA, Asofsky R, Sher FA: Cutaneous leishmaniasis in anti-IgM treated mice: enhanced resistance due to functional depletion of a B cell dependent T cell involved in the suppressor pathway. J Immunol 132:2072, 1984
21. Howard JG, Nicklin S, Hale C, Liew FY: Prophylactic immunization against experimental leishmaniasis. I. Protection in mice genetically vulnerable to fatal *Leishmania tropica* infection. J Immunol 129:2206, 1982
22. Howard JG, Liew FY, Hale C, Nicklin S: Prophylactic immunization against experimental leishmaniasis. II. Further characterization of the protective immunity against fatal *Leishmania tropica* infection induced by irradiated promastigotes. J Immunol 132:450, 1984
23. Liew FY, Howard JG, Hale C: Prophylactic immunization against experimental leishmaniasis. III. Protection against fatal *Leishmania tropica* infection induced by irradiated promastigotes involves $Ly1^+2^-$ T cells which do not mediate cutaneous DTH. J Immunol 132:456, 1984
24. North RJ: Cellular mediators of anti-*Listeria* immunity as an enlarged population of short-lived, replicating T cells. J Exp Med 138:342, 1973
25. Zinkernagel RM, Doherty PC: MHC-restricted cytotoxic T cells: studies on the biological role of polymorphic major transplantation antigens in determining T cell restriction-specificity, function, and responsiveness. Adv Immunol 27:51, 1979
26. Mackaness GB: The influence of immunologically committed lymphoid cells on macrophage activity in vivo. J Exp Med 129:973, 1969
27. Mackaness GB: The immunological basis of acquired cellular resistance. J Exp Med 120:105, 1964

28. Simon HB, Sheagren JN: Cellular immunity in vitro. I. Immunologically mediated enhancement of macrophage bacterial capacity. J Exp Med 133:1377, 1971
29. Simon HB, Sheagren JN: Enhancement of macrophage capacity by antigenically stimulated immune lymphocytes. Cell Immunol 4:163, 1972
30. Fowles RE, Fajardo IM, Leibowitch JL, David JR: The enhancement of macrophage bacteriosis by products of activated lymphocytes. J Exp Med 138:952, 1973
31. Mauël J, Buchmüller Y, Behin R: Studies on the mechanism of macrophage activation. I. Destruction of intracellular *Leishmania enrietti* in macrophages activated by co-cultivation with stimulated lymphocytes. J Exp Med 148:393, 1978
32. Buchmüller Y, Mauël J: Studies on the mechanism of macrophage activation: II. Parasite destruction in macrophages activated by supernatants from concanavalin A-stimulated lymphocytes. J Exp Med 150:359, 1979
33. Berman JD, Dwyer DM, Wyler DJ: Multiplication of *Leishmania* in human macrophages in vitro. Infect Immun 26:375, 1979
34. Nacy CA, Diggs CL: Intracellular replication of *Leishmania tropica* in mouse peritoneal macrophages: comparison of amastigote replication in adherent and non-adherent macrophages. Infect Immun 34:310, 1981
35. Nacy CA, Meltzer MS, Leonard EJ, Wyler DJ: Intracellular replication and lymphokine-induced destruction of *Leishmania tropica* in C3H/HeN mouse macrophages. J Immunol 127:2381, 1981
36. Wyler DJ: In vitro parasite-monocyte interactions in human leishmaniasis: evidence for an active role of the parasite in attachment. J Clin Invest 70:82, 1982
37. Panosian CB, Wyler DJ: Acquired macrophage resistance to in vitro infection with *Leishmania*. J Infect Dis 148:1049, 1983
38. Oster CN, Nacy CA: Macrophage activation to kill *Leishmania tropica:* kinetics of macrophage response to lymphokines that induce antimicrobial activities against amastigotes. J Immunol 132:1494, 1984
39. Hoover DL, Nacy CA: Macrophage activation to kill *Leishmania tropica:* defective intracellular killing of amastigotes by macrophage elicited with sterile inflammatory agents. J Immunol 132:1487, 1984
40. Adams DO, Hamilton TA: The cell biology of macrophage activation. Annu Rev Immunol 2:283, 1984
41. Murray HW: Susceptibility of *Leishmania* to oxygen intermediates and killing by normal macrophages. J Exp Med 158:670, 1983
42. Murray HW, Cartelli DM: Killing of intracellular *Leishmania donovani* by human mononuclear phagocytes. J Clin Invest 72:32, 1983
43. Scott P, James S, Sher A: The respiratory burst is not required for killing of intracellular and extracellular parasites by a lymphokine-activated macrophage cell line. Eur J Immunol 15:553, 1985
44. Nathan CF, Murray HW, Wiebe ME, Rubin BY: Identification of interferon γ as the lymphokine that activates human oxidative metabolism and antimicrobial activity. J Exp Med 158:670, 1983
45. Murray HW, Spitalny GL, Nathan CF: Activation of mouse peritoneal macrophages in vitro and in vivo by interferon-γ. J Immunol 134:1619, 1985
46. Nacy CA, Fortier AH, Meltzer MS, et al: Macrophage activation to kill *Leishmania major:* activation of macrophages for intracellular destruction of amastigotes can be induced by both recombinant interferon-γ and non-interferon lymphokines. J Immunol 135:3505, 1985
47. Sadick MD, Locksley RM, Tubbs C, Raff HV: Murine cutaneous leishmaniasis: resistance correlates with the capacity to generate interferon-γ in response to *Leishmania* antigens in vitro. J Immunol 136:655, 1986

48. Sharpe AH, Gaulton GN, McDade KK, et al: Syngeneic monoclonal antiidiotype can induce cellular immunity to reovirus. J Exp Med 160:1195, 1984
49. Bray RS, Bryceson ADM: Cutaneous leishmaniasis of the guinea pig. Action of sensitized lymphocytes on infected macrophages. Lancet 2:898, 1968
50. Panosian CB, Sypek JP, Wyler DJ: Cell contact-mediated macrophage activation for antileishmanial defense. I. Lymphocyte effector mechanism that is contact dependent and noncytotoxic. J Immunol 133:3358, 1984
51. Sypek JP, Panosian CB, Wyler DJ: Cell contact-mediated macrophage activation for antileishmanial defense. II. Identification of effector cell phenotype and genetic restriction. J Immunol 133:3351, 1984
52. Sypek JP, Panosian CB, Wyler DJ: Antigen recognition by effector T cells in antileishmanial defense. J Infect Dis 152:1057, 1985
53. Sypek JP, Wyler DJ: Cell contact-mediated macrophage activation for antileishmanial defense: mapping of the genetic restriction to the I region of the MHC. Clin Exp Immunol 62:449, 1985
54. Scott P: Impaired macrophage leishmanial activity at cutaneous temperature. Parasite Immunol 7:277, 1985
55. Wyler DJ, Beller DI, Sypek JP: Macrophage activation for antileishmanial defense by an apparently novel mechanism. J Immunol 138:1246, 1987
56. Granelli-Piperno A, Inaba K, Steinman RM: Stimulation of lymphokine release from T lymphocytes. Requirement for mRNA synthesis and inhibition by cyclosporin A. J Exp Med 160:1792, 1984
57. Wiskocil R, Weiss A, Imboden J, et al: Activation of a human T cell line: a two-stimulus requirement in the pretranslational events involved in the coordinate expression of interleukin 2 and interferon-γ genes. J Immunol 134:1599, 1985
58. Herold KC, Lancki DW, Moldwin RL, Fitch FW: Immunosuppressive effects of cyclosporin A on cloned T cells. J Immunol 136:1315, 1986
59. Alexander J, Phillips RS: *Leishmania tropica* and *Leishmania mexicana:* cross immunity in mice. Exp Parasitol 45:93, 1978
60. Pérez H, Arrendondo B, Machado R: *Leishmania mexicana* and *Leishmania tropica:* cross immunity in C57BL/6 mice. Exp Parasitol 48:9, 1979
61. Bloom BR, Mehra V: Immunological unresponsiveness in leprosy. Immunol Rev 80:5, 1984
62. Handman E, Ceredig R, Mitchell GF: Murine cutaneous leishmaniasis: disease patterns in intact and nude mice of various genotypes and examination of some differences between normal and infected macrophages. Aust J Exp Biol Med Sci 57:9, 1979
63. Howard JG, Hale C, Liew WLC: Immunological regulation of experimental cutaneous leishmaniasis. I. Immunogenetic aspects of susceptibility to *Leishmania tropica* in mice. Parasite Immunol 2:203, 1980
64. Bradley DJ, Taylor BA, Blackwell JM, et al: Regulation of *Leishmania* populations within the host. III. Mapping of the locus controlling susceptibility of visceral leishmaniasis in the mouse. Clin Exp Immunol 37:7, 1979
65. Plant J, Glynn AA: Genetics of resistance to infection with *Salmonella typhimurium* in mice. J Infect Dis 133: 72, 1976
66. Skamene E, Gros P, Forget A, et al: Genetic regulation of resistance to intracellular pathogens. Nature 297:506, 1982
67. Blackwell JM, Freeman JC, Bradley DJ: Influence of H-2 complex on acquired resistance to *Leishmania donovani* infection in mice. Nature 283:72, 1980
68. Blackwell JM, Hale C, Roberts MB, et al: An H-11-linked gene has a parallel effect

on *Leishmania major* and *L. donovani* infections in mice. Immunogenet 21:385, 1985

69. DeTolla LJ, Semprevivo LH, Palczuk NC, Passmore HC: Genetic control of acquired resistance to visceral leishmaniasis in mice. Immunogenet 10:353, 1980
70. Blackwell JM, Howard JG, Liew FY, Hale C: Mapping of the gene controlling susceptibility to cutaneous leishmaniasis. Mouse News Lett 70:86, 1984
71. Bardaró R, Jones TC, Lorenco R, et al: A prospective study of visceral leishmaniasis in an endemic area of Brazil. J Infect Dis 154:639, 1986
72. Haldar JP, Ghose S, Saha KC, Ghose AC: Cell-mediated immune response in Indian kala azar and post-kala azar dermal leishmaniasis. Infect Immun 42:702, 1983
73. Carvalho EM, Teixeira RS, Johnson WD: Cell-mediated immunity in American visceral leishmaniasis: reversible immunosuppression during acute infection. Infect Immun 33:498, 1981
74. Petersen EA, Neva FA, Oster CN, Diaz HB: Specific inhibition of lymphocyte-proliferation responses by adherent suppressor cells in diffuse cutaneous leishmaniasis. N Engl J Med 306:387, 1982
75. Wyler DJ: Circulating factor from a kala azar patient suppresses in vitro anti-leishmanial T cell proliferation. Trans R Soc Trop Med Hyg 76:304, 1982
76. Carvalho EM, Andrews BS, Martinelli R, et al: Circulating immune complexes and rheumatoid factor in schistosomiasis and visceral leishmaniasis. Am J Trop Med Hyg 32:61, 1983
77. Pearson RD, De Alencar JE, Romito R, et al: Circulating immune complexes and rheumatoid factors in visceral leishmaniasis. J Infect Dis 147:1102, 1983
78. Galvão-Castro B, Ferreira JAS, Marzochi KR, et al: Polyclonal B cell activation, circulating immune complexes and autoimmunity in human American visceral leishmaniasis. Clin Exp Immunol 56:58, 1984
79. Barral A, Carvalho EM, Badaró R, Barral-Netto M: Suppression of lymphocyte proliferative responses by sera from patients with American visceral leishmaniasis. Am J Trop Med Hyg 35:735, 1986
80. Carvalho EM, Badaró R, Reed SG, et al: Absence of gamma interferon and interleukin 2 production during active visceral leishmaniasis. J Clin Invest 76:2066, 1985
81. Howard JG, Hale C, Liew FY: Immunological regulation of experimental cutaneous leishmaniasis. III. Nature and significance of specific suppression of cell-mediated immunity in mice highly susceptible to *Leishmania tropica*. J Exp Med 152:594, 1980
82. Liew FY: Specific suppression of responses to *Leishmania tropica* by a cloned T cell line. Nature 305:630, 1983
83. Howard JG, Hale C, Liew FY: Immunological regulation of experimental cutaneous leishmaniasis. IV. Prophylactic effect of irradiation as a result of abrogation of suppressor T cell generation in mice genetically susceptible to *Leishmania tropica*. J Exp Med 153:557, 1981
84. Milon G, Titus RG, Cerottini JC, et al: Higher frequency of *Leishmania major*-specific $L3T4^+$ T cells in susceptible BALB/c as compared with resistant CBA mice. J Immunol 136:1467, 1986
85. Titus RG, Ceredig R, Cerottini JC, Louis JA: Therapeutic effect of anti-L3T4 monoclonal antibody GK1.5 on cutaneous leishmaniasis in genetically susceptible BALB/c mice. J Immunol 135:2108, 1985
86. Behforouz NC, Wenger CD, Mathison BA: Prophylactic treatment of BALB/c

mice with cyclosporine A and its analog B-5-49 enhances resistance to *Leishmania major*. J Immunol 136:3067, 1986
87. Solbach W, Forberg K, Kammerer E, et al: Suppressive effect of cyclosporin A on the development of *Leishmania tropica*-induced lesions in genetically susceptible BALB/c mice. J Immunol 137:702, 1986
88. McMahon-Pratt D, David JR: Monoclonal antibodies recognizing determinants specific for the promastigote stage of *Leishmania mexicana*. Mol Biochem Parasitol 6:317, 1982
89. Handman E, Hocking RE: Stage-specific, and cross-reactive antigens of *Leishmania* species identified by monoclonal antibodies. Infect Immun 37:28, 1982
90. Jaffe CL, McMahon-Pratt D: Monoclonal antibodies specific for *Leishmania tropica*. I. Characterization of antigens associated with stage- and species-specific determinants. J Immunol 131:1987, 1983
91. McMahon-Pratt D, David JR: Monoclonal antibodies that distinguish between New World species of *Leishmania*. Nature 291:581, 1981
92. McMahon-Pratt D, Bennet E, David JR: Monoclonal antibodies that distinguish subspecies of *Leishmania braziliensis*. J Immunol 129:926, 1982
93. Jaffe CL, Bennet E, Grimaldi G, McMahon-Pratt D: Production and characterization of species-specific monoclonal antibodies against *Leishmania donovani* for immunodiagnosis. J Immunol 133:440, 1984
94. McMahon-Pratt D, Bennett E, Grimaldi G, Jaffe CL: Subspecies- and species-specific antigens of *Leishmania mexicana* characterized by monoclonal antibodies. J Immunol 134:1935, 1985
95. Handman E, Greenblatt CL, Goding JW: An amphipathic sulphated glycoconjugate of *Leishmania:* characterization with monoclonal antibodies. EMBO J 3:1206, 1984
96. Handman E, Goding JW: The *Leishmania* receptor for macrophages is a lipid containing glycoconjugate. EMBO J 4:329, 1985
97. Etges RJ, Bouvier J, Hoffman R, Bordier C: Evidence that the major surface proteins of three *Leishmania* species are structurally related. Mol Biochem Parasitol 14:141, 1985
98. Russell DG, Wilhelm H: The involvement of the major surface glycoprotein (gp63) of *Leishmania* promastigotes in attachment to macrophages. J Immunol 136:2613, 1986
99. Chang CS, Chang K-P: Monoclonal antibody affinity purification of a *Leishmania* membrane glycoprotein and its inhibition of *Leishmania*-macrophage binding. Proc Natl Acad Sci USA 83:100, 1986
100. Anderson S, David JR, McMahon-Pratt D: In vivo protection against *Leishmania mexicana* mediated by monoclonal antibodies. J Immunol 131:1616, 1983
101. Handman E, Mitchell GF: Immunization with *Leishmania* receptor for macrophages protects mice against cutaneous leishmaniasis. Proc Natl Acad Sci USA 82:5910, 1985
102. Berman JD, Dwyer DM: Expression of *Leishmania* antigen on the surface membrane of infected human macrophages in vitro. Clin Exp Immunol 44:342, 1981
103. de Ibarra AAL, Howard JG, Snary D: Monoclonal antibodies to *Leishmania tropica major:* specificities and antigen location. Parasitology 85:523, 1982
104. Williams KM, Sacci JB, Anthony RL: Identification and recovery of *Leishmania* antigen displayed on the surface membrane of mouse peritoneal macrophages infected in vitro. J Immunol 136:1853, 1986

14 Recent Advances in the Diagnosis and Management of Leishmaniasis and American Trypanosomiasis

Franklin A. Neva

Although basic research in parasitology has produced exciting new insights into the fundamental biology of *Leishmania* and the trypanosomes, unfortunately few of these results have so far been translated into clinically useful approaches. The fact of the matter is that there have been few, if any, significant advances in the diagnosis and management of infections caused by *Leishmania* and by *Trypanosoma cruzi*. There has, however, been a good deal of activity and many publications that claim or imply advances on these subjects. I will therefore try to survey this activity critically with the following purposes in mind:

1. Hopefully, to identify a few items that actually constitute advances (in either diagnosis or management)
2. To comment upon certain developments that could turn out to be advances

3. In the process of this search and evaluation mission, possibily to illuminate and even clarify some of the important issues concerning diagnosis and management

LEISHMANIASIS

Diagnosis

Specimen Collection in Cutaneous Leishmaniasis

Many of the points that I wish to make simply involve the difference in the perspective of a clinician facing a lesion of uncertain causation from that of a laboratory research worker whose focus is purely upon the leishmanial parasite. For example, two innovations in diagnostic techniques that have been widely promoted are needle aspiration of the edges of cutaneous lesions for culture[1] and the use of liquid media containing insect hemolymph for growth of leishmania.[2] Neither technique is really new, but there seems to be new interest in advocacy for their use.

Let us first consider the pros and cons of the needle aspiration technique versus other methods for obtaining diagnostic specimens. This will be restricted to cutaneous and mucocutaneous leishmaniasis (CL and MCL) now, with the consideration of the visceral disease later. There is no doubt that even the small amount of tissue juice and cells obtained by the aspiration technique is often sufficient for recovery of organisms by culture and sometimes enough for a stained smear. However, since growth of the parasite on primary isolation and subsequent passage can vary greatly, depending upon species and even upon strains within species, a small inoculum may seriously compromise the chances of growing the parasite. The big advantage of needle aspiration is that it is so simple and can generally be done in the field or in a primary health care facility, the only requirements being a needle, syringe, skin disinfectant, sterile saline, and culture medium containing antibiotics.

If, however, there is any question about the etiologic diagnosis and the patient is encountered in a secondary or referral type of health care facility, then I believe a different approach is indicated. This is the circumstance under which these patients are generally encountered in the United States and Europe, so a wider spectrum of differential diagnoses should then be considered. Specimens for bacterial, mycobacterial, and fungal culture and tissue for histopathologic examination should be obtained. In some clinical settings, such as lesions on mucous membranes, cultures for herpes simplex virus should also be obtained. Tissue pathology is sometimes helpful even if *Leishmania* are later obtained by culture. An additional consideration is that if tissue rather than an aspirate is obtained for culture, a larger inoculum can be used and the chances of obtaining a positive culture are enhanced, regardless of the organism present. The procedure that we follow at the National Institutes of Health (NIH) in suspected cases of CL seen for the first time is as follows.

Under local anesthesia a biopsy specimen is obtained from the intact edge of the lesion; this may be either a punch (preferably at least 4 mm in diameter) or an elliptical specimen depending upon the site of the lesion. A slice of up to one-half the biopsy specimen is taken for impression smears plus fixation for tissue sections. The other half is ground in a mortar with cell culture medium without antibiotics to make a 0.5 to 1 percent suspension. We frequently allow coarse particles to settle out of the suspension for about 30 seconds and use the supernate for culture; in either event, half of the suspension is brought promptly to the clinical microbiology laboratory for Gram, acid-fast, and fungal stains, routine bacteriologic culture, and culture for acid-fast organisms and for fungi. Antibiotics, either gentamicin at 50 μg/ml or penicillin and streptomycin at 100 units/ml or 100 μg/ml, respectively, in final concentration are added to the remaining half of the suspension, and this is used as inoculum for leishmanial cultures.

Specimen Collection in Mucocutaneous Leishmaniasis

The patient with mucocutaneous lesions often presents a real problem, particularly when the lesion is deep in the nose or otherwise not readily accessible. Without assistance from an experienced otolaryngologist it may be difficult even to assess the nature and extent of the pathology, let alone obtain tissue for diagnostic studies. In such situations needle aspirates are sometimes the only specimens that can be obtained. If at all possible however, a generous specimen should be obtained in mucocutaneous cases because: (1) the causative organism is usually a member of the most difficult to grow *Leishmania braziliensis* complex; (2) affected tissues contain relatively few organisms; and (3) the site of the other makes it especially important to rule out lesion pathology, such as Wegener's granulomatosis or mid-line granuloma, or other causative organisms. Even though our experience with MCL has been very small, I have been impressed with the importance of adequate visualization of the affected area so that an optimum site can be biopsied. In two instances proliferative or papillomatous-appearing nasal lesions were present in the nose, as well as ulcerative destructive lesions. Positive cultures were obtained from the proliferative lesions, suggesting that the pathology may not be uniform and that organisms are more likely to be found before ulceration occurs. In view of these considerations an adequate diagnostic evaluation of suspected MCL in the field or in a health center is very difficult—a hospital is almost essential.

Leishmanial Culture for Cutaneous and Mucocutaneous Disease

Although glowing reports have appeared of the advantages of liquid media containing insect cell culture constituents for leishmanial culture,[1,2] the comparisons with conventional diphasic media are not really adequate. In one study[1] the tiny volume of inoculum from aspirated specimens could not possibly have been sufficient without dilution to compare growth in two types of cultures. There is great variation among different species of *Leishmania* in their capacity to grow in any medium on primary isolation, and this variation may even extend to isolates within the species. In general, *Leishmania braziliensis braziliensis* and other members of this complex are the most fastidious.[3] Isolates of *L. major* and *L. donovani* generally grow well, as do members of the *L. mexicana* complex. For those laboratories dealing with patients from a restricted geographic region, where growth characteristics of the most prevalent leishmanial strain(s) are known from past experience, use of a specialized medium, such as one of the liquid media, is justified. However, a referral center seeing patients from any part of the world should use a growth medium best suited to a wide variety of leishmanial isolates. Even in some patients with diffuse cutaneous leishmaniasis (DCL), in whom the parasite load in lesions is extraordinarily high (10^5 to 10^6 per milligram of tissue), I have encountered relative difficulty in primary isolation and maintenance of an isolate. This was the case in Venezuela and Ethiopia. From serial 10-fold dilutions of the inoculum, the estimated number of organisms required to initiate growth was 100 or more rather than the 1 to 10 organisms required with isolates that grow easily, as those from the Dominican Republic.

Other considerations for choice of culture medium in primary isolation of *Leishmania*, as I have emphasized elsewhere,[4] are the variability in different lots of fetal bovine serum, the unknown shelf life of commercial media, and the suggestion that 30 percent defibrinated or hemolyzed rabbit blood is superior to 15 percent or less blood. Therefore, we are reluctant to use the liquid insect cell culture media and prefer to use NNN diphasic media with 30 percent defibrinated rabbit blood for primary isolation of *Leishmania* from patients. Incidentally, the solid-phase slants can be prepared in optically clear screw-cap tubes (Nunclon tissue culture tube, PGC Scientifics Corp., Gaithersburg, MD) to which the inoculum and 1.5 ml of fluid overlay can be added, which still permits examination of the culture under an inverted microscope for motile flagellates. This obviates the need for opening the tube to sample the overlay for organisms and thus reduces the chances for contaminating the cultures.

The results of several isolation attempts comparing NNN with Schneider's medium are presented in Table 14-1. Similar results comparing NNN with liquid 199 medium are summarized in Table 14-2, including one trial with two different lots of fetal bovine serum (FBS). In all instances 0.5 percent tissue suspensions prepared from biopsy specimens were used as inoculum with equal volumes inoculated into the cultures.

New Technology for Detection and Speciation of *Leishmania*

The last few years have seen a great deal of effort and a number of publications in which the new technology of molecular biology has been applied to leishmaniasis. Most of this work has dealt with basic issues, such as structure

Table 14.1. Primary Isolation of *Leishmania* from Patients in NNN Media versus Schneider's with 30 Percent FBS

Leishmanial Species	Medium	Result
L. tropica	NNN	Positive at 10° only[a]
(M.N-Afghanistan)	Schneider's	Negative
L. major	NNN	Positive at 10°, $10^{-1.0}$, and $10^{-2.0}$ [a]
(M.F.-Isreal)	Schneider's	Positive for 1 of 2 at 10°, negative at $10^{-1.0}$ and $10^{-2.0}$
L. b. braziliensis[b]	NNN	Negative
(L.E.-Peru)	Schneider's	Negative
	199 medium with 30% FBS	Negative

[a] 10° = undiluted sample; $10^{-1.0}$ = sample diluted 1 : 10; $10^{-2.0}$ = sample diluted 1 : 100.
[b] This lesion from same patient was positive in NNN 2 months earlier.

and function of kinetoplast DNA, classification and evolutionary relationships of species, antigenic analysis, etc.[5–7] However, some of the work has been directed specifically to use of molecular probes to detect leishmanial DNA for diagnosis of the infection, and to differentiation between species of *Leishmania* by these techniques.[8] Wirth and McMahon-Pratt at Harvard[8] and investigators at Walter Reed Army Institute of Research have been among the first to use these techniques. Dot blots of about 100 cultured promastigotes can be detected with k DNA probes. However, it is doubtful if a similar degree of sensitivity can be readily achieved with clinical specimens that contain white cells and other tissue components. Impression smears and dot blots from clinical specimens contain very small volumes of material unless a concentration technique can be used. The critical question in comparing the relative sensitivity of culture and of other methods is the minimum number of parasites required for detection. Culture techniques have the advantage of permitting a much larger inoculum. On the other hand, many species of *Leishmania* require, on primary isolation, more than one—perhaps even a hundred or more—organisms before growth can be initiated. Yet, on balance it would seem that molecular probes at the very best can only match and do not currently exceed

Table 14-2. Primary Isolation of *Leishmania* from patients in NNN Media versus Medium 199 with 20 to 30 Percent FBS

Leishmanial Species	Medium	Result
L. major	NNN	Positive at 10° and $10^{-1.0}$ [a]
(E.H.-Jordan)	199 with 20% FBS	Negative
L.b. braziliensis	NNN	at 10° only
(L.E.-Peru)	199 with 30% FBS	Negative
L.b. braziliensis	NNN	Positive at 10° and $10^{-1.0}$ [a]
(R.S.-Bolivia)	199 with 30% FBS	Negative
L. aethiopica	NNN	Positive up to $10^{-2.0}$ [a]
DCL case	199 with 30% FBS Lot 1	Positive up to $10^{-2.0}$
Ethiopia	199 with 30% FBS Lot 2	Negative

[a] 10° = undiluted sample; $10^{-1.0}$ = sample diluted 1 : 10; $10^{-2.0}$ = sample diluted 1 : 100

the sensitivity of culture techniques for diagnosis of leishmaniasis. They do have the advantage of speed and the potential for easy analysis of numerous specimens. However, the requirement for radioisotopes with molecular probes is a serious disadvantage, which restricts their use to fairly sophisticated laboratory facilities. Unless the molecular probe technology can be adapted to detection systems that do not require radioisotopes, it will remain a specialized research tool rather than a routine procedure.

Rapid species identification of a leishmanial isolate is another problem for which new technology has been advocated. The implication here is that knowing the species of infecting parasite will influence the patient's treatment. Interestingly, this argument seems to be more important to laboratory research workers than to the clinicians who care for the patient. The only *Leishmania* to which this consideration applies are the New World species because of their association with MCL. In fact, there seems to be a widely prevalent belief that only *L. brasiliensis brasiliensis* causes mucocutaneous disease. While the majority of MCL cases may very well be caused by *L.b. braziliensis,* other members of the *L. braziliensis* complex, namely *L.b. panamensis* and/or *L.b guyanesis,* were found in the majority of eight MCL isolates reported recently from Colombia.[9] Also, although infrequent, members of the *L. mexicana* complex have been isolated from MCL patients.[10] Furthermore, we still do not understand the role of factors other than the parasite in the pathogenesis of MCL. The geographic origin of the disease is probably as significant a risk factor as is the species of the parasite. Therefore, it is doubtful that a patient with CL due to *L.b. brasiliensis* should be treated any differently from one with CL caused by other members of the *L. braziliensis* complex or even the *L. mexicana* complex. Speciation of *Leishmania* is very important for epidemiologic purposes, and it may eventually provide useful clues to the pathogenesis of late sequelae, but it is not really needed in management of the individual patient at present.

Delayed Hypersensitivity Skin Test

While there has been movement and even a few advances in diagnosis and treatment of leishmaniasis, the situation with regard to availability of antigens for use in the delayed hypersensitivity (DTH) skin test has actually retrogressed. Years ago individual investigators prepared their own antigens for the Montenegro or the leishmanin test for DTH, as the skin tests are called in Latin America and the Old World, respectively. But now the detailed procedures for characterization and tests of safety required for injectable drugs or reagents by government agencies, plus the restrictions imposed by clinical research committees before approval of clinical protocols using investigational drugs, has effectively choked off use of the leishmanial skin test. The only skin test antigen that, to my knowledge, has been commercially available (produced by Burroughs Wellcome in England) will disappear from the market because it will no longer be manufactured. Apparently, the commercial market for it is too small. In my experience (F.A. Neva, unpublished observations), the Burroughs Wellcome leishmanial antigen was active and gave consistently positive DTH responses in proven cases of cutaneous disease that we tested.

I believe it is unfortunate that a commercial skin test antigen is not available to authorized users. While the results of the leishmanin skin test are not essential in diagnosis and management of patients, the presence or absence of DTH responsiveness can provide useful information to the clinician in several different situations. First, in patients from known endemic areas with lesions that are clinically and histopathologically compatible with leishmaniasis but in whom cultures are negative, a negative skin test would provide further confirmatory evidence that the lesion is not leishmanial in etiology. In such a situation, a negative skin test might even obviate the need for doing leishmanial cultures, especially if the anergic state can be ruled out by other skin tests. In just the opposite situation, namely, parasitologic evidence of leishmanial infection by histology or culture, a negative skin test to leishmanin might indicate the need for longer or more intensive chemotherapy or might indicate DCL. Finally, the general availablity of a standardized reagent to assess previous sensitization to leishmanial antigens would make it easier to compare epidemiologic studies in different geographic areas of the world. It is ironic that at a time when numerous possible "high-tech" answers are being offered to clinical problems, the proven "low-tech" procedures are being abandoned. This seems to be a general phenomenon—not confined to medicine.

Serology in Diagnosis

There have been no significant innovations in the use of serologic tests for diagnosis of CL and MCL. When this subject was reviewed four years ago, serologic tests for diagnosis were not considered particularly useful by themselves,[4] and I do not believe the situation has changed. One reason for this is that the antibody levels are relatively low regardless of the test used, which increases the likelihood of cross-reactions. The frequency of false positive reactions has not been carefully evaluated. Another reason for the limited usefulness of serology is that more definitive parasitologic diagnostic tests can generally be done. In visceral leishmaniasis, by contrast, antibody levels are very high, so that the serology test is a useful tool.

Special Considerations in Diagnosis of Visceral Leishmaniasis (Kala-Azar)

Giemsa-stained smears and/or culture of aspirated bone marrow or spleen specimens are still the methods of choice for diagnosis of visceral leishmaniasis. The causative organism, *L. donovani,* does not appear to be especially difficult to grow, so various types of media are probably equally suitable for primary isolation and maintenance. Aspiration and culture of material from peripheral lymph nodes has also been recommended as an alternative source of specimens in diagnosis of kala-azar. Since peripheral lymphadenopathy is not a prominent clinical feature in kala-azar patients, lymph nodes would not seem to be a good site for recovery of organisms. On the other hand, where even simple equipment and hospital support facilities to check platelet counts and prothrombin times are lacking, lymph node aspiration may be the only alternative to splenic or bone marrow aspiration. Only a needle, syringe, and culture medium are needed. In a recent study in the Sudan, Petersen was able to obtain positive smears or cultures from lymph node aspirates in about 60 percent of clinically suspected cases of kala-azar (E. Petersen, M.D., personal communication).

As mentioned earlier, patients with active visceral leishmaniasis almost always have high levels of antileishmanial antibodies. The serologic test generally used is an enzyme-linked immunosorbent assay (ELISA) procedure.[11,12] Since specific antibody levels are high, even a field ELISA test that is read visually has been described.[13]

Evaluation of Response to Treatment of Kala-Azar, with Particular Reference to Splenic Aspiration. Although the individual components are not new, the overall protocol developed for following kala-azar patients during treatment by several groups in Nairobi, Kenya, merits special comment. This was a collaboration of Anthony Bryceson, a group from Walter Reed Institute of Research, and workers at Kenyatta National Hospital.[14,15] The plan is simply a weekly evaluation of key clinical and laboratory measurements, including splenic aspiration for smear and culture for parasitologic examination. Disappearance of fever, decrease in spleen size, and increases in white blood count and hemoglobin were among the most useful simple criteria for evaluating response to treatment. Another critical parameter to follow was the estimate of relative numbers of organisms in smears of splenic aspirates. Perhaps the most important contribution of this group of workers has been the detailed description of their technique of splenic aspiration.[16,17] Several factors that contribute to the relative safety of their method of splenic aspiration are (1) the nature of the pathologic process in the spleen, which makes it firm and less likely to tear, and (2) the speed (<1 second) of the procedure using a No. 21 needle. Additional criteria in selection of patients include a definitely palpable spleen, the absence of ascites, a platelet count above 40,000/mm^3 and a prothrombin time no greater than 5 seconds over the control. Use of this protocol, including splenic aspiration, provides a systematic way to follow the course of the patient to determine whether there is response to treatment. Use of such a plan is especially important to establish a baseline of experience and is then indispensable if different treatment regimens are to be compared.

Treatment

New Use of Old Drug—Pentostam

One definite advance in the treatment of leishmaniasis is the realization that pentavalent antimony can be given in larger daily doses and for longer periods than was formerly appreciated. This was the consequence of the finding that kala-azar in Kenya frequently required 30 days of Pentostam treatment to achieve cure[18] and of a reevaluation of the rapid renal excretion of antimony.[19] Based upon this information Chulay et al.[14] showed in a group of 10 patients that Pentostam could be given in a dose of 10 mg of antimony per kilogram of body weight as often as three times a day for 10 days intravenously without significant toxicity or ill effects. In Brazil Marsden has used pentavalent antimony (Glucantime) in a dosage of 28 mg antimony per kilogram per day for 15 days for treatment of MCL.[20] A rest period between courses of treatment is not considered necessary if no toxicity has occurred.[20] The dose of Pentostam now generally recommended for treatment of leishmanial disease is 20 mg/kg/day for up to 20 days, with continuation of the course if clinical response has not occured.[21] This same recommendation, however, suggests that an individual dose be limited to no more than 8.0 ml. If the 8.0-ml dose limitation is followed, it would mean that only individuals weighing 90 lb or less would receive 20 mg/kg of the drug, a 125-lb person would receive 15 mg/kg, and a husky 187-lb adult male would be getting the old dose of 10 mg/kg. The pharmacologic reasoning behind the 8.0-ml single dose limitation, which seems to be an arbitrary value, is not clear. The main point is that the permissible total dosage of pentavalent antimony for treatment of leishmaniasis has been increased to two to four times the amount originally recommended, and this is accomplished mainly by increasing the duration of treatment. Incidentally, with the increased daily dosage of 8.0 ml or more, it is usually necessary to administer either Pentostam or Glucantime intravenously rather than intramuscularly.

Toxic and untoward effects attributed to pentavalent antimony, even in the larger doses or for longer durations, are generally characterized as minimal or not constituting "a major problem" in the reports from Kenya.[14,15] In contrast, Marsden's paper on experience with 89 cases of cutaneous and mucocutaneous disease in Brazil cites a rather high frequency of arthralgias, myalgias, and anorexia, as well as reversible, minimal liver function and electrocardiographic (ECG) abnormalities in patients receiving large-dose or prolonged pentavalent antimony treatment.[20] In our own experience at the NIH involving 25 patients, most of whom received the old dose of 10 mg/kg per day for 10 days, but often two or three courses, untoward effects were limited to local discomfort at the injection site (IM), mild general weakness, and sometimes anorexia, with mild, reversible liver function abnormalities or transient T-wave ECG changes. More recently, using 15 mg/kg per day for longer periods, we have observed significant arthralgias and myalgias more commonly. We have seen leukopenia down to 1,800/mm^3 in one patient, which was clearly associated with Pentostam administration. As the experience with larger dosage increases, it is likely that the frequency and severity of untoward effects will also increase.

Other Drugs in Treatment of Leishmaniasis

For nearly half a century pentavalent antimony was the only effective drug for leishmaniasis, but since the late 1970s several new classes of compounds have been introduced that show activity in human infections. The idea of using allopurinol and related analogues was developed by Marr and coworkers.[22] Allopurinol alone was found to be useful in a few cases of kala-azar in Kenya,[23] but more commonly it has been used in conjunction with Pentostam treatment in patients not responding to Pentostam alone.[24] Allopurinol was used in doses of 21 to 24 mg/kg/day for periods of 23 to 54 days. Results with an analogue, allopurinol riboside, which was more active in vitro than allopurinol, have been somewhat disappointing in humans. A trial of the riboside for CL due presumably to *L.b. panamensis* in Panama has not been more effective than Pentostam (R. Saenz, personal communication). Nevertheless, interest in and further work on these related compounds is justified since they represent drugs with a new mechanism of action against hemoflagellate parasites against which chemotherapeutic innovations have been meager. An additional advantage of this group of drugs is that they are administered orally, an important consideration in endemic areas of leishmaniasis.

Ketoconazole, an imidazole antifungal agent, is another orally administered drug that appears to be reasonably effective against both Old and New World CL. In one group of six patients from the Atlantic coast of Nicaragua (parasite species not identified) healing occurred in 8 to 12 weeks on 400 mg of ketoconazole per day, but the follow-up period was only 3 months.[25] Six of eight patients with *L. major* cutaneous disease in Israel were apparently cured on the same dose given for 4 weeks.[25] This second study was more thorough than the first because lesions were checked at 2-week intervals by smears and cultures. Ketoconazole is currently under evaluation for CL in Panama, but it is still too early for conclusions about efficacy (R. Saenz, M.D., personal communication). The duration of treatment and cost of the drug would be deterrents to wider use of ketoconazole.

Local Treatment of Cutaneous Leishmaniasis

The focal nature of CL and the fact that usually only one or a few lesions are present make the possibilities of locally applied medication especially attractive. Injection of antimonial or other drugs is mentioned in textbooks and in anecdotal reports, but I am unaware of any controlled studies involving substantial numbers of patients. An Israeli group at Hadassah University Hospital, headed by El-On, has carried out studies of topical treatment in experimental animals and in humans using an ointment containing 15 percent paromomycin sulfate and 12 percent methylbenzethonium chloride in soft paraffin. A recent publication by this group[27] summarizes their experience in treating 67 patients with *L. major* cutaneous infections by twice daily applications of the ointment to lesions. They reported 72 percent of treated patients became free of parasites at the end of the 10-day treatment period, and 15 percent were parasite-free within an additional 20 days without further treatment. While these results sound impressive on the surface, several points must be taken into account. First, *L. major* infections often heal spontaneously; in fact, in those patients with multiple lesions, a high percentage of untreated lesions were also parasite-free by 30 days after the start of treatment. Next, the treated lesions were described as appearing worse clinically during and at the end of treatment than at the start, with various degrees of inflammation associated with treatment. Therefore, this treatment may depend in part upon a local, nonspecific inflammatory response. At any rate, these efforts, as well as other studies on topical therapy of cutaneous leishmaniasis, offer some hope that effective topical therapy may be developed for certain types of patients.

Our experience at the NIH in the use of local heat treatment for selected cases of CL is even more restricted. A recent report[28] described the results of applying local heat at a minimum of 39 to 40°C for a total period of at least 24 hours over 3 to 4 days to lesions of patients with DCL from the Dominican Republic. The infecting organism in these casis is a member of the *L. mexicana* complex and is killed in vitro by exposure to 35°C for 24 to 48 hours. The lesions of three patients treated in this way were clinically and parasitologically cured by local heat; after 2 years one patient had a local recurrence, but the other two remained clinically free of disease for at least 3 to 4 years. The lesions from two subsequent DCL cases from the Dominican Republic were also rendered parasite-free by local heat. A Mexican DCL patient has recently been found to have a temperature-sensitive parasite as well. However, we were unable to demonstrate either a clinical or a significant parasitologic response to local heat treatment in several Ethiopian patients with DCL, even though their organisms were destroyed in vitro in 48 hours at 35°C. Except for the Ethiopian DCL cases, response to local heat correlates quite well with in vitro heat sensitivity of the infecting parasite. Use of heat treatment for CL is only applicable to those patients who do not respond to conventional chemotherapy (such as DCL) and whose organism is heat-sensitive.

AMERICAN TRYPANOSOMIASES AND CHAGAS' DISEASE: DEFINITION OF ISSUES

This portion of my chapter has deliberately been subtitled ". . . Trypanosomiases *and* Chagas' disease" rather than ". . . Trypanosomiases or Chagas' disease" to emphasize that infection with *T. cruzi* is not synonymous with the disease named after the discoverer of the parasite. Even though many of our Latin American colleagues use these terms interchangeably, I believe the distinction is more than academic. Even in highly endemic areas, no more than about half of infected individuals develop clinical manifestations of chronic Chagas' disease, and in some geographic areas of Latin America the proportion of those with a positive serology who go on to develop chronic Chagas' disease is much lower.[29,30] This distinction between infection with *T. cruzi* and Chagas' disease is therefore important also as a reminder that the pathogenesis of the chronic disease is still unknown. One of the most important advances that could be made in Chagas' disease would be an elucidation of the pathogenesis of the cardiomyopathy and the megadisease that characterize the chronic phase. The pros and cons for the hypothesis that chronic Chagas' disease is an autoimmune phenomenon have recently been summarized by Kierzenbaum and Hudson,[31,32] but the concept has been set back by the finding that the putative autoimmune antibodies in infected individuals bind to animal and not to human tissues.[33]

In view of this continuing uncertainty over the pathogenesis of Chagas' disease, what are the issues or problems on the basis of which advances can be evaluated? Even though volumes have been written about serodiagnosis of infection by the parasite, the lack of specificity of diagnostic tests is still a perennial problem. Detection of low-level parasitemia for definitive diagnosis of infection and for following response to drug therapy depends currently upon the rather archaic process of feeding "clean" vector insects upon the patient, the procedure called *xenodiagnosis*. Increased sensitivity and simplification of this slow and labor-intensive process, which can yield very useful information, would be a distinct advance. Since diagnosis of chronic Chagas' disease is still a diagnosis of exclusion, development of laboratory tests that would reliably indicate disease as well as infection caused by the parasite also would constitute an advance. Better yet would be development of means of identifying those infected individuals at greater risk of developing chronic Chagas' disease, of which the majority of infected people, those in the indeterminate state, show no signs. Finally, more effective and less toxic drugs than the two that are currently available would be highly desirable. These, then, are what I consider to be the main problems or issues in Chagas' disease that would benefit from advances.

Serodiagnosis

With regard to the subject of serodiagnosis of *T. cruzi* infection, there are a variety of serologic tests, primarily indirect hemagglutination, direct parasite agglutination, and indirect fluorescent antibody tests, which are adequate for routine screening purposes in blood banks, etc.[34] However, individual instances arise from time to time in which specificity approaching the absolute in a serologic test is desirable. There is now accumulating evidence that antibodies to specific antigenic components of *T. cruzi* can be consistently demonstrated in the serum of chronically infected individuals. The two most prominent of these antigens are cell-surface glycoproteins of about 90,000 and 72,000 molecular weight.[35] The most convincing evidence that I have seen for a specific serologic test for *T. cruzi* infection is a radiolabeled immunoprecipitation test developed by Kirchhoff et al.[36] With this test these investigators were consistently able to show antibodies in the sera of proven *T. cruzi* infections from diverse geographic areas of the Americas. There were no cross-reactions with a variety of other sera that are likely to cross-react in other serologic tests for antibodies to *T. cruzi*. I think such a serologic test to specific *T. cruzi* antigens will likely become a "gold standard" in those few situations in which greatest specificity is required.

Is Chronic Chagas' Disease Caused by Certain Varieties of *T. cruzi*?

A great degree of heterogeneity has been demonstrated among different strains or stocks of *Trypanosoma cruzi*. On the basis of isoenzyme profiles Miles has grouped isolates of *T. cruzi* into three broad groups, or *zymodemes* (Z), which correspond roughly to geographic regions of South America, as well as into types of tramsmission cycles.[37] For example, isolates of Z2 are common in southern and central Brazil, where megadisease occurs. However, all three zymodemes can infect humans and can cause acute disease. Kinetoplast DNA analysis of *T. cruzi* stocks shows groupings that conform broadly with zymodemes but also shows a distinct number of subgroups. Single-cell isolates, or clones, of *T. cruzi* recovered from the same patient have been shown by Dvorak and coworkers[38] to differ in growth rate, DNA content, and virulence for experimental animals. However, none of this information as yet will permit identification of strains of *T. cruzi* that either will or will not cause chronic disease. The fact that certain zymodemes, such as Z1 and Z3, are not associated with megadisease can be predicted just as well from their geographic location. Although certain molecular or immunologic markers may ultimately be useful in identifying parasites with or without chronic disease potential, they are not yet available.

Antigen Detection as an Aid to Diagnosis

Low-level parasitemia is commonly present in apparently normal individuals during the indeterminate phase of chronic infection with *T. cruzi*. The only methods currently available for demonstrating such low-level parasitemias are by culture of the blood, preferably after some type of concentration procedure, or by xenodiagnosis. This latter method involves allowing multiple "clean" laboratory-reared insects to partake of a blood meal on the patient or to ingest the patient's blood through an artificial membrane. It is generally conceded that xenodiagnosis, especially if 40 or more insects are used per feeding, is a more sensitive method than culture for detecting very small numbers of circulating parasites. The sensitivity probably approaches detection of 1 to 10 organisms in the total volume of blood taken up by the insects because the trypanosomes multiply in the insect's gut and can be detected when the intestinal contents are examined 2 to 4 weeks later. The only problem with xenodiagnosis is that it is a very time-comsuming and tedious procedure.

It is very unlikely, I think, that molecular probes, such as k DNA, can achieve the sensitivity of xenodiagnosis. Therefore, direct detection of parasite DNA in the blood of chronic patients is probably not very realistic. Antibody probes for detecting parasite antigens in the blood may be more sensitive but will still probably not equal the sensitivity of xenodiagnosis. However, the use of molecular probes to detect parasite material from pooled intestinal contents of insects used in xenodiagnosis would be much more feasible. If successful, it would also be a time- and labor-saving technique. Even though this innovation would still require the reduviid insects, xenodiagnosis could be utilized to a greater extent. Such simplification of xenodiagnosis would make it easier to monitor the effect of chemotherapy on parasitemia in indeterminate cases of infection.

Chemotherapy of Chagas' Disease

Unfortunately, there have been no recent developments as far as new or more effective drugs for this disease are concerned. Nifurtamox, a nitrofuran derivative, and Radonil, a benzimidazole compound, are still the two drugs recommended for treatment of the acute disease. Only the former drug is available in the United States through the Centers for Disease Control. These two drugs are of approximately equal efficacy, which is not of dramatic degree, and they are also relatively toxic.

One issue concerning chemotherapy of Chagas' disease that is still very much unresolved is whether the chronically infected individual should be treated. In those with manifest signs and symptoms of chronic disease, antiparasitic treatment would seem pointless—the damage, whatever its pathogenesis, has already been done. A more reasonable question is whether the patient with a positive serology but in the indeterminate phase should be treated. The argument here is whether elimination of existing parasites will prevent future disease. Since the pathogenesis of chronic disease is not known and the available drugs are probably not totally effective against intracellular parasites, the benefits of a long course of therapy with a toxic drug is uncertain. Here a controlled clinical trial would be useful to evaluate the effect of treatment on long-term outcome. A careful assessment of toxicity and morbidity of the chemotherapy would also be useful. Unfortunately, such a controlled trial is not likely to be carried out. Many, perhaps most, physicians in Latin America are treating their indeterminate phase patients, but nobody knows whether such treatment is worthwhile.

REFERENCES

1. Hendricks L, Wright N: Diagnosis of cutaneous leishmaniasis by in vitro cultivation of saline aspirates in Schneider's Drosophila medium. Am J Trop Med Hyg 28:962, 1979
2. Childs GE, Foster KA, McRoberts MJ: Insect cell culture media for cultivation of New World *Leishmania*. Int J Parasitol 8:255, 1978
3. Lainson R, Shaw JJ: Leishmaniasis of the New World: taxonomic problems. Br Med Bull 28:44, 1972
4. Neva FA: Diagnosis and treatment of cutaneous leishmaniasis. p. 364. In Remington JS, Swartz MN (eds): Current Clincial Topics in Infectious Diseases. Vol. 3. McGraw-Hill, New York, 1982
5. Barker DC, Butcher J: The use of DNA probes in the identification of leishmaniasis:

discrimination between isolates of the *Leishmania mexicana* and *L. braziliensis* complexes. Trans R Soc Trop Med Hyg 77:285, 1983

6. Spithill TW, Grumont RJ: Identification of species, strains and clones of *Leishmania* by characterization of kinetoplast DNA minicircles. Mol Biochem Parasitol 12:217, 1984
7. Lawrie JM, Jackson PR, Stiteler JM, Hockmeyer WT: Identification of pathogenic *Leishmania* promastigotes by DNA: DNA hybridization with kinetoplast DNA cloned into *E. coli* plasmids. Am J Trop Med Hyg 34:257, 1985
8. Wirth DF, McMahon-Pratt D: Rapid identification of *Leishmania* species of specific hybridization of kinetoplast DNA in cutaneous lesions. Proc Natl Acad Sci 79:6999, 1982
9. Saravia NG, Holgium AF, McMahon-Pratt D, D'Alessandro A: Mucocutaneous leishmaniasis in Colombia: *Leishmania braziliensis* subspecies diversity. Am J Trop Med Hyg 34:714, 1985
10. Sampaio RN, Marsden PD, Cuentas EAL, et al: *Leishmania mexicana amazonensis* isolated from a patient with fatal mucosal leishmaniasis. Rev Soc Brasil Med Trop 18:273, 1985
11. Hommel M, Peters W, Ranque J: The micro-ELISA technique in the serodiagnosis of visceral leishmaniasis. Ann Trop Med Parasitol 72:213, 1978
12. Edrissan GH, Darabian P: A comparison of enzyme-linked immunosorbent assay and indirect fluorescent antibody test in the serodiagnosis of cutaneous and visceral leishmaniasis in Iran. Trans R Soc Trop Med Hyg 73:289, 1979
13. Ho M, Leeuwenburg J, Mbugua G: An enzyme-linked immunosorbent assay (ELISA) for field diagnosis of visceral leishmaniasis. Am J Trop Med Hyg 32:943, 1983
14. Chulay JD, Bhatt SM, Muigai R, et al: A comparison of three dosage regimens of sodium stibogluconate in the treatment of visceral leishmaniasis in Kenya. J Infect Dis 148:148, 1983
15. Kager PA, Rees, PH, Manguyu FM, et al: Clinical hematological and parasitological response to treatment of visceral leishmaniasis in Kenya. A study of 64 patients. Trop Geog Med 36:21, 1984
16. Chulay JD, Bryceson ADM: Quantitation of amastigotes of *Leishmania donovani* in smears of splenic aspirates from patients with visceral leishmaniasis. Am J Trop Med Hyg 32:475, 1983
17. Kager PA, Rees, PH, Manguyu FM, et al: Splenic aspiration; experience in Kenya. Trop Geog Med 35:125, 1983
18. Manson-Bahr PEC: East African kala-azar with special reference to the pathology, prophylaxis and treatment. Trans R Soc Trop Med Hyg 53:123, 1959
19. Rees PH, Keating MI, Kager PA, Hockmeyer WT: Renal clearance of pentavalent antimony (sodium stibogluconate). Lancet 2:226, 1980
20. Marsden PD: Pentavalent antimonials: old drugs for new diseases. Rev Soc Brasil Med Trop 18:187, 1985
21. Abramowicz M (ed): Handbook of Antimicrobial Therapy—the Medical Letter. Rev. Ed. The Medical Letter, Inc. New Rochelle, NY, 1986
22. Marr JJ, Berens RL: Pyrazolopyrimidine metabolism in the pathogenic *Trypanosomatidae*. Mol Biochem Parasitol 7:339, 1983
23. Kager PA, Rees PH, Wellde BT, et al: Allopurinol in the treatment of visceral leishmaniasis. Trans R Soc Trop Med Hyg 75:556, 1981
24. Chunge CN, Gachihi G, Muigai R, et al: Visceral leishmaniasis unresponsive to

antimonial drugs. III. Successful treatment using a combination of sodium stibogluconate plus allopurinol. Trans R Soc Trop Med Hyg 79:715, 1985
25. Urcuyo FG, Zais N: Oral ketoconazole in the treatment of leishmaniasis. Int J Dermatol 21:414, 1982
26. Weinrauch L, Livshin R, Evan-Paz Z, El-On J: Efficacy of ketoconazole in cutaneous leishmaniasis. Arch Dermatol Res 275:353, 1983
27. El-On J, Livshin R, Evan-Paz, Z, et al: Topical treatment of cutaneous leishmaniasis. J Invest Dermatol 87:284, 1986
28. Neva FA, Petersen EA, Corsey R, et al: Observations on local heat treatment for cutaneous leishmaniasis. Am J Trop Med Hyg 33:800, 1984
29. Macedo V: Chagas' disease (American trypanosomiasis). p. 1783. In Wyngaarden JB, Smith H (eds): Cecil Textbook of Medicine. 17th Ed. WB Saunders, Philadelphia, 1985
30. Kirchoff LV, Neva FA: Trypanosoma species (Chagas' disease). p. 1531. In Mandell GE, Douglas GR, Bennett JE (eds): Principles and Practice of Infectious Diseases. 2nd Ed. John Wiley & Sons, New York, 1985
31. Kierszenbaum F: Is there autoimmunity in Chagas' disease? Parasitol Today 1:4, 1985
32. Hudson L: Autoimmune phenomena in chronic chagasic cardiopathy. Parasitol Today 1:6, 1985
33. Khoury EL, Diez C, Cossio PM, et al: Heterophile nature of EVI antibody in *Tyrpanosoma cruzi* infection. Clin Immunol Immunopathol 28:283, 1983
34. VanMeirvenne N, LeRay D: Diagnosis of African and American trypanosomiasis. Br Med Bull 41:156, 1985
35. Snary D: Biochemistry of surface antigens of *Trypanosoma cruzi*. Br Med Bull 41:144, 1985
36. Kirchoff LV, Gam AA, d'AGusmào R, et al: Increased specificity of serodiagnosis of Chagas' disease (American trypanosomiasis) by detection of antibody to the 72 and 90 kDa glycoproteins of *Trypanosoma cruzi*. J Infect Dis 155:561, 1987
37. Gibson WC, Miles MA: Application of new technologies to epidemiology. Br Med Bull 41:115, 1985
38. Dvorak JA: The natural heterogeneity of *Trypanosoma cruzi:* biological and medical implications. J Cell Biochem 24:357, 1984

15 Molecular Approaches to the Study of *Toxoplasma gondii*

John C. Boothroyd
J. Lawrence Burg
Susana D. Nagel
Dalia Perelman

Toxoplasma gondii is a protozoan parasite which has long been known as an important pathogen of humans and animals.[1,2] Until recently its greatest notoriety has come from its ability to cause severe disease in the developing fetus or late sequelae in the children of women who acquire their first infection in their first trimester of pregnancy. Since about 1968 to 1978, however, this opportunistic pathogen has become an important factor in the management of patients who are immunocompromised.[3] This latter group includes those receiving immunosuppressive drugs (e.g., transplant recipients) and, most recently, patients with the acquired immunodeficiency syndrome (AIDS).[4] In such patients a disseminated infection can occur with potentially fatal consequences.

Currently, control of this disease is largely exercised after the fact, with little if any direct prophylaxis. Following diagnosis (see Ch. 16), drugs are prescribed, but these drugs are not without some toxicity and potential side effects and so their use is limited, particularly in pregnant women. Therefore, one important goal for scientists working on *T. gondii* is to identify unusual biochemical processes in the parasite, which might be exploited in the development of novel chemotherapeutic strategies. Such goals are very long-range, and although many such pathways have been identified in other pathogens, the leap from their identification to their exploitation in treatment has proved very difficult owing to limitations in our understanding of structure versus function relationships in the relevant molecules (see Ch. 6 and 7). That is, simply identifying a novel enzymatic or other pathway does not enable one to design an inhibitory drug, let alone one that will have a low toxicity for the host.

Vaccines, on the other hand, have been developed for many important bacterial and viral pathogens. Although the adaptation of vaccine technology to the protozoan parasites has been slow, this has been more for political and economic reasons than for technical ones. With the increase in importance of *T. gondii* as a human pathogen, it is clear that the time has come for development of a vaccine that would safely and effectively reduce the number of infected and diseased individuals. One potential problem in achieving this goal is that, as with any vaccine, it is important to identify those at risk and administer the vaccine prior to exposure to the pathogen. Recent surveys indicate that about 15 to 30 percent of adults in the United States are seropositive[5] while in some other countries, such as France, where the eating of incompletely cooked meat is more common, this figure rises to as much as 80 percent.[6] Any vaccination program would be to reduce the incidence of infection in the human dren if it is to have the maximal effect. The most likely effect of such a vaccination program would be to reduce the incidence or infection in the human population, and the most likely benefit would be to prevent sequelae in the offspring of mothers exposed to *T. gondii* during pregnancy. However, a vaccine administered to humans would not affect the animal reservoirs of the organism, and the risk of infection would persist for the unvaccinated and for those whose immunity has waned. It is unpredictable whether individuals vaccinated as children would remain immune to infection if a subsequent immunosuppressive illness occurred or if immunosuppressive drugs were given.

A second major goal for basic scientists is to apply the recently developed techniques of molecular biology and immunology to the diagnosis and prevention of toxoplasmosis, including the possibility of devising novel vaccine strategies. In the following sections, we will discuss three subjects that are pertinent to this goal. The first will be an introduction to the basic biology of the organism and the pathogenesis of the disease it causes; the second will be a description of the starting questions underlying our work and our accomplishments to date; and the third will be a discussion of one novel strategy that has been developed by others and that we hope to exploit in the development of safe and effective vaccines against toxoplasmosis.

Some of the work described has been previously published in collaboration with Lloyd Kasper and Pat Ware of Dartmouth Medical School and Jeffrey Prince, Somesh Sharma, and Jack Remington of the Palo Alto Medical Foundation.

BIOLOGY OF THE ORGANISM

Toxoplasma gondii (from Greek words meaning "arc form," because of its shape, and "gundi," the African rodent from which it was first isolated) is a protozoan parasite within the order *Eucoccidia*. It is a close cousin of *Eimeria*, the causative agent of chicken coccidiosis, a disease well studied because of its economic impact on the poultry industry. The life cycle of *T. gondii* is schematically presented in Figure 15-1. Members of the cat family are the definitive hosts (hosts to the parasites sexual cycle), and many other species of mammals may be incidental hosts (hosts to asexual cycle only). Oocysts shed in cats' feces can remain viable in the soil for long periods. They are ingested by humans and other incidental hosts who consume contaminated food or water. Each oocyst contains two sporocysts, each of which contain four sporozoites. These are released when oocysts encounter the gastric juices, following which they penetrate into intestinal epithelial cells. Here, several divisions occur, resulting in the generation of the life cycle form known as *tachyzoites* (''speedy animals'') (Fig. 15-2). Tachyzoites migrate throughout the body and invade many tissues, most notably muscle and brain. In a healthy adult animal little if any disease results from this stage of the infection. There follows, however, a latent phase of the disease due to the formation of cysts in host tissues. The cysts persist, frequently for the life of the animal, and may occasionally rupture, releasing many *bradyzoites* (''slow animals''). The pathogenesis of disease in the fetus and the immunosuppressed individual differs. Since it is almost exclusively the fetuses of women experiencing a primary infection who are at risk, it appears that the bradyzoites of chronically (latently) infected mothers pose little threat to the developing fetus. However, in immunosup-

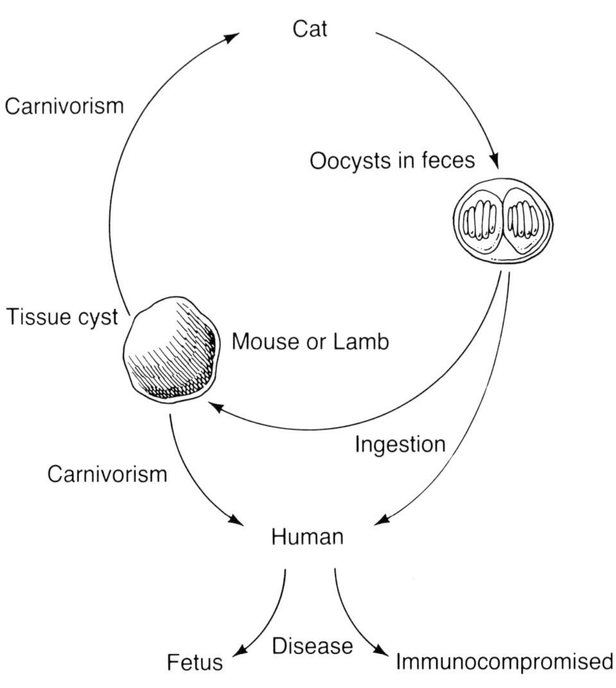

Fig. 15-1. Life cycle of *Toxoplasma gondii* (described in detail in the text).

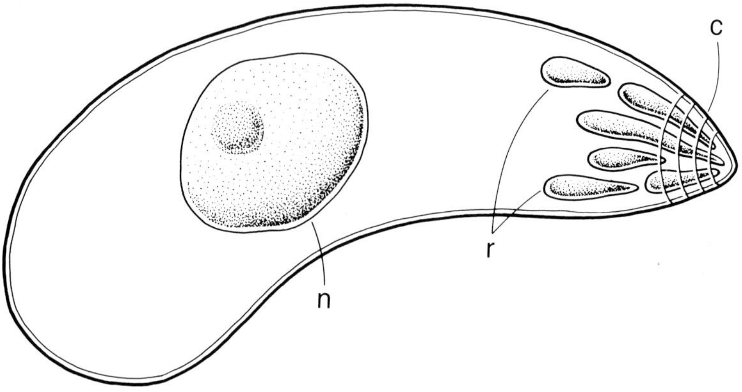

Fig. 15-2. Schematic diagram of a tachyzoite. This trophozoite form of the parasite is the product of asexual division within an infected cell. Infection of a cell by a single tachyzoite results in the release of upwards of 64 daughter tachyzoites by a binary process known as *endodyogeny*.[2] The main features of the tachyzoite are the conoid (c) and vesicular rhoptries (r) at the apical end and the nucleus (n). The arclike form of the tachyzoite gives rise to the genus name (see text). The parasites are about 6 to 8 μm long and 2 μm across.

pressed patients, the rupturing cyst may be responsible for many, if not most, cases of disseminated disease (see Ch. 16.)

The life cycle is completed when cats eat the cyst-containing tissue of infected animals. These cysts rupture in the cats' digestive system, and the bradyzoites invade the intestinal epithelium. In cats, unlike other animals, a cycle of sexual differentiation of the parasites ensues. Following fusion of the gametes and zygote formation, meiosis occurs, and an unsporulated oocyst is produced. Oocysts are excreted in the cats' feces and mature in the soil, resulting in the generation of the eight sporozoites discussed above. All forms of the parasite except the zygote and unsporulated oocyst are apparently haploid, with a genomic complexity of about 7×10^7 base pairs (bp).

A subcycle within this life cycle can occur when animals other than cats ingest raw flesh (or other tissue) of an infected animal harboring tissue cysts. As in cats, these cysts rupture and the bradyzoites invade the intestinal epithelium; however, no sexual cycle ensues and only tachyzoites are generated. As described above, these can ultimately lead to the formation of tissue cysts. The result of this is that such a subcycle leads to propagation of the parasites up through the food chain, but, unless the parasites are ingested by a cat, the life cycle is not completed. One of the most common modes of transmission to humans is the eating of undercooked red meat.

Control of toxoplasmosis in humans can be effected by blocking virtually any of the parts of the life cycle, particularly those involving ingestion of tissue cysts or oocysts by a human.

Very little is known about the pathogenesis of toxoplasmosis. In healthy adults *T. gondii* is clearly not very pathogenic, as evidenced by the infrequent and mild symptoms (resembling those of mononucleosis) that it causes. This argues against a potent toxin. The disease in the fetus involves primarily the nervous system, with blindness, hydrocephaly, and severe mental retardation as some of the major manifestations. In immunosuppressed individuals a disseminated disease is observed, with the central nervous system again the principal target organ. Disease, at least in infants and immunosuppressed individuals, thus seems to be largely a direct consequence of the destruction of invaded tissue. This aspect of the disease is discussed further in Chapter 16.

RESEARCH GOALS AND ACCOMPLISHMENTS TO DATE AT STANFORD

Aims of Studies

Our approach is to investigate the molecular details of *Toxoplasma gondii* in an effort to understand its antigenic structure and basic molecular processes. Our hope is that this information will contribute to the development of novel diagnostic, chemotherapeutic, and vaccination strategies.

The specific questions being addressed are:

1. What is the relative position of the Coccidia, particularly *T. gondii,* on the evolutionary tree and with regard to the other protozoa? Information about the relationship of *T. gondii* to other organisms may yield insights into potential points of vulnerability. We are approaching this question through the study of tubulin genes.
2. What is the mechanism of invasion into nonphagocytic cells, and how do the parasites defend themselves against the killing activity of the macrophage?
3. How are genes expressed and regulated in *T. gondii?*
4. What is the structure and function of the major surface antigens?
5. Can we use cloned genes for generating large quantities of the surface antigens for use as immunogens and/or in diagnosis?
6. Can we use a combination of recently developed techniques to rapidly determine genetic linkage maps and investigate meiosis in these organisms?

In this section we will describe some of our initial experiments that address these questions.

Studies on the Tubulin Genes

There are two major sorts of tubulin found in virtually every eukaryotic cell: α-tubulin and β-tubulin (for review, see Cleveland[7]). These molecules form heterodimers, which can be assembled into polymeric structures called *microtubules*. The microtubules are critical for many cellular functions, most notably meiosis, motility, and maintenance of the cell's shape through the cytoskeleton. In most other organisms these proteins are each encoded by multiple genes. In the Kinetoplastida (including trypanosomes and *Leishmania*) these multiple genes are tandemly repeated.

We have shown that in *T. gondii* there is only one complete gene coding for each of the two sorts of tubulin.[10] This indicates that if different tubulins are required for the different microtubules, they must be modified post-translationally. Such post-translational modification has been observed with other protozoa and seems likely to explain how only one α- and one β-tubulin gene can suffice in *T. gondii*.

We have sequenced both *T. gondii* tubulin genes and made the following observations. First, unlike the vast majority of all other genes so far studied in other protozoa, the tubulin genes of *T. gondii* are broken up by the presence of several intervening sequences or *introns* (Fig. 15-3). Only a few genes in *Plasmodium* have previously been found to possess introns, and then typically only one. In the Kinetoplastida, no introns have yet been observed. Kinetoplastida also apparently possess the novel ability to splice in trans two discrete messenger RNA transcripts (Sutton and Boothroyd, submitted). It may be that these trans splicing mechanisms preclude cis splicing in the Kinetoplastida. We are currently investigating whether a similar phenomenon exists in *T. gondii*.

Second, the predicted amino acid sequences of the tubulins of *T. gondii* are well conserved, retaining considerable homology with the tubulins of other eukaryotes. Table 15-1 presents a matrix of the percent homology among tubulins of different organisms. As yet, the complete tubulin structure has been determined for only three protozoa. It will clearly be of interest to investigte tubulin structure in other coccidia, particularly *Plasmodium* and *Eimeria*. Such investigations might help to establish the precise evolutionary relationships

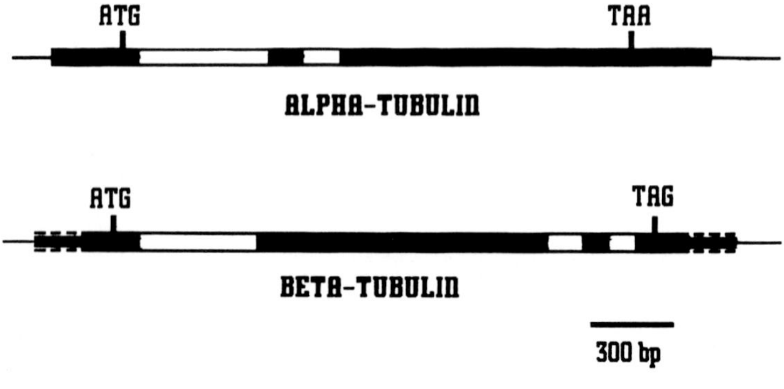

Fig. 15-3. Schematic representation of the structure of the tubulin genes. The portions of the gene that are represented in the final, mature mRNA are shown as dark boxes while the intervening sequences (introns), which are removed from the primary transcript, are shown as open boxes. The start (ATG) and stop (TAA) codons for each gene are also shown. The maps are drawn to the scale shown.

Table 15-1. Percentage Homology among α-Tubulins

	Toxo.	Chlamy.	Tryp.	Rat	Schizo.	Ref.
Toxo.	100	94	89	86	72	Boothroyd[10]
Chlamy.		100	91	86	72	Silflow[13]
Tryp.			100	85	71	Kimmel[9]
Rat				100	78	Lemischka[14]
Schizo.					100	Toda[15]

Toxo. = *Toxoplasma gondii*; Chlamy. = *Chlamydomonas reinhardi*; Tryp. = *Trypanosoma brucei;* Schizo. = *Schizosaccharomyces pombe*.

among these organisms. This sort of information helps one to apply the knowledge derived for one organism to its close relatives.

ISOLATION OF ANTIGEN GENES

Potential Use of Cloned Antigen Genes

Since about 1982 there has been an explosion of activity aimed at identifying the major protein antigens of various protozoan pathogens and then using molecular biology to isolate the genes coding for these proteins. Such work has the following potential uses:

1. Determination of the primary structure of polypeptide antigens, enabling correlations to be made between structure and function
2. Generation of materials for use as vaccines, either by expression in other cell systems (e.g., bacteria or yeast) or by synthesis of short peptides in vitro
3. Identification of molecular probes for use as diagnostic tools, which might be recombinant proteins (generated as described in item 2) or nucleic acid probes
4. Studies on the extent of strain variation at the molecular level and comparison of strain-specific molecular markers with virulence or pathogenicity of different strains (see Ch. 9 for a discussion of this approach with *Giardia lamblia*)

Generation of Recombinant Gene Libraries

There are two methods commonly used for generating gene libraries. The first of these is to randomly shear genomic DNA and insert this into expression vectors. This method assumes that if enough recombinants are generated, the probability is good of having at least one recombinant in the population that expresses a fusion protein corresponding to the antigen of interest. (The term *recombinant* refers to expression vectors (viruses or plasmids) whose DNA contains an "insert" of foreign DNA, in this case a stretch of genomic DNA of

T. gondii.) In practice, for a genome the size of *T. gondii,* at least 5×10^6 independent recombinants are needed. This allows for the entire genome to be represented by the recombinants with at least one insert having one of its ends falling within any 10-base-pair region of the genome. Allowing for only one in six insertions of *T. gondii* DNA into the expression vector being in the correct orientation and reading frame for expression of the corresponding polypeptide, functional recombinants should exist in such a library, with fusions corresponding to every 60 base pairs.

We generated one such library and screened it with serum from an infected mouse.[10] Among the recombinants expressing peptides reactive with this serum was one that was found at above average frequency. This recombinant, arbitrarily termed B1, has been characterized as follows:

The B1 gene is 2.2-kilobase (kb) long and is tandemly repeated about 50 times in a head-to-tail manner (Fig. 15-4). There are no extensive open reading frames based on the complete sequence of the gene. This suggests that either only a short polypeptide product is encoded or that there are introns in this gene, as described for the tubulin genes above. Unfortunately, we have not been able to identify the protein product encoded by this gene as it exists in the parasite. This is in progress.

The second strategy is to make complementary DNA (cDNA) copies of the total mRNA population of the parasite and clone these cDNA copies as recombinant molecules in expression vectors. Such a library has been generated by us and by Prince, Sharma, and Remington. This library has been screened using polyclonal antisera raised against a purified *T. gondii* surface antigen[10] termed p22 to reflect its apparent molecular weight in kilodaltons. p22 is one of four major surface antigens.[11]

The recombinant corresponding to this antigen contains an insert of about 520 base pairs, which has been completely sequenced and seems to be coding for about 16 kilodaltons of polypeptide.[10] This is not the complete gene as only a fragment has been inserted, and hence this size is a minimal estimate of the total coding potential of the gene.

Use of monospecific antiserum to identify a particular gene is obviously open to the artifact of obtaining a gene coding for a cross-reacting antigen. To determine whether this is the case, it is necessary to purify the fusion material

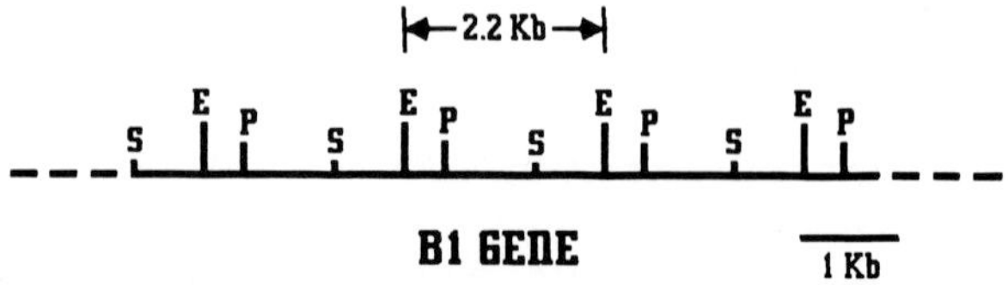

Fig. 15-4. Schematic map showing the tandem repetition of the B1 gene. This gene was identified as described in the text. It is about 2.2 kilobase-pairs long and is tandemly repeated. It codes for an immunogen in natural infections, but the identity of this polypeptide is not yet known. (E = EcoRI; P = PstI; S = SacI.)

from the recombinant and use this to generate an antiserum in rabbits. This has been done for the putative p22 recombinant, and the antiserum thus generated is currently being tested against a lysate of *T. gondii* to determine the identity of the cloned gene, whose definitive identification, however, is best obtained by direct comparison of sequences derived from the protein and cloned gene independently. Our collaborators at Dartmouth are currently trying to obtain sufficient amounts of the purified p22 for direct sequence analysis.

The Potential of *Salmonella* as a Novel Vaccine Carrier

Obtaining a cloned gene corresponding to a protective antigen is only one step in the process leading to the development of an effective vaccine. The next step is to generate sufficient amounts of the recombinant protein to administer in effective doses. This, too, is not particularly difficult for most proteins, given the facilities and resources at the command of any major pharmaceutical company.

However, once the material has been generated, there is still a major hurdle that must be cleared—administration of the immunogenic material in a safe and efficacious manner. Although our knowledge of this area is growing rapidly, we are still not able to predict accurately which form of the material or which route of administration will be most effective.

In collaboration with Bruce Stocker of Stanford University we are exploring the possible use of *Salmonella* as a carrier of recombinant antigens for administration as an effective vaccine.[12] The advantages to using such a system can be summarized as follows:

1. Safe and effective vaccine strains of *Salmonella* have already been developed. These are live strains attenuated through the possession of nonreversible mutations in essential metabolic pathways. In addition, it is possible to position the desired determinants on the surface of the bacterium by using knowledge based on work with *Escherichia coli.* This may be important in the presentation of the antigens by the macrophage or other presenting cell. Currently too little information is available to predict the relative importance of this latter point in eliciting an effective response.

2. *Salmonella* is a gram-negative bacterium closely related to *E. coli,* which has been studied in enormous detail for decades, and the information is generally transferable between the two. As a result, it is possible to do all preliminary experiments on the development of good expression and presentation methods in *E. coli* and to transfer the results to the *Salmonella* strains at a later stage.

3. *Salmonella* is an enteric pathogen with many similarities to *T. gondii.* For example, it can penetrate into cells (including macrophages) and first makes intimate contact with the host in the digestive system. It too must penetrate throughout the intestinal epithelium before spreading through the body. It is reasonably clear that the sort of immunity elicited is dependent on

the route of administration, with, for example, mucosal immunity being best stimulated by contact of a vaccine with mucosal surfaces. Hence, the mimicry of the route of infection of *Toxoplasma* by *Salmonella* is likely to elicit good levels of immunity.

4. Vaccination of humans has traditionally been especially difficult because of the shortage of safe and effective adjuvants. The *Salmonella* bacterium is, in some ways, an adjuvant itself, and so the use of additional materials may prove unnecessary.

The discussion on *Salmonella* is intended to inform the reader of a possible future direction of vaccine delivery, especially for vaccines against organisms with an intestinal portal of entry. As yet, the development of this potential has just begun to be explored, but we predict that this sort of strategy may prove particularly important in the next stage of developing vaccines against parasites.

CONCLUSION

We have tried to present an overview of the approaches we have adopted in trying to effect better control of an increasingly important disease. It will be clear to any brave soul who has made it this far that our work is in its infancy. Yet, we feel that there is an enormous potential for applying the remarkable technological tools now available to the modern researcher to achieve this goal. Exciting times lie ahead.

ACKNOWLEDGMENTS

We appreciatively acknowledge our collaborators in this work, Lloyd Kasper and Pat Ware at Dartmouth Medical School and Jeffrey Prince, Somesh Sharma, and Jack Remington at the Palo Alto Medical Foundation. This work was supported by grants to J.C.B. from the National Institutes of Health (AI21025), March of Dimes, and the MacArthur Foundation. J.C.B. holds a special fellowship in molecular parasitology from the Burroughs Wellcome fund. S.D.N. was supported in part by a grant from the Johnson & Johnson Co. J.L.B. holds a Giannini Foundation fellowship in medical research.

REFERENCES

1. Babudieri B, Desmonts G, Garnham PCC, et al: Toxoplasmosis: Report of a WHO Meeting of Investigators. World Health Organization, Geneva, 1969
2. Dubey JP: *Toxoplasma, Hammondia, Besnoita, Sarcocystis,* and other tissue cyst-forming coccidia of man and animals. p. 101. In Kreier JP (ed): Parasitic Protozoa. Academic Press, New York, 1977
3. Vietzke WM, Gelderman AH, Grimley PM, et al: Toxoplasmosis complicating malignancy. Experience at the National Cancer Institute. Cancer 21:816, 1968

4. Luft BJ, Brooks RG, Conley FK, et al: Toxoplasmic encephalitis in patients with acquired immune deficiency syndrome. JAMA 252:913, 1984
5. Feldman HA: A nationwide serum survey of United States military recruits, 1962. Am J Epidemiol 81:385, 1965
6. Desmonts G, Couvreur J: Congenital toxoplasmosis. A prospective study on 378 pregnancies. N Engl J Med 290:1110, 1974
7. Cleveland DW, Sullivan KF: Molecular biology and genetics of tubulin. Annu Rev Biochem 54:331, 1985
8. Landfear SM, McMahon-Pratt D, Wirth DF: Tandem arrangement of tubulin genes in the protozoan parasite *Leishmania enriettii*. Mol Cell Biol 3:1070, 1983
9. Kimmel BE, Samson S, Hirschberg R, et al: Tubulin genes of the African trypanosome *Trypanosoma brucei rhodesiense*: nucleotide sequence of a 3.7-kb fragment containing genes for alpha and beta tubulins. Gene 35:237, 1985
10. Boothroyd JC, Burg JL, Nagel SD, et al: Antigen and tubulin genes of *Toxoplasma gondii*. (in press.) In Agabian N, Goodman H, Noguiera N (eds): UCLA Symposia on Molecular and Cellular Biology: Molecular Strategies of Parasitic Invasion. Alan R. Liss, New York, 1986
11. Kasper LH, Crabb JH, Pfefferkorn ER: Purification of a major membrane protein of *Toxoplasma gondii* by immunoabsorption with a monoclonal antibody. J Immunol 130:2407, 1983
12. Hoiseth SK, Stocker BAD: Aromatic-dependent *Salmonella typhimurium* are non-virulent and effective as live vaccines. Nature 291:238, 1981
13. Silflow CD, Chisholm RL, Conner TW, et al: The two alpha-tubulin genes of *Chlamydomonas reinhardi* code for slightly different proteins. Mol Cell Biol 5:2389, 1985
14. Lemischka I, Sharp PA: The sequences of an expressed rat alpha tubulin gene and a pseudogene with an inserted repetitive element. Nature 300:330, 1982
15. Toda T, Adachi Y, Hiraoka Y, et al: Identification of the pleiotropic cell division cycle gene NDA2 as one of two different alpha-tubulin genes in *Schizosaccharomyces pombe*. Cell 37:233, 1984

16 Diagnosis and Management of Cerebral Toxoplasmosis in Patients with Acquired Immunodeficiency Syndrome

J. Louise Gerberding

Toxoplasma gondii is now recognized as a major cause of morbidity and mortality in patients with the acquired immunodeficiency syndrome (AIDS). In immunologically normal adults it usually produces an asymptomatic or mildly symptomatic infection. However, like many other opportunistic pathogens, it causes a serious, rapidly progressive, and often fatal disease in immunocompromised hosts. Because toxoplasmosis responds to appropriate therapy in most afflicted patients, prompt diagnosis and treatment are crucial. Here we review the pathogenesis, epidemiology, and clinical manifestations of toxoplasmosis and outline a rational approach to managing AIDS patients with this disease. The biology and life cycle of *T. gondii* are discussed in Chapter 15.

DIFFERENTIAL DIAGNOSIS OF CEREBRAL TOXOPLASMOSIS IN AIDS

The spectrum of neurologic disease associated with AIDS and AIDS-related conditions (ARC) continues to expand (Table 16-1). Unfortunately, the neurologic findings in patients with toxoplasmosis are not specific and can be seen in association with many conditions.

In addition to *T. gondii,* other opportunistic pathogens such as *Mycobacterium avium-intracellulare,* cytomegalovirus, and papovavirus have been found in the brains of AIDS patients. *Mycobacterium tuberculosis* has also been isolated, particularly in Haitian patients and intravenous drug users. Fungi such as *Cryptococcus neoformans, Aspergillus fumigatus, Coccidioides immitis, Histoplasma capsulatum,* and *Candida albicans* have been isolated from brain abscesses and other parenchymal lesions. Bacterial meningitis with encapsulated organisms should be considered in the differential diagnosis.

Infection with human immunodeficiency virus (HIV), even in the absence of secondary infection, is now known to account for a large percentage of the neuropsychiatric manifestations of AIDS and ARC.[19] Diagnosis of opportunistic infection is complicated by the significant overlap in the neurologic sequelae of HIV infection with those of other pathogens, including *T. gondii.* Alterations in mental status, focal neurologic deficits, and psychiatric disturbances are common to many of these infections.

In addition to infection, other diseases may involve the brain in AIDS patients. Malignancies such as primary CNS lymphoma, metastatic systemic lymphoma, and, rarely, metastatic Kaposi's sarcoma have been diagnosed. Cerebrovascular accidents from marantic endocarditis, hypoxemia, or hemorrhage can occur. Reactive psychological disturbances related to the stresses inherent in coping with a fatal disease may mimic organic disease and confuse the diagnosis even further.

Table 16-1. Central Nervous System Manifestations of HIV Infection

	UCSF (n = 128)	Total Reported (n = 320)
Viral Syndromes		
Subacute encephalitis	35 (27%)	54 (17%)
Aseptic meningitis	17	21
HSV encephalitis	8	9
Other	6	10
Nonviral infections		
Toxoplasma gondii	18 (14%)	103 (32%)
Cryptococcus neoformans	16 (13%)	41 (13%)
Candida albicans	2	6
Other	3	12
Neoplasms		
Primary CNS lymphoma	9 (7%)	15 (5%)
Systemic lymphoma	2	12
Kaposi's sarcoma	2	3
Other/Unknown	10	34

(From Levy, et al,[17] with permission.)

DIAGNOSTIC STRATEGY

Despite the long list of potential pathophysiologic processes in AIDS patients with CNS disease, infection with *T. gondii* is by far the most common etiology for which specific effective treatment is available. In a comprehensive review of HIV-infected patients with neurologic dysfunction, 103 of 315 (33 percent) were found to have cerebral toxoplasmosis.[17] For this reason the approach to determining the etiology of neurologic AIDS should be directed toward diagnosing or excluding *T. gondii* infection. Patients presenting with headache, focal neurologic signs, or seizures are at highest risk for cerebral toxoplasmosis and should be promptly evaluated.

Computed Tomographic Scan

A CT scan should be obtained in any patient suspected of having toxoplasmosis. Delayed scanning after a double dose of iodine contrast material provides the best diagnostic information.[26–28] Abnormal CT scans are found in nearly all patients with documented cerebral toxoplasmosis, although, rarely, a completely normal scan will be obtained. Lesions are typically focal, multiple, and located in the basal ganglia, in the gray matter, or in the interface between the gray and white matter.[17,21,24–28] Three patterns have been described: ring enhancement with surrounding edema, nodular enhancement with edema, and focal edema without enhancement. Not infrequently, large lesions produce mass effect with midline shift suggestive of impending herniation. Calcification is unusual. Although the presence of typical ring-enhancing lesions is highly suggestive of toxoplasmosis, the diagnosis cannot be definitively established by CT criteria alone since other opportunistic infections and CNS lymphomas can produce similar CT findings.

Magnetic Resonance Imaging

In certain instances magnetic resonance imaging (MRI) scanning may demonstrate lesions not seen on CT scan. Even with the increased sensitivity of this technique, a diagnosis of toxoplasmosis cannot be definitively established without tissue confirmation.

Lumbar Puncture

A lumbar puncture should be performed in patients with neurologic manifestations of AIDS. However, if toxoplasmosis is suspected, this procedure should be delayed until a CT scan has been performed to exclude large lesions with mass effect even when the physical examination does not suggest focal neurologic deficits or elevated intracranial pressue. The cerebrospinal fluid

(CSF) cell count, glucose concentration, and protein concentration should be measured. The CSF may be entirely normal in toxoplasmosis. The protein is slightly elevated in up to 50 percent of cases, although extreme elevations are distinctly unusual.[13,17] A mononuclear pleiocytosis is seen in 15 percent. The glucose is usually normal. A Gram stain should be performed to exclude bacterial meningitis. In addition, an India ink preparation and a cryptococcal antigen test should be performed to detect infection with *Cryptococcus neoformans*.

Serologic Evidence of Toxoplasmosis

Available Antibody Tests

Although it is possible to culture *T. gondii* by inoculating tissue cultures or mouse peritoneal cavities, these methods are time-consuming and cumbersome.[33] For this reason serologic tests to demonstrate specific antibody to *T. gondii* are used to establish a diagnosis of acute infection or to document prior infection in immunocompetent hosts. A variety of tests to measure immunoglobulin G or M antibodies have been developed.[1] Because these tests vary in sensitivity, specificity, and the type of antibody detected, they must be interpreted with caution.

The Sabin-Feldman (SF) dye test for IgG antibody to *T. gondii* is the reference serologic test for diagnosing toxoplasmosis. The patient's serum is incubated with complement and live tachyzoites. If specific IgG antibody is present, the tachyzoites lyse and do not take up alkaline methylene blue stain. The titer is defined as the dilution of serum at which half of the organisms are stained. In normal hosts the antibodies measured in this test appear 1 to 2 weeks after infection, reach a peak titer in 6 to 8 weeks, and decline over 1 to 2 years.[1] The indirect fluorescent antibody (IFA) test measures the same antibodies as the SF test and is more convenient and economical to perform. Quantitative titers are more difficult to obtain and false positive results occur with sera that contain antinuclear antibodies.[1] The agglutination (AG) test is another convenient method, which is useful for screening but not readily available in the United States. Of the tests to measure IgM antibody, the double-sandwich IgM enzyme-linked immunosorbent assay (DS-IgM-ELISA) is the most sensitive and specific.[1]

Diagnostic Utility

In immunocompetent hosts acute acquired toxoplasmosis is reliably diagnosed when seroconversion from a negative titer to a positve titer occurs or when a fourfold increase in titer over 3 weeks is observed. A single high titer measured by the SF or IFA test is suggestive of acute infection. A stable SF or IFA titer less than 1 : 1,024 is unusual in acute toxoplasmosis in normal adults; a negative SF or IFA test excludes the diagnosis. A low titer of IgM antibody by the DS-IgM-ELISA method makes acute infection extremely unlikely, whereas a high titer with a single high IgG titer by the SF or IFA test makes acute infection highly probable.[1]

Serologic tests for specific antibody are somewhat less reliable in establishing a diagnosis of acute toxoplasmosis in immunocompromised than in immunocompetent hosts, owing, at least in part, to the depressed antibody responses in these patients. However, establishing a diagnosis by serologic tests is even more difficult in patients with AIDS. In the first large series reported, only 1 of 37 patients had a positive titer in the IgM ELISA test[2] (Table 16-2). Although the SF test was always positive, titers were greater than 1 : 1,024 in only eight patients and greater than 1 : 2,048 in only one. A diagnostic fourfold rise in titer was demonstrated in only 2 of 16 patients. In this same series, 17 of 29 patients with an SF titer of 1 : 512 or lower had titers measured by AG that were 5 to 20 times higher than in the SF test. The ratio of titers measured by these two methods was much lower in immunologically normal hosts with toxoplasmosis or in AIDS patients without toxoplasmosis.[2]

The diagnostic utility of measuring titers of CSF antibody to *T. gondii* has not been fully evaluated but does not appear promising. In 12 patients with cerebral toxoplasmosis, 4 had negative CSF titers by SF, 6 had titers that were lower than corresponding serum titers, and 2 had titers equal to serum titers.[2]

In summary, serologic studies are rarely diagnostic of toxoplasmosis in AIDS patients. A negative SF or IFA test makes the diagnosis of acute toxoplasmosis extremely unlikely but does not exlude it altogether, since at least one patient with documented toxoplasmosis has had a negative SF test. A high titer or antibody measured by AG in association with a low titer measured by SF or a stable SF or IFA titer greater than 1 : 1,024 is strongly suggestive of the diagnosis. The absence of IgM antibody does not exclude the diagnosis of acute infection.

Demonstration of *Toxoplasma* Antigen in Body Fluids

Tests to measure *T. gondii* antigens in sera are currently undergoing evaluation and appear to be sensitive and specific in preliminary studies.[34] If these methods are reliable in other body fluids or tissues, the ability to diagnose toxoplasmosis in AIDS patients without employing invasive procedures may be greatly enhanced.

Table 16-2. Clinical Utility of Toxoplasma Serology in AIDS

SF dye test usually positive but in low titer; rarely diagnostic
Rising titers rarely demonstrated
AG titer/SF titer > 5 suggests diagnosis
Negative SF dye test reduces probability of toxoplasmosis but does not exclude diagnosis
IgM rarely present even in acute disease
CSF titers not helpful

Histologic Diagnosis

In many AIDS patients intracranial pathology can be diagnosed with certainty only by tissue examination. Brain biopsy has been proved to establish a diagnosis in at least 85 percent of cases.[17] The diagnostic yield of brain biopsy can be improved if care is taken to ensure adequate sampling and processing of involved tissue. In patients with accessible focal lesions on CT scan, directed needle biopsy or excisional biopsy is preferred. An attempt should be made to sample the margins of the lesions and surrounding brain tissue. Blind biopsy is less sensitive, but has provided useful information in patients with normal CT scans, focal lesions that are not accessbile to biopsy, or diffuse parenchymal disease.

Characteristically, histopathologic examination of brain tissue from AIDS patients with toxoplasmosis demonstrates a profoundly destructive but well-demarcated necrotizing encephalitis.[2,35,36] The process may be focal or diffuse. Astrocytosis is evident at the periphery of the lesion. Productive arteritis with fibrosis of the adventitial and medial tunicae is typically present and is usually associated with monocytic perivascular cuffing. Although no characteristic clearly distinguishes the histopathology of toxoplasmosis in AIDS patients from that found in other immunocompromised patients, neutrophils comprise a greater proportion of the inflammatory cells in the latter group.[2]

The diagnosis of toxoplasmosis requires the demonstration of organisms in inflamed brain tissue. Tissue cysts are often not detected, but when present they are located in the noninflamed brain tissue bordering necrotic foci. Both free and vacuolated forms of tachyzoites can be found in the margins of the lesion. Free tachyzoites and remnants of phagocytized tachyzoites can also be identified in the central necrotic debris.

Conventional staining techniques, including hematoxylin-eosin (HE) and Wright-Giemsa (WG), may fail to demonstrate organisms in up to 50 percent of cases.[2] A rapid diagnosis can sometimes be may be made by examining touch smears stained with WG, but distortion and artifacts frequently interfere with the interpretation of these preparations. Frozen sections are also occasionally positive, but formalin-fixed, paraffin-embedded specimens stained with HE or WG are more likely to demonstrate the organism.

A direct immunofluorescence assay performed with monoclonal anti-*Toxoplasma* antibodies labeled with fluorescein isothiocyanate appears to be a useful method for demonstrating tachyzoites in touch preparations and should be routinely performed.[37] The peroxidase antiperoxidase (PAP) method is also very sensitive for demonstrating free tachyzoites, tissue cysts, and phagocytized organisms.[38] This method can be used on formalin-fixed, paraffin-embedded tissue specimens prepared for light microscopy. Cellular detail is preserved so that the presence of *Toxoplasma* organisms can be interpreted in the context of the histopathologic findings. The PAP method should be used in cases of necrotizing encephalitis when conventional stains and immunofluorescence assay fail to identify the organism or when toxoplasmosis is not suspected until the specimen has been processed for permanent sections.

TREATMENT

Recommendations for treatment of toxoplasmosis in AIDS patients are based on clinical observations in other patient populations, data obtained from murine models of *T. gondii* infection, and retrospective analysis of treatment outcomes. No prospective randomized controlled trials comparing therapeutic regimens in AIDS patients have been reported to date.

Combination therapy with pyrimethamine and sulfadiazine is usually instituted. Synergism between pyrimethamine and sulfadiazine or other trisulfapyrimidines has been demonstrated in mice.[39] Because AIDS patients appear to be particularly susceptible to sulfa allergies and bone marrow suppression, these drugs are usually administered at lower dosages than those used in other patients (Table 16-3).

For sulfadiazine we recommend a loading dose of 2 g followed by a maintenance dose of 1 g every 6 hours. In addition to severe allergic reactions, side effects attributed to this drug include interstitial nephritis, nausea, vomiting, and diarrhea. Pyrimethamine is given concurrently at a dose of 25 mg/day after a 50-mg loading dose. Bone marrow suppression with severe pancytopenias, gastrointestinal (GI) complaints, and headache are the most common toxic effects seen with this drug. Folinic acid (10 mg/day) should be administered to minimize the bone marrow suppressive effects of these folic acid antagonists (see Chapter 6 for discussion of folinic acid). Folinic acid does not interfere with therapeutic efficacy since *T. gondii* does not take up this drug.[1]

Both pyrimethamine and sulfadiazine penetrate the blood-brain barrier. Both are active against free tachyzoites as well as phagocytized organisms. However, neither drug is active against tissue cysts, and they should not be used for primary prophylaxis in individuals with latent infections.[1] The potential teratogenic effect of pyrimethamine precludes its use in the first trimester of pregnancy.

Not infrequently, major toxicities develop that necessitate adjustments in the therapeutic regimen. Successful desensitization to sulfadiazine by gradually increasing the dose from 250 mg/day after pretreatment with dexamethasone

Table 16-3. Treatment of CNS Toxoplasmosis

Drug	Dose	CNS Penetration	Toxicity
Sulfadiazine[a]	ld : 2 g md : lg/q6h	40–80%	GI/renal/ rash/marrow
Pyrimethamine	ld : 50 mg/2day md : 25 mg/day or qod	10–25%	Marrow/GI/ha
Folinic acid	10 mg/day		

ld = loading dose; md = maintenance dose; ha = headache; qod = every other day, (alternate days).

[a] Long-term maintenance:? sulfadiazine (500 mg every 6 h).

has been reported.[40] We have successfully reinstituted therapy at lower dosages (250 to 500 mg every 6 hours) in some patients after resolution of pancytopenia. Pyrimethamine alone (50 mg/day) has been recommended by some authorities since single-agent therapy appears to be efficacious in the murine model.[2]

Spiramycin, a macrolide antibiotic with good CNS penetration, is used in Europe to treat pregnant women with toxoplasmosis. The drug is not approved for use in the United States. Animal studies suggest that clindamycin may be efficacious even though CSF levels are extremely low.[41,42] This drug is not currently recommended for use in human cerebral toxoplasmosis, although it is beneficial in chorioretinitis. Experience with other folic acid antagonists is limited. Trimethoprim-sulfamethoxazole is less active in animal models than sulfadizine and pyrimethamine.[2] Therapeutic success with trimethoprim-sulfamethoxazole in one AIDS patient has been reported.[13]

The response rate in AIDS patients treated with a combination of sulfadiazine and pyrimethamine is at least 80 percent in most reports. Symptomatic improvement is usually evident by day 10 of treatment, followed by resolution of CT scan abnormalities after 2 to 4 weeks. Cure is uncommon; most patients relapse after therapy is discontinued. This is not surprising, given the permanent immunosuppression in AIDS patients and the inability of currently available drugs to eradicate latent tissue cysts. Treatment for a minimum of 8 to 10 weeks with both drugs is recommended. Prolonged suppressive therapy to prevent relapse is warranted. Although suppressive regimens are largely empiric, we have used sulfadiazine (500 mg every 6 hours) in several patients and have found a low incidence of relapse.

Survival in AIDS patients with cerebral toxoplasmosis is influenced by the severity of the disease at presentation and the incidence of other opportunistic infections. Prolonged survival has been reported, but up to 70 percent of patients die within 1 year of diagnosis.[13]

INDICATIONS FOR BRAIN BIOPSY

The approach to the diagnosis and treatment of AIDS patients with suspected cerebral toxoplasmosis remains controversial. Proponents of the use of brain biopsy in all suspected cases argue that the clinical presentation and radiographic findings are not specific for toxoplasmosis and that mixed infections, lymphoma, and other potentially treatable diseases may be present.[44] On the other hand, many authorities recommend empiric anti-*Toxoplasmosis* therapy in patients with typical symptoms, signs, and CT scan features of toxoplasmosis to avoid the potential morbidity from invasive diagnostic procedures. Although other opportunistic infections and malignancies may produce similar neurologic abnormalities, toxoplasmosis is by far the most common treatable infection diagnosed. Furthermore, a delay in therapy of cerebral lymphoma is unlikely to significantly influence survival.

To help resolve this controversy we have developed a protocol outlining our diagnostic approach to AIDS patients suspected of having cerebral toxoplasmosis. The following patients are treated empirically for toxoplasmosis with pyrimethamine, sulfadiazine, and folinic acid: (1) patients with a high probability of having toxoplasmosis; (2) patients who refuse brain biopsy; (3) patients with no accessible lesions on CT scan; and (4) patients with a negative brain biopsy (Table 16-4). Our criteria for a high probability of toxoplasmosis include: (1) the simultaneous presence of neurologic symptoms or signs consistent with toxoplasmosis; (2) preexisting evidence of HIV infection (Centers for Disease Control (CDC)–defined AIDS, ARC, positive HIV culture, or documented HIV antibody); (3) no evidence of disseminated opportunistic infection or systemic lymphoma; (4) low probability of reactivation tuberculosis; (5) the presence of focal lesions consistent with toxoplasmosis on CT or MRI scan *or* a rising titer of antitoxoplasmosis antibody. Patients with evidence of elevated intracranial pressure may be treated for 5 days with decadron. Those with a history of seizures are also treated with dilantin.

A follow-up CT scan is performed after 2 weeks of empiric therapy or at any time that clinical deterioration occurs. If the CT scan suggests progressive disease, brain biopsy is performed. If the CT scan demonstrates improvement, therapy is continued. If the scan is unchanged, therapy is continued for an additional 2 weeks and another CT scan is obtained. If improvement is still not evident, brain biopsy is performed.

Brain biopsy is recommended at the time of initial presentation in patients who do not meet all the criteria for high-probability toxoplasmosis, for those with a negative SF (or other equally sensitive) antibody test, and in those whose initial CT scan suggests impending herniation.

The value of this approach is currently under investigation at our institution. By identifying a subset of patients with the highest probability of toxoplasmosis, we hope to obviate the need for brain biopsy in all patients presenting with neurologic manifestations of AIDS. We believe the incidence of other treatable conditions in which a 2-week delay in therapy would significantly alter outcome is low enough in our population to justify this approach (Table 16-1).

Table 16-4. Empiric Treatment of Toxoplasmosis in AIDS

Patients with high-probability toxoplasmosis
CNS symptoms or signs
CDC-defined AIDS, ARC, or HIV antibody
No evidence of disseminated disease
Focal lesions on CT (or MRI) consistent with toxoplasmosis or a rising titer of anti-*Toxoplasma* antibody
Patients who refuse brain biopsy
Patients with inaccessible lesions on CT scan
Patients with a negative brain biopsy

REFERENCES

1. McCabe RE, Remington JS: *Toxoplasma gondii*. p. 1540. In Mandell GE, Douglas GR, Bennett JE (eds): Principles and Practices in Infectious Diseases. John Wiley & Sons, New York, 1985
2. Luft BJ, Brooks RG, Conley EK, et al: *Toxoplasma* encephalitis in patients with acquired immune deficiency syndrome. JAMA 252:913, 1984
3. Nathan CR, Murray HW, Cohn ZA: Current concepts: the macrophage as an effector cell. N Engl J Med 303:622, 1980
4. Unanue ER: Cooperation between mononuclear phagocytes and lymphocytes in immunity. N Engl J Med 303:977, 1980
5. Lane HC, Masur H, Edgar LC, et al: Abnormalities of B-cell activation and immunoregulation in patients with the acquired immunodeficiency syndrome. N Engl J Med 309:153, 1983
6. Murray HW, Rubin BY, Masur H, et al: Impaired production of lymphokines and immune (gamma) interferon in the acquired immunodeficiency syndrome. N Engl J Med 310:883, 1984
7. Vollmer TL, Walder MK, Steinman L, Conley FK: Depletion of T_4 lymphocytes with monoclonal antibody reactivates toxoplasmosis in the central nervous system: a model of superinfection in AIDS. J Immunol 138:3737, 1987
8. Krick JA, Remington JS: Toxoplasmosis in the adult: an overview. N Engl J Med 298:550, 1978
9. Ryning FW, McLeod R, Maddox JC, et al: Probable transmission of *Toxoplasma gondii* by organ transplantation. Ann Intern Med 90:47, 1979
10. Siegel SE, Lunde MN, Gelderman AH, et al: Transmission of toxoplasmosis by leukocyte transmission. Blood 37:388, 1971
11. Feldman HA, Miller LT: Serologic study of *Toxoplasma* prevalence. Am J Hyg 64:320, 1956
12. Moskowitz LB, Kory P, Chan JC, et al: Unusual causes of death in Haitians residing in Miami: high prevalence of opportunistic infections. JAMA 250:1187, 1983
13. Wong B, Gold JW, Brown AE, et al: CNS toxoplasmosis in homosexual men and parenteral drug abusers. Ann Intern Med 100:36, 1984
14. Blaser MJ, Cohn DL: Opportunistic infections in patients with AIDS: clues to the epidemiology of AIDS and the relative virulence of pathogens. Rev Infect Dis 8:21, 1986
15. Chernik NL, Armstrong D, Posner JB, et al: Central nervous system infections in patients with cancer. Medicine 52:563, 1973
16. Hakes TB, Armstrong D: Toxoplasmosis: problems in diagnosis and treatment. Cancer 52:1535, 1983
17. Levy RM, Bredesen DE, Rosenblum ML: Neurological manifestations of the acquired immune deficiency syndrome: experience at UCSF and review of the literature. J Neurosurg 62:475, 1985
18. Horowitz SL, Bentson JR, Benson F, et al: CNS toxoplamosis in acquired immunodeficiency syndrome. Arch Neurol 40:649, 1983
19. Danziger A, Leibman AJ: Cerebral toxoplasmosis in a patient with acquired immunodeficiency syndrome. Surg Neurol 20:477, 1983
20. Snider WD, Simpson DM, Nielsen S, et al: Neurologic complications of acquired immune deficiency syndrome: analysis of fifty patients. Ann Neurol 14:403, 1983

21. Snow RB, Lavyne MH: Intracranial space-occupying lesions in acquired immune deficiency patients. Neurosurgery 16:148, 1985
22. Armstrong D: Central nervous system infections in the immunocompromised host. Infection 12:suppl. 1, S58, 1984
23. Navia BA, Petitio CK, Gold JW, et al: Cerebral toxoplasmosis complicating the acquired immune deficiency syndrome: clinical and neuropathologic findings in 27 patients. Ann Neurol 19:224, 1986
24. Post MJ, Chan JC, Hensley GT: Toxoplasma encephalitis in Haitian adults with acquired immunodeficiency syndrome: a clinical-pathologic-CT correlation. AJR 140:861, 1983
25. Kelly WM, Brant-Zawadzki M: Acquired immunodeficiency syndrome: neuroradiologic findings. Radiology 149:485, 1983
26. Whelan MA, Kricheff II, Handler M, et al: Acquired immunodeficiency syndrome: cerebral computed tomographic manifestations. Radiology 149:477, 1983
27. Handler M, Ho V, Whelan M, Budzilovich G: Intracerebral toxoplasmosis in patients with acquired immunodeficiency syndrome. J Neurosurg 59:994, 1983
28. Post MJ, Kursunoglu SJ, Hensley GT, et al: Cranial CT in acquired immunodeficiency syndrome: spectrum of diseases and optimal contrast technique. AJR 145:929, 1985
29. Parke DW, Font RL: Diffuse toxoplasmic retinochoroiditis in a patient with AIDS. Arch Ophthalmol 104:571, 1986
30. Tourani JM, Israel BD, Venet A, Andrieu JM: Unusual pulmonary infection in a puzzling presentation of AIDS (letter). Lancet 1:989, 1985
31. Nistal M, Santana A, Paniaqua R, Palacios J: Testicular toxoplasmosis in two men with the acquired immunodeficiency syndrome (AIDS). Arch Pathol Lab Med 110:744, 1986
32. Farthing CF, Henry K, Shansin DC, et al: Clinical investigation of lymphadenopathy, including lymph node biopsies, in 24 homosexual men with antibodies to the human T-cell lymphotropic virus type III (HTLV-III). Br J Surg 73:180, 1986
33. Hofflin JM, Remington JS: Tissue culture isolation of *Toxoplasma* from blood of a patient with AIDS. Arch Intern Med 145:925, 1985
34. Lindenschmidt EG: Enzyme-linked immunosorbent assay for detection of soluble *Toxoplasma gondii* antigen in acute-phase toxoplasmosis. Eur J Clin Microbiol 4:488, 1985
35. Millard PR: AIDS: histopathological aspects. J Pathol 143:223, 1984
36. Moskowitz LB, Hensley GT, Chan JC, et al: Brain biopsies in patients with acquired immune deficiency syndrome. Arch Pathol Lab Med 108:368, 1984
37. Sun T, Greenspan J, Tenenbaum M, et al: Diagnosis of cerebral toxoplasmosis using fluorescein-labeled antitoxoplasma monoclonal antibodies. Am J Surg Pathol 10:312, 1986
38. Conley FK, Jenkins KA, Remington JS: *Toxoplasma gondii* infection of the central nervous system: use of the peroxidase-antiperoxidase method to demonstrate *Toxoplasma* in formalin fixed, paraffin embedded tissue sections. Hum Pathol 12:690, 1981
39. Eigles DE, Coleman N: An evaluation of pyrimethamine and sulfadiazine alone and in combination in experimental mouse toxoplasmosis. Antibiot Chemother 5:529, 1955
40. Bell ET, Tapper ML, Pollock AA: Sulfadiazine densitization in AIDS patients. (Letter). Lancet 1:163, 1985

41. Araujo FG, Remington JS: Effect of clindamycin on acute and chronic toxoplasmosis in mice. Antimicrob Agents Chemother 5:647, 1974
42. Hofflin JM, Remington JS: Clindamycin and murine intracerebral toxoplasmosis. In Intersci Congr Antimicrob Agents Chemother, 1985
43. Lakhanpal V: Clindamycin in the treatment of toxoplasmic retinochoroiditis. Am J Ophthalmol 95:605, 1983
44. Levy RM, Pons VG, Rosenblum ML: Intracerebral mass lesions in the acquired immunodeficiency syndrome (AIDS). N Engl J Med 309:1454, 1984

17 Perspectives on Immunization Against Malaria

Terence J. Hadley
Jeffrey D. Chulay

Malaria continues to be a major health and economic problem in many developing countries and a common cause of infection among travelers. Efforts to control the disease by the use of drugs and insecticides have achieved only limited success. In many areas malaria parasites have become resistant to drugs, mosquitoes have become resistant to insecticides, and the cost of control measures are prohibitively high. Over the past decade there has been renewed interest in developing a malaria vaccine. Clyde et al. demonstrated that humans can be effectively vaccinated against malaria by using irradiated sporozoites,[1] and many other studies have demonstrated that various animals can be successfully vaccinated against malaria with crude antigen preparations of blood-stage parasites or gametes (sexual-stage parasites).[2,3] Useful animal models include *Plasmodium berghei* and *Plasmodium yoelli* in mice, *Plasmodium gallinaceum* in chickens, *Plasmodium lophurae* in ducks, *Plasmodium knowlesi* in rhesus monkeys, and *Plasmodium falciparum* in *Aotus* monkeys or squirrel monkeys. Monoclonal antibodies, recombinant DNA technology, and the in vitro culture of malaria parasites provide the tools needed to examine specific antigens as potential immunogens. Some of the problems encountered in research on malaria vaccines are: (1) there is no in vitro test that correlates with or predicts effective immunity; (2) the mechanisms of naturally acquired immunity are still not well understood and the relative importance of humoral and cellular immunity has not been clearly defined; (3) immunization trials in monkeys are limited by the expense and scarcity of monkeys; also the immunology of human malarias in monkeys may differ significantly from that in humans; and (4) malaria parasites display a striking degree of antigenic poymorphism and also undergo antigenic variation under immune pressure.[4] Despite these problems, information obtained from in vitro experiments and animal models points to certain antigens that may be effective immunogens. Some of these have already been purified and tested. Successful vaccination of monkeys has involved the use of Freund's complete adjuvant, which is too toxic for human use. Work is now being done to identify safe and effective adjuvants for use in humans.[5]

LIFE CYCLE AND GENETICS OF MALARIAL PARASITES

Life Cycle

Malaria infections are initiated when the female *Anopheles* mosquito takes a blood meal and injects sporozoites into subcutaneous capillaries. Sporozoites rapidly enter hepatocytes and develop over 1 to 2 weeks into exoerythrocytic schizonts. Merozoites emerge from exoerythrocytic schizonts and infect erythrocytes, thereby initiating the erythrocytic stage of the infection. The erythrocytic stage is associated with the clinical manifestations of the disease. After invading an erythrocyte, a merozoite develops from a small ring form into a trophozoite, then divides asexually to produce a schizont. Schizont-infected erythrocytes rupture and release newly formed merozoites, which invade other erythrocytes. Some merozoites develop into gametocytes rather than asexual parasites. Male and female gametocytes are ingested by the mosquito in a blood meal. Gametes emerge from gametocyte-infected erythrocytes in the gut of the mosquito and fertilization occurs. Fertilized gametes (zygotes) develop into invasive forms (ookinetes), which penetrate the gut wall of the mosquito and form oocysts. Sporozoites develop within oocysts and subsequently emerge and migrate to the salivary glands of the mosquito. When the mosquito takes a blood meal, sporozoites enter the bloodstream and initiate an infection.

Genetics

Malaria parasites are haploid in the intermediate host (e.g., man).[6] Diploid stages, chromosomal reassortment, and meiosis occur in the mosquito.[6] It is not known, however, at what mosquito stage meiosis occurs. Genetic cross experiments with cloned lines of *P. falciparum* have recently been carried out in chimpanzees.[6] Such experiments allow analysis of the genetic "behavior" of antigens, enzymes, and biologic phenotypes (e.g., drug resistance). For example, Wellems et al. recently analyzed a genetic cross and demonstrated that a histidine-rich protein (HRP III) of *P. falciparum,* previously shown to have arisen through gene duplication from HRP II, is not genetically linked to HRP

II and is in fact located on a different chromosome.[7,8] This finding indicated that the HRP III gene had undergone interchromosomal transposition (see section on histidine-rich proteins). It is possible that genetic crosses will produce unique variants, which will be useful in studying the function of certain malarial proteins.

Plasmodium Falciparum

There are four species of *Plasmodium* that infect man; *P. falciparum, P. vivax, P. ovale,* and *P. malariae*. Each species has its own characteristic morphology and biology. *P. falciparum* causes high parasitemias and most malaria-associated deaths; *P. vivax* causes considerable morbidity and probably is also responsible for some malaria-related deaths. In this chapter we will discuss primarily *P. falciparum,* as that is the focus of our research at the Walter Reed Army Institute of Research. Some reference will also be made to *P. berghei* in mice and *P. knowlesi* in rhesus monkeys. In addition to causing most malaria-related mortalities, *P. falciparum* also presents the therapeutic problem of drug resistance in many areas of the world. Recent work by Martin et al. demonstrated that chloroquine resistance can be reversed by exposing parasitized erythrocytes to a calcium channel blocker.[9] This suggests that chloroquine resistance may involve a pump, which extrudes the drug through a mechanism similar to that described in multidrug-resistant cancer cell lines. This observation may prove to be extremely important to our understanding of chloroquine resistance.

An important feature of the life cycle of *P. falciparum* is that asexual parasites undergo *sequestration,* the process by which trophozoite- and schizont-infected erythrocytes bind to endothelial cells of postcapillary venules. Sequestration may benefit parasites by preventing them from circulating through the spleen, which is a site of parasite destruction. The molecular basis of sequestration is an area of active investigation and will be discussed subsequently in this chapter.

ACQUIRED IMMUNITY

Features of Naturally Acquired Immunity

Naturally acquired immunity to malaria develops after repeated infections, usually only after many years.[10–12] The age at which an individual becomes effectively immune is related to the incidence of malaria in the area in which the person lives. Children in hyperendemic areas, such as West Africa, become immune by around age 5. Immunity is often not "sterile," that is, individuals may have parasites in their blood without having overt symptoms of malaria. Parasitemias in children are often at levels that would cause severe illness in nonimmune individuals. In addition to immune mechanisms that prevent rising parasitemia, there appear to be immune mechanisms that prevent disease despite significant parasitemia. The latter may involve immunity to a toxin or soluble pathogenic factor, tolerance to antigens that produce destructive immune responses in the nonimmune individuals, or the emergence of less pathogenic parasites. Adults in West Africa usually have immunity that suppresses parasitemia to very low, often undetectable, levels. Even in adults, however, immunity may not be completely effective, and intermittent bouts of malaria can occur. In areas of the world where malaria is less endemic, immunity takes longer to develop, and adolescents and adults may suffer from severe malaria. The major complications of malaria, such as renal failure, cerebral malaria, and severe hemolytic anemia are usually associated with high parasitemias. If *P. falciparum* malaria is left untreated and fatal complications do not occur, clinical symptoms may subside after several weeks, but parasitemia may persist for many months and clinical recrudescence can occur.

Immunity to malaria is stage-specific and strain-specific. For example, immunity against sporozoites does not confer immunity against blood-stage parasites.[1] The strain specificity of blood-stage malarial immunity has been demonstrated in experimental infections in humans and animals.[13–16] Many of the studies in humans were done in patients with neurosyphilis who were treated with malaria infections, a form of therapy that was effective in up to two-thirds of these patients (M. Young, personal communication). Strains of malaria are often designated by their geographic origin, a designation that does not reflect the true extent of antigenic polymorphism. If defined by serologic methods or by reactivity with monoclonal antibodies, many strains (or serotypes) can be detected within a single geographic area.[17–19] Conversely, antigenically related strains can be found in geographically different areas (see section on acquired immunity and vaccine design). Although immunity to one strain does not confer protection against other strains, individuals living in endemic areas eventually become immune to many or all strains in that area. It is not known whether this represents the overall effect of many different strain-specific effector mechanisms or whether individuals also develop immunity directed against antigenic epitopes common to all strains. Serologic data from experiments in Gambia suggest that there may be important antigenic epitopes on the surface of infected erythrocytes that are common to many or all strains.[17]

Another feature of antimalarial immunity is that it is rapidly lost when an immune individual leaves a malarious area. The maintenance of immunity may require constant boosting by infection. The cellular and molecular mechanisms underlying this phenomenon are unknown.

Mechanisms of Immunity

The subject of immunity in malaria has been previously reviewed.[20,21] Both antibody-mediated and cell-mediated mechanisms appear to be involved. Cohen et al. demonstrated that parasitemias in infected children can be reduced by infusion of immunoglobulin from immune adults,[22] and similar results have been obtained in rodent and primate models.[16,23] The mechanism of action of the immunoglobulin is unclear. Immune sera cause agglutination of merozoites as they emerge from schizont-infected erythrocytes in vitro.[24–26] Agglutinated merozoites are unable to invade erythrocytes. Whether this occurs in vivo is not known. Merozoites may also be targets of antibody-dependent or antibody-independent cell-mediated immunity, a mechanism that would not be reflected in the typical in vitro growth inhibition or invasion assay (see section on anti-merozoite immunity).

Howard et al. demonstrated that malaria parasites incorporate parasite proteins into the erythrocyte membrane, some of which form antigenic determinants on the surface of infected erythrocytes.[27,28] It is highly probable that these antigens are targets of protective immunity as they are directly exposed to the immune system for prolonged periods of time. Antibodies to parasite proteins on the surface of an infected erythrocyte could affect the normal physiology of the parasite or could be involved in killing the parasite by antibody-dependent cell-mediated mechanisms in the spleen. For example, antibodies against antigens on the surface of *P. falciparum*–infected erythrocytes prevent binding of these erythrocytes to endothelial cells and thereby prevent sequestration.[29,30] Interference with sequestration appears to have an adverse effect on parasite survival as the parasite is forced to circulate through the spleen[31] (see section on endothelial-binding ligands).

The spleen is clearly required for optimal immunity to malaria. Rhesus monkeys previously immunized with merozoites of *P. knowlesi* in Freund's complete adjuvant lost their ability to resist infection following splenectomy.[32] Loss of immunity occurred despite the fact that the titer of growth-inhibitory antibodies in the monkeys' sera did not fall after splenectomy. This suggests that antimerozoite antibodies may work in conjunction with cell-mediated mechanisms in the spleen. In the rodent malaria caused by *P. berghei* passive transfer of immunity with sera was less effective in protecting splenectomized rats than intact rats.[33] Thus, protective antiparasite antibodies appear to work in concert with a cellular mechanism present in the spleen in rodents.

Cellular mechanisms in the spleen may also operate independently of antibody. Interferon-activated, monocyte-derived macrophages are capable of killing intracellular *P. falciparum* parasites in vitro.[34] Both oxygen-dependent and oxygen-independent effector mechanisms appear to be operative. Grun and Weidanz reported that immunity to the rodent malarial parasite *P. chabaudi adami* could develop in B cell–deficient mice.[35] The effector mechanisms involved have not yet been determined.

A monoclonal antibody against the circumsporozoite protein (CSP) of *P. berghei* was shown in passive transfer experiments to confer protection against sporozoite initiated infections in mice.[36,37] Anti-CSP antibodies were shown to develop in West Africans in an age-dependent fashion, which generally correlated with the onset of immunity.[38,39] However, a correlation between the titer of anti-CSP antibodies and immunity to malaria was not apparant in a more recent study in East Africa.[40] In this study, individuals were treated with cura-

tive doses of Fansidar and tetracycline and then followed with frequent examination of blood smears for evidence of infection with *P. falciparum*. These subjects were also tested for antibodies against the CSP. Reinfection occurred in some subjects and not in others. There was no correlation between the titer of anti-CSP antibodies and protection from reinfection. Similarly, in rodents vaccinated with the CSP, protection against infection after intravenous inoculation of sporozoites did not correlate with the titer of anti-CSP antibodies.[41] These experiments indicate that there are immune mechanisms other than anti-CSP antibodies that afford protection against sporozoite-initiated infections. In rodents immunized with irradiated sporozoites, immunity could be passively transferred with spleen cell populations enriched in T cells.[41–44] Chen et al. demonstrated that B cell–deficient mice can be successfully vaccinated against sporozoites.[45] It appears likely that immunization with sporozoites induces cell-mediated immunity directed against intrahepatic parasites in addition to antibodies directed against the CSP. γ-Interferon has been shown to inhibit development of intrahepatic parasites, and this may be an important nonantibody mediator of immunity.[46]

Acquired Immunity and Vaccine Design

Understanding mechanisms of naturally acquired immunity should aid in designing a vaccine. However, a vaccine will have to improve upon nature in terms of the time it takes to induce immunity. Naturally acquired immunity takes years to develop and occurs only after repeated infections, whereas a vaccine must be able to induce immunity after two or three inoculations. Designing such a vaccine may take further understanding of why repeated infections are necessary to induce immunity.

A major factor in the slow rate at which malarial immunity develops is the striking degree of antigenic polymorphism among malarial parasites.[4] Clinical immunity may develop only after exposure to a large number of antigenically distinct strains. Not only do antigenic differences exist among different strains, but antigenically variant parasites can also arise within a single strain during the course of an infection.[47,48] This phenomenon has recently been demonstrated with cloned parasites and may account for the chronicity of malaria infections.[49,50] The capability of the parasite to vary its antigenic makeup may pose a major obstacle to vaccine development against blood-stage parasites. Hopefully, it will be possible to identify common regions of antigenically diverse molecules that are capable of inducing protective immunity.

It is also possible that the epitopes that are targets of protective immunity are poorly immunogenic and that host immune mechanisms recognize these epitopes only after repeated infection. Also, malaria infections may cause suppression of immune responses to important epitopes.[51] For example, the normal antibody response to irradiated sporozoites in mice was suppressed during an active blood-stage infection.[52] Mechanisms of immunosuppression are poorly understood and may be associated with polyclonal B cell activation, macrophage dysfunction, and/or induction of suppressor T cells.[51]

VACCINE DEVELOPMENT

Several approaches are being taken to develop a malaria vaccine. One approach is to first identify molecules of the parasite that are directly exposed to the immune system of the host, including molecules on the surface of sporozoites, on the surface of merozoites, and on the surface of infected erythrocytes. Parasite receptors are also considered to be potentially effective immunogens since antibodies against receptors may interfere with important parasite–host cell interactions. Such receptors include merozoite receptors for erythrocytes and endothelial-binding ligands that mediate binding of *P. falciparum*–infected erythrocytes to endothelial cells of postcapillary venules during sequestration (see sections on life cycle and on endothelial-binding ligand). It is not known whether receptor molecules for binding to erythrocytes are targets of naturally acquired immunity. However, a molecule that is not a target of naturally acquired immunity may induce a protective immune response if presented as a purified antigen together with an effective adjuvant in a vaccine.

Another approach, developed by Kemp et al., is to clone malarial genes in expression systems and analyze expressed antigens using polyspecific and monospecific antisera.[53] Deciding which cloned antigen to pursue can be difficult and often depends on some prior knowledge of antigen. For example, McCutcheon et al. developed a method for preparing a genomic DNA expression library using mung bean nuclease.[54] The library was screened with monoclonal antibodies against the CSP of *P. falciparum* based on prior knowledge of the importance of this antigen.[55]

In the following sections we will focus on a few antigens that we consider interesting and that may exemplify some of the approaches and problems discussed above. Our major interests at the Walter Reed Army Institute of Research have been in developing a sporozoite vaccine and a blood-stage vaccine. We have focused on the CSP of *P. falciparum* sporozoites and the major surface glycoprotein (Pf 195) of *P. falciparum* merozoites and have also attempted to identify parasite molecules that function as receptors during invasion.

Antisporozoite Immunity

In 1969 Nussenzweig et al. demonstrated that immunity to rodent malaria could be achieved in mice by the inoculation of sporozoites from irradiated mosquitoes.[56–58] Clyde et al. showed that similar immunity could be achieved in man.[1] Immunity against sporozoites was shown to be species-specific but not strain-specific and to be stage-specific in that immunized individuals were not protected against blood-stage parasites (introduced by inoculation of infected blood).[1,58] Infectivity of sporozoites in mice could be neutralized by preincubating sporozoites with antisporozoite antisera.[58] Monoclonal antibodies produced against the CSP of *P. berghei* were shown to confer protection in passive transfer experiments.[36,37] Monoclonal antibodies were used to characterize the CSP, which is the major protein on the surface of the sporozoite[59,60] (no other sporozoite surface protein has yet been identified). Analogous CSPs were identified on sporozoites of *P. falciparum, P. vivax,* and *P. knowlesi*. The gene for the CSP of *P. knowlesi* (a monkey parasite) was cloned by Ellis et al. and Ozaki et al. and was shown to contain an area of tandemly repeated sequences.[61,62] The gene for the CSP of *P. falciparum* subsequently cloned by Dame et al. and Enea et al,[55,63] consists of an NH_2-terminal signal peptide and a COOH-anchor region. It has a large central region, which codes for tandemly repeated Asn-Ala-Asn-Pro sequences interspersed with a few Asn-Val-Asp-Pro sequences. This repeat region is immunodominant in that all monoclonal antibodies against the CSP recognize epitopes in the repeat, as do most of the anti-CSP antibodies found in serum of infected individuals.[64] Synthetic peptides coupled to carriers and recombinant peptides of the repeat region of the CSP were both shown to be immunogenic in rabbits and mice.[65,66] Antisera against repeat peptides were shown to react with intact sporozoites and inhibit their invasion into human hepatic cells and a hepatoma cell line in vitro.[67,68] Anti-CSP antisera, preincubated with sporozoites, may also interfere with their subsequent development as intrahepatic schizonts.[67] Both synthetic and recombinant peptides, recently tested for immunogenicity in man in two studies[69,70] induced antisporozoite antibodies. They afforded protection against subsequent infection in one of six individuals challenged in one study and in one of seven in the other. These first trials demonstrated that an antisporozoite subunit vaccine can elicit anti-CSP antibodies in man and confer protection from subsequent challenge in some individuals. However, most of the individuals tested were not protected against subsequent infection, and it is clear that other constructs will need to be tested.

The immunogen tested at Walter Reed Army Institute of Research and the National Institutes of Health was a peptide (designated R32Tet32) produced by Young et al. using recombinant DNA techniques[71] and consisting of 32 amino acids from the repeat region of the CSP and 32 amino acids coded for by the tetracycline resistance gene read out of frame. Good et al. focused attention on the importance of malaria-specific T-cell epitopes within this recombinant peptide.[72] An optimal primary response requires that an immunogen have a T-cell site on the same molecule as B-cell epitopes, so that T-cell "help" can be elicited when B cells and T cells interact by binding to different regions of the same antigen. In the case of R32Tet32, a T-cell site was found in both the repeat and the Tet32 tail when tested in certain inbred strains of mice. However, few of the several mouse strains tested recognized a T-cell site within the repeat. Some of these strains mounted an antirepeat antibody response because of help produced by the T-cell site within the Tet32 tail, but such a response would not be boosted by subsequent infection with sporozoites, as boosting would require the T-cell site on the vaccine to be the same as the T-cell site on the sporozoite.

These studies raised two questions that are now being addressed: whether the genetically determined nonresponsivness to T-cell sites within the repeat will be observed in man and whether a more optimal immune response can be obtained by including other T-cell sites from the CSP in the vaccine. In a recent study Good et al. identified the major immunodominant T-helper cell epitope of the CSP (which is outside the repeat region).[73] This epitope coupled to the major B-cell epitope (from the tandem repeat region) elicited very high antibody responses when used as an immunogen in mice. This study illustrates an important approach in the rational design of synthetic or recombinant fragment (subunit) vaccines.

A potential problem in the development of an effective sporozoite vaccine is antigenic polymorphism, which has been identified in the circumsporozoite genes from the simian malarial parasites *P. knowlesi* and *P. cynomolgi*.[74–76] The polymorphism was marked in the repeat region and antisera against the CSP of one *P. knowlesi* strain (the Nuri strain) did not cross-react with the CSP of another strain (the H strain).[75] Although such polymorphism has not been detected in the many strains of *P. falciparum* examined to date, low-incidence variants may exist, which could be selected for by vaccine-induced immunity in a population.[77,78]

For an antisporozoite vaccine to be effective, the development of all sporozoites into viable hepatic schizonts needs to be inhibited. Theoretically, if a single sporozoite escapes antisporozoite immunity, a blood-stage infection will be initiated. A blood-stage vaccine, in contrast, may afford protection even if it is only partially effective, since protection may not require total prevention of parasitemia but rather its suppression to nonthreatening levels. As immunity to malaria is short-lived, both a sporozoite vaccine and a blood-stage vaccine may require boosting by natural infection. We therefore feel that an effective antimalarial vaccine will need to combine blood-stage antigens with antigenic sites of the CSP.

Antimerozoite Immunity

Serum from some immune individuals inhibits invasion of erythrocytes by merozoites in vitro as a result of agglutination of merozoites as they emerge from schizont-infected erythrocytes. It is unclear which merozoite surface-associated antigens are the targets of invasion-blocking antibodies. Several laboratories have produced monoclonal antibodies that block invasion in vitro. Some of these have been against Pf 195, the major glycoprotein on the merozoite surface of *P. falciparum*. In some studies the concentration of antibody required to block invasion in vitro has been relatively high (200 μg/ml),[79] and such high concentrations of specific antibodies may not be achievable in vivo. It is possible, however, that anti–Pf 195 antibodies in vivo work in concert with splenic cells. Dvorak showed that invasion of an erythrocyte by a merozoite in vitro takes 10 to 20 seconds.[80] Prior to invasion an interaction occurs between merozoite and erythrocyte, which causes a wave of deformation of unknown cause and function and of about 5 to 10 seconds duration throughout the erythrocyte. Thus a merozoite may be exposed to the immune system for at least 15 to 30 seconds prior to its invasion of an erythrocyte. During this time the merozoite could circulate through the spleen, where it would be susceptible to cell-mediated immunity, either as a free unattached merozoite or as a merozoite in the process of invading an erythrocyte. This type of antimerozoite immunity would not be detected in the typical in vitro growth or invasion assay.

Merozoite receptors for the erythrocyte may be effective immunogens if antireceptor antibodies can block invasion. The concept of erythrocyte and parasite receptors and their importance in invasion was developed by Miller and colleagues and has recently been reviewed.[81]

The 195-kD Protein of *P. falciparum*

The major component on the surface of merozoites of *P. falciparum* is a 195,000-molecular-weight (195-kD) glycoprotein.[82] Analogous proteins are present on other species of malaria.[83] The analogous antigen of *P. knowlesi* is synthesized during schizogony and is inserted into the membrane of schizonts as an intact protein.[84,85] At or near the time of erythrocyte rupture and merozoite release, the 230-kD protein of *P. knowlesi* or the 195-kD protein of *P. falciparum* is proteolytically degraded to lower-molecular-weight peptides, which appear on the surface of the merozoite.[86–88] The functional significance of this proteolytic processing is unknown.

Murine monoclonal antibodies against this glycoprotein can block invasion in vitro, but high concentrations of antibody are required.[79,84] A murine monoclonal antibody against the analogous protein of *P. yoelli* (a murine malarial parasite) protected animals on passive transfer.[89] Specific domains of this large protein may be more important than other domains as targets of immunity; specific subclasses of immunoglobulins may be more protective than others; and/or the mechanism of protection on passive transfer may involve antibody-dependent, cell-mediated immunity. Human monoclonal antibodies against Pf 195 appear to block invasion at low concentrations (10 μg/ml).[90] It is possible that these human monoclonal antibodies recognize more crucial epitopes than most murine monoclonal antibodies.

Mice immunized with the analogous protein of *P. yoelli* were protected against subsequent infection,[91] but protection could not be passively transferred with serum and was probably due to cell-mediated mechansims.[92] Immunization of *Aotus* monkeys with the 195-kD protein produced partial protection.[93–96] The 195-kD protein has been shown to be highly variant among strains, and immunity induced with this antigen appears to be strain-specific.[96]

Genes coding for the Pf 195 protein of different strains have been cloned and sequenced.[97,98] These genes have repeat regions, which vary from strain to strain, and constant regions, which are shared among strains. Experiments with synthetic peptides corresponding to different regions of the molecules should clarify which, if any, region is involved in invasion-blocking immunity and whether regions shared among strains can induce protective immunity.

An Antigen of Ring-Infected Erythrocytes

Perlman et al. identified and characterized a 155-kD antigen by immunofluorescence using immune sera and glutaraldehyde-fixed, air-dried infected erythrocytes.[99] The antigen appears in the erythrocyte membrane of ring-infected cells and in micronemes of merozoites.[100] (*Micronemes* are small apical organelles adjacent to the larger organelles called *rhoptries* and may play a role in invasion.) Morphologic studies indicate that the contents of rhoptries are released into the erythrocyte membrane at the time of invasion, during which the 155-kD antigen is thought also to be inserted into erythrocyte membrane during invasion. Human oligospecific antisera and human monoclonal antibodies against the 155-kD antigen inhibit invasion in vitro at low concentrations (below 10 μg/ml).[101] The gene for this antigen has been cloned and sequenced by Coppel et al. and consists in part of tandemly repeated sequences.[102] In the strains studied thus far this antigen does not appear to be variant. Recombinant 155-kD protein was used to immunize *Aotus* monkeys, which were subsequently challenged with blood-stage parasites of *P. falciparum*.[103] Some of the immunized monkeys but none of the control monkeys were protected against overwhelming infection.

A Glycophorin-Binding Antigen

Sialic acid on the erythrocyte membrane is important for optimal invasion by *P. falciparum* parasites.[81] Glycophorin A is the major sialoglycoprotein of the erythrocyte membrane and as such provides a large number of sialic residues with which the parasite can interact. En(a-) erythrocytes, which lack glycophorin A, are partially resistant to invasion.[104,105] Glycophorin A coupled to aminoethyl polyacrylamide beads has been used by Perkins for affinity purification of a 130-kD protein of *P. falciparum*.[106] The gene for the 130-kD antigen has been cloned and sequenced and consists of tandemly repeated sequences of 50 amino acids, which appear to contain the domain necessary for binding to glycophorin A.[107] A recent study indicates that the 130-kD antigen may bind to aminoethyl polyacrylamide without coupled glycophorin A because of charge-charge interactions.[108] The specificity of binding of the 130-kD protein to glycophorin A requires further clarification. It is not yet known whether this protein binds to intact erythrocytes. Other glycophorin-binding antigens prepared by glycophorin A coupled to Sepharose,[109] have been described; they include 140-kD, 70-kD, and 35-kD proteins. Specific antisera to these proteins are not yet available, and it is also unknown whether they bind to intact erythrocytes.

Erythrocyte-Binding Antigens

Intact erythrocytes have been used as affinity substrates to identify potential parasite receptors. A 175-kD antigen binds to erythrocytes of humans, *Aotus* monkeys, squirrel monkeys, and chimpanzees, all of which are susceptible to invasion by *P. falciparum*[110]; it does not bind to erythrocytes of rabbits or guinea pigs, both of which are resistant to invasion by *P. falciparum*. Binding of the 175-kD antigen to human erythrocytes can be prevented by pretreating the erythrocytes with neuraminidase or trypsin, both of which reduce invasion.

Chymotrypsin treatment of human erythrocytes, which does not reduce invasion, has no effect on the binding of this antigen. Further evaluation of the 175-kD antigen as a possible receptor for sialic acid–dependent ligands on the erythrocyte membrane will require a monospecific antiserum against this antigen.

Many malarial proteins of one species have analogous proteins in other species. For example, all malarial species examined thus far have a CSP and a major protein on the surface of the merozoite (e.g., Pf 195 in *P. falciparum* is analogous to Pk 230 in *P knowlesi*). If the 175-kD protein of *P. falciparum* is a receptor, it seems reasonable that *P. knowlesi* should have an analogous protein but with a different receptor specificity. Merozoites of *P. knowlesi* invade sialic acid–deficient erythrocytes with normal or increased efficiency but are unable to invade human erythrocytes that lack the Duffy blood group antigens. It has been hypothesized that *P. knowlesi* produces a protein (analogous to the 175-kD protein of *P. falciparum*) that binds specifically to Duffy-positive erythrocytes (including those treated with neurominidase or trypsin) but not to Duffy-negative erythrocytes or chymotrypsin-treated erythrocytes that lack the Duffy antigens. Such a molecule (135-kD) was recently identified by Haynes et al,[111] and was also shown to bind specifically to the Duffy glycoprotein immobilized on nitrocellulose. The studies on the 175-kD protein of *P. falciparum* and the 135-kD protein of *P. knowlesi* complement one another in suggesting that these proteins may be receptors.

Two Receptors

Although sialic acid on the erythrocyte membrane is required for optimal invasion by *P. falciparum* parasites, Mitchell et al. identified a strain of *P. falciparum* that can invade erythrocytes by a sialic acid–independent pathway.[112] This strain, designated the Thai-Tn strain, showed only a 50 percent reduction in invasion with neurominidase-treated erythrocytes, in contrast to the usual 90 percent or greater reduction obtained with the Camp strain and other strains reported in the literature. The 7G8 clone of the Brazilian IT strain is similar to the Thai-Tn strain in that it invades neurominidase-treated erythrocytes with 50 percent efficiency compared with normal erythrocytes.

The 7G8 strain and the Camp strain were used to study invasion of M^kM^k erythrocytes, which lack glycophorins A and B.[113] Glycophorins A and B have been proposed as ligands on the erythrocyte membrane involved in invasion. Invasion rates with 7G8 parasites and M^kM^k erythrocytes were 50 percent of those with normal erythrocytes; whereas invasion rates with Camp parasites and M^kM^k were 20 percent of those with normal erythrocytes. Similar results were obtained with En(a-) erythrocytes, which lack only glycophorin A. Thus, both 7G8 and Camp parasites are able to invade in the absence of glycophorins A and B. When M^kM^k erythrocytes were treated with neuraminidase, invasion by Camp parasites was reduced by 90 percent compared with untreated M^kM^k erythrocytes, whereas invasion by 7G8 parasites was unaffected. When M^kM^k

erythrocytes were treated with trypsin, invasion by 7G8 parasites was reduced by 90 percent, whereas invasion by Camp parasites remained unaffected.

In summary, Camp parasites are heavily dependent on sialic acid for invasion. Optimal invasion occurs in the presence of the sialic acid on glycophorins A (and possibly B); however, in the absence of both glycophorins the parasite is able to utilize sialic acid elsewhere on the membrane. These other sites are not sensitive to degradation by trypsin and may be located on glycolipids. 7G8 parasites also utilize the sialic acid of glycophorins A (and possibly B) but are able to invade efficiently in the absence of both sialic acid and glycophorins A and B. 7G8 parasites may have two receptors, one for silaic acid and another for a sialic acid–independent site that is sensitive to degradation by trypsin and is located on a protein other than glycophorin A or B. Recent invasion studies with glycophorin C–deficient cells suggest that the sialic acid–independent ligand is not located on glycophorin C either (F. Klotz, unpublished data). The sialic acid–independent trypsin-sensitive site has not yet been identified.

The data indicating that parasites have more than one receptor have implications for vaccine development. If parasite receptors are to be used as immunogens, both the sialic acid–dependent and the sialic acid–independent receptors must be identified.

Rhoptry Components

Rhoptries are apical organelles of the merozoite, which secrete components into the erythrocyte membrane during invasion. Prior to invasion the erythrocyte membrane undergoes a wave of deformation, and a vacuole is formed into which the parasite moves. Rhoptry components appear to play a role in these processes, and they are accessible to antibody, they may be targets of invasion-blocking immunity. Monoclonal antibodies have been produced that react with rhoptry components. Some monoclonal antibodies react with an 80- to 40-kD doublet by immunoprecipitation; others react with a 150- to 140-kD doublet.[114] Further work is required to evaluate these antigens as immunogens.

Endothelial-Binding Ligand

Udeinya et al. developed an in vitro model for sequestration whereby trophozoite- and schizont-infected erythrocytes bind to cultured endothelial cells and melanoma cells.[115,116] Only strains that produce knobs on the erythrocyte membrane bind. This in vitro observation correlates with electron microscopic studies showing that in infected *Aotus* monkeys knobs constituted the points of attachment between infected erythrocytes and endothelial cells.[117,118] Knobless strains, which have been produced in the laboratory by long-term in vitro culture, do not bind to endothelial or melanoma cells. Some knobby strains also do not bind, which indicates that a membrane component, termed the *endothelial-binding ligand,* is necessary for binding, in addition to knobs. Immune sera had previously been shown to react with knob-associated antigen by immunoelectron microscopy.[120,121] Udeinya et al. showed that binding of infected erythrocytes to endothelial cells could be inhibited or reversed by sera from immune monkeys.[30] This effect was strain-specific, that is, immune sera from a monkey infected with one strain of *P. falciparum* inhibited binding of the homologous strain but not of heterologous strains. This finding indicated that the endothelial binding ligand is strain-variant.

A major component of knobs is the 88kD histidine-rich protein (HRP) identified by Kilejian and shown to be present in strains that produce knobs but not in strains that do not produce knobs.[122] Leech et al. showed that knobs, as defined by electron microscopy, and the 88-kD histidine-rich protein behaved similarly in terms of their extractability in various detergents.[123] Both were present in the insoluble pellet after extraction in Triton X 100 and appear to be associated with the erythrocyte cytoskeleton. There is no clear evidence that the histidine-rich protein is exposed on the surface of infected erythrocytes, and although it appears to be a component of knobs, it does not per se appear to be the endothelial-binding ligand.

Leech et al. also demonstrated that treatment of trophozoite- and schizont-infected erythrocytes with low concentrations of trypsin (1 μg/ml) prevents their binding to melanoma cells.[29] In the same study a 250- to 300-kD protein was identified, which is located on the surface of infected trophozoites and schizonts, is sensitive to degradation by low concentrations of trypsin, and is strain-variant. Aley et al. demonstrated that this protein could be labeled by surface iodination on erythrocytes infected with knob-forming but not knobless parasites.[124] The evidence thus far is consistent with this molecule being the endothelial-binding ligand.

Although the endothelial-binding ligand is variant, it may have a constant domain which is the site of interaction with endothelial cells. Antibodies against such a domain should block binding by all strains. If binding of infected erythrocytes to endothelial cells can be prevented, parasites would have to circulate through the spleen, which would adversely affect the parasites and probably lower parasitemia.

David et al. showed that reversal of sequestration occurred in infected squirrel monkeys infused with immune sera and was accompanied by a drop in parasitemia.[31] They also observed that parasites passaged in splenectomized monkeys lost their ability to bind to melanoma cells.[31] The endothelial-binding ligand therefore not only is a promising candidate for a vaccine but also may be useful in investigating the ability of the parasite to modulate expression of its antigens.

Barnwell et al. showed that monoclonal antibodies against a 88-kD antigen on the surface of endothelial cells blocks binding in vitro.[125] It appears likely that this antigen is the molecule to which parasitized erythrocytes bind in vivo. Parasitized erythrocytes also bind specifically to thrombospondin, a molecule present in various cells, including endothelial cells and platelets.[126] Only parasites that produce knobs bind; knobless variants do not. The precise role of thrombospondin in the binding of parasitized erythrocytes to endothelial surfaces has not yet been defined.

Marsh and Howard recently used immune sera from individuals in west Africa and an agglutination assay with infected erythrocytes to demonstrate antigenic diversity among isolates of a trypsin-sensitive antigen on the surface of infected erythrocytes.[17] Convalescent sera from recently infected children agglutinated their own parasitized erythrocytes but not those of other children in the village. In contrast, immune sera from adults agglutinated most children's parasitized erythrocytes. Antibodies from adult immune sera that had been bound and eluted from parasitized erythrocytes of one child reacted with infected erythrocytes from all children. This finding suggests that adult immune sera contain antibodies against a domain shared by all parasites. If so, such a constant domain may be a target of protective immunity. The antigen responsible for agglutination in this study may be the endothelial-binding ligand, although this has not yet been established.

S Antigens

Wilson[129] identified and characterized S antigens, which are found in the sera of infected individuals and in culture supernatants and are heat-stable and antigenically diverse. They have been further characterized by Anders et al. and Winchell et al., and the gene coding for an S antigen was cloned and sequenced by Coppel et al.[128–130] The sequence was the first demonstration of a tandem repeat in a malarial antigen and was soon followed by demonstration of tandem repeats in the CSP of *P. knowlesi*, and tandem repeats have now been demonstrated in many malarial antigens. Antigens with tandem repeats may be more readily identified by screening DNA libraries because they give strong signals when probed with antisera or DNA probes. However, tandemly repeated sequences (and therefore epitopes) appear to be so characteristic of malarial antigens that they must have some as yet undetermined function important to parasite survival.

The function of S antigens, like the function of most malarial antigens identified to date, is unknown. The S antigens appear to be located within the parasitophorous vacuole and may be released at the time of rupture. Their antigenic diversity suggests they may be a target of immunity. A monoclonal antibody against a 220-kD S antigen of a strain from Papua New Guinea blocked invasion when incubated with mature schizont-infected erythrocytes of the same strain.[131] The mechanism of blockade is unknown, but this effect suggests that some S-antigen molecules may bind to the surface of the merozoite.

Histidine-Rich Proteins

Three HRPs are synthesized by *P. falciparum* parasites; these have been designated HRP I, HRP II, and HRP III.[7,8,123,132] HRP I was first identified by Kilejian and shown to be associated with knobs on the membrane of infected erythrocytes involved in cytoadherence (see section on endothelial-binding ligands).[122] Both HRP II and HRP III are soluble and can be detected in the medium of cultured parasites.[7,8,123,132] The genes for HRP II and HRP III have been cloned, and their high degree of homology indicates that they arose through gene duplication.[7,8] The functions of HRP II and III are unknown although there are indications that parasites that possess HRP II multiply more effectively in vitro than variants that lack it.[8]

Transmission-Blocking Immunity

Carter and Gwadz developed the concept and the experimental evidence for transmission-blocking immunity.[133–135] They immunized animals with gametes, then infected them with malaria and found that when mosquitos fed on these animals, oocysts did not appear in the guts of the mosquitoes. Further studies showed that antigamete antibodies ingested by the mosquito with the blood meal interfered with fertilization or with subsequent development of the gamete. These experiments form the basis of a potentially important way of interfering with the transmission of malaria. Transmission-blocking immunity would not protect against malaria once an individual is infected, but it would prevent transmission of the infection to other individuals. Antigenic diversity of gamete antigens appears to be very limited, probably because these antigens have not been under the kind of immune pressure exerted on many blood-stage antigens. Transmission-blocking immunity can be boosted by blood-stage infections, and recent evidence indicates that target antigens of transmission-blocking immunity are present in gametocytes.[136,137] Mendis et al. demonstrated that transmission-blocking immunity against *P. vivax* can result from naturally acquired infections, suggesting that gametocytes contain the effective immunogens.[137] Target antigens of transmission-blocking immunity have been identified by monoclonal antibodies, and current investigation is directed towards cloning the genes for these antigens. In addition to decreasing the incidence of malaria in a population, transmission-blocking immunity may also prevent transmission of mutant blood-stage parasites that have become resistant to a drug or to vaccine-induced immunity.

Antigenic Variation

P. knowlesi parasites incorporate a protein into the erythrocyte membrane that is exposed on the erythrocyte surface and forms the schizont-infected cell surface antigen (SICA). This protein clearly undergoes antigenic variation during the course of *P. knowlesi* infections in rhesus monkeys, as has been demonstrated with cloned parasites.[49] Furthermore, expression of this protein is lost when cloned parasites are introduced into splenectomized monkeys.[49] Loss of the antigen occurs rapidly and may be due to an induced genotypic switching rather than to selection of a random mutation. Antigenic variation of SICAs has also been demonstrated during the course of chronic infections with *P. falciparum* in squirrel monkeys.[47] Furthermore, *P. falciparum*–infected erythrocytes that bind to endothelial cells in vitro lose their capacity for cytoadherence when passaged in splenectomized squirrel monkeys.[31] The cytoadherence molecule, which may be the high-molecular-weight protein identified by Leech et al., appears to be analogous to the SICA of *P. knowlesi*.[29] It is important to note that both *P. knowlesi* and *P. falciparum* can alter erythrocyte surface antigens during the course of infections, and this provides the parasite with a mechanism for circumventing immunity targeted against these antigens.

There is now evidence that malaria parasites can also alter merozoite-associated antigens in response to immune pressure. Miller et al. demonstrated that antibodies against the 140-kD merozoite surface protein of *P. knowlesi* (a monkey parasite) could block invasion in vitro.[138] David et al. immunized rhesus monkeys with purified 140-kD antigen and demonstrated that this antigen undergoes alteration in response to immune pressure so that it is no longer recognized by protective antibodies.[48] Two of four immunized monkeys developed a chronic low-level parasitemia when infected with *P. knowlesi,* in contrast to control animals (and two immunized animals), which developed high parasitemias requiring treatment. Parasites obtained from the partially protected monkeys with chronic parasitemias were antigenically different from parasites of the parent isolate used to infect the monkeys and were termed *variants*. Sera from monkeys and rabbits immunized with the 140-kD protein blocked invasion of erythrocytes by the parent isolate but not by the variant isolate. Further immunochemical analysis revealed that variant parasites did not possess the 140-kD antigen but instead had several alternate forms of this antigen of various molecular weights. The multiplicity of variants probably reflected the presence of multiple different clones within the variant population. Whether these variants were present at low levels in the parent isolate, whether they arose by mutation and selection during the course of the infection, or whether they were induced by immune pressure has not yet been determined. The study by Klotz et al. using cloned parasites suggests that the 140-kD variants arise by mutation and selection during the infection.[50] This variation occurs independently of the variation of the SICA and probably by a different genetic mechanism. These studies make it clear that potential targets of immunity can vary under immune pressure, a fact that will greatly complicate development of a vaccine. Based on the work of Miller et al., David et al., and Klotz et al., the 140-kD antigen of *P. knowlesi* now affords a model system in which the genetic mechanisms of antigenic variation by the parasite can be studied.[37,48,50]

Summary

Our overall perspective on a malaria vaccine is that it will include regions of the CSP and determinants on merozoites, on infected erythrocytes, and on gametes. Our optimism regarding the development of a vaccine has been tempered by emerging data on polymorphism and antigenic variation in malaria antigens, especially blood-stage antigens. Blood-stage parasites have had to survive in the mainstream of the host's immune system, and antigenic polymorphism and antigenic variation are probably two of several strategies that they have developed to evade host defense mechanisms.[4] It will be important to define constant domains of variant molecules and to determine whether such domains can be targets of effective immunity. Domains involved in cell-cell interaction (e.g., domains that bind to erythrocytes during invasion or to endothelial cells during sequestration) are likely to be constant and need to be identified. Constant domains of the endothelial binding ligand may be especially promising as this molecule is exposed to the immune system for prolonged periods during the life cycle. Constant domains of Pf 195 also need to be explored, as this is the major antigen on the surface of the merozoite and its polymorphism suggests that it is a target of immune pressure.

Recent studies have emphasized the importance of T-helper cell epitopes in the induction of immunity.[72,73] Also, recent data from field studies and work with a mouse malaria model have underscored the importance of cell-mediated immunity in protection against sporozoite-induced infection. Most in vitro work has centered on inhibitory effects of antibodies (e.g., inhibition of growth and of parasite invasion of erythrocytes or hepatocytes). Such assays do not detect antibody-independent immunity or antibody-dependent cell-mediated immunity. Optimal in vitro assays have not yet been developed for detecting cell-mediated immunity in malaria, which may best be studied in rodent malarias at present. Also, little is known of immunity against hepatic stages, and work is now beginning to explore this "neglected" stage.

Because of the complexities in developing an antimalaria vaccine, it is imperative that research efforts be continued in the field of antimalarial chemotherapy. The increasing prevalence of chloroquine-resistant *P. falciparum* represents a major threat to developing countries. Recent work on the reversal of chloroquine resistance by verapamil may be an important step in understanding this problem.[9]

Ultimately, control of malaria will probably require a multifaceted approach, involving immunization, chemotherapy, mosquito eradication, and perhaps even the genetic manipulation of mosquito populations to make them resistant to malaria.[139] Methods of modern biology are just beginning to give us new insights into this ancient disease.

REFERENCES

1. Clyde DF, McCarthy VC, Miller RM, Woodward WE: Immunization of man against falciparum and vivax malaria by use of irradiated sporozoites. Am J Trop Med Hyg 24:397, 1975
2. Miller LH, David PH, Hadley TJ: Perspectives for malaria vaccination. Philos Trans R Soc Lond [Biol] 307:99, 1984
3. Miller LH, Howard RJ, Carter R, et al: Research toward malaria vaccines. Science 234:1349, 1986

4. Howard RJ: Vaccination against malaria: recent advances and the problems of antigenic diversity and other parasite evasion mechanisms. Int J Parasitol 17:17, 1987
5. Siddiqui WA, Kan SC, Kramer K, et al: Use of a synthetic adjuvant in an effective vaccination of monkeys against malaria. Nature 289:64, 1981
6. Walliker D, Quakyi IA, Wellems TE: Genetic analysis of the human malaria parasite *Plasmodium falciparum*. Science 236:1661, 1987
7. Wellems TE, Howard RJ: Homologous genes encode two distinct histidine-rich proteins in a clone isolate of *Plasmodium falciparum*. Proc Natl Acad Sci USA 83:6065, 1986
8. Wellems TE, Howard RJ: Homologous genes encode two distinct histidine-rich proteins in a clone isolate of *Plasmodium falciparum*. Proc Natl Acad Sci USA 83:6065, 1986
9. Martin SK, Osuola AM, Milhous WK: Reversal of chloroquine resistance in *Plasmodium falciparum* by verapamil. Science 235:899, 1987
10. McGregor IA, Gilles HM, Walters JH, et al: Effects of heavy and repeated malarial infections in Gambian infants and children: effects of erythrocytic parasitization. Br Med J 2:686, 1956
11. Maegraith BH: Malaria. p. 27. In Woodruff AW (ed): Medicine in the Tropics. Churchill Livingstone, Edinburgh, 1974
12. Wyler DJ: Malaria—resurgence, resistance and research. N Engl J Med 308:934, 1983
13. James SP, Nicol WD, Shate PG: A study of induced malignant tertial malaria. Proc R Soc Med 25:1153, 1932
14. Boyd MF, Stratman-Thomas WK, Kitchens SF: On acquired immunity to *Plasmodium falciparum*. Am J Trop Med Hyg 16:139, 1936
15. Boyd MF, Stratman-Thomas WK: Studies on benign tertian malaria. I. On the occurrence of acquired tolerance to *Plasmodium vivax*. Am J Hyg 17:55, 1933
16. Sadun EH, Hickman RL, Wellele BT, et al: Active and passive immunization of chimpanzees infected with west African and southeast Asian strains of *Plasmodium falciparum*. Milit Med 131:1250, 1966
17. Marsh K, Howard RJ: Antigens induced on erythrocytes by *P. falciparum:* expression of diverse and conserved determinants. Science 231:150, 1985
18. McBride JS, Walliker D, Morgan G: Antigenic diversity in the human malaria parasite *Plasmodium falciparum*. Science 217:254, 1982
19. McBride JS, Newbold CS, Arnand R: Polymorphism of a high molecular weight schizont antigen of the human malaria parasite *Plasmodium falciparum*. J Exp Med 161:160, 1985
20. Taylor DW, Siddiqui WA: Recent advances in malarial immunity. Annu Rev Med 33:64, 1982
21. Perrin LH, Dayal R: Immunity to asexual erythrocytic stages of *Plasmodium falciparum:* role of defined antigens in the humoral response. Immunol Rev 61:245, 1982
22. Cohen S, McGregor IA, Carrington SC: Gamma globulin and acquired immunity to human malaria. Nature 192:733, 1961
23. Diggs CL, Osler AG: Humoral immunity in rodent malaria. II. Inhibition of parasitemia by serum antibody. J Immunol 102:298, 1969
24. Cohen S, Butcher GA, Crandall RB: Action of malaria antibody in vitro. Nature 223:368, 1969
25. Miller LH, Aikawa M, Dvorak JA: Malaria (*Plasmodium knowlesi*) merozoites: immunity and the surface coat. J Immunol 114:1237, 1975

26. Chulay JD, Aikawa MK, Diggs C, Haynes JD: Inhibitory effects of immune monkey serum on synchronized *Plasmodium falciparum* cultures. Am J Trop Med Hyg 30:12, 1981
27. Howard RJ, Barnwell JW, Kao V: Antigenic variation in *Plasmodium knowlesi* malaria: identification of the variant antigen on infected erythrocytes. Proc Natl Acad Sci USA 80:4129, 1983
28. Howard RJ: Alteration in the surface membrane of red blood cells during malaria. Immunol Rev 61:67, 1982
29. Leech JH, Barnwell JW, Miller LH, Howard RJ: Identification of a strain-specific malarial antigen exposed on the surface of *Plasmodium falciparum* infected erythrocytes. J Exp Med 159:1567, 1984
30. Udeinya IJ, Miller LH, McGregor IA, Jensen JB: *Plasmodium falciparum* strain-specific antibody blocks binding of infected erythrocytes to amelonotic melanoma cells. Nature 303:429, 1983
31. David PH, Hommel M, Miller LH, et al: Parasite sequestration in *Plasmodium falciparum* malaria: spleen and antibody modulation of cytoadherence of infected erythrocytes. Proc Natl Acad Sci USA 80:5075, 1983
32. Butcher GA, Mitchell GH, Cohen S: Antibody-mediated mechanisms of immunity to malaria induced by vaccination with *Plasmodium knowlesi*. Immunology 34:77, 1978
33. Quinn TC, Wyle DJ: Mechanisms of action of hyperimmune serum in mediating protective immunity to rodent malaria (*Plasmodium berghei*). J Immunol 123:2245, 1979
34. Ockenhouse CF, Schulman S, Shear HL: Induction of crisis forms in the human malaria parasite *Plasmodium falciparum* by γ-interferon-activated, monocyte-derived macrophages. J Immunol 133:1601, 1984
35. Grun JL, Weidanz WP: Immunity to *Plasmodium chabaudi adami* in the B-cell deficient mouse. Nature 290:143, 1981
36. Yoshida N, Nussenzweig RS, Potocnjak P, et al: Hybridoma produces protective antibodies directed against the sporozoite stage of malaria parasite. Science 207:71, 1980
37. Potocnjak R, Yoshida N, Nussenzweig RS, Nussenzweig V: Monovalent fragments (Fob) of monoclonal antibodies to a sporozoite surface antigen (Pb44) protect mice against malarial infection. J Exp Med 151:1504, 1980
38. Nardin EH, Nussenzweig RS, McGregory IA, Bryan JH: Antibodies to sporozoites: their frequent occurrence in individuals living in an area of hyperendemic malaria. Science 206:597, 1979
39. Hoffman SL, Wistar R, Ballou WR, et al: Immunity to malaria and naturally acquired antibodies to the circumsporozoite protein of *Plasmodium falciparum*. N Engl J Med 315:601, 1986
40. Hoffman SL, Oster CN, Plowe CV, et al: Naturally acquired antibodies to sporozoites do not prevent malaria: vaccine development implications. Science 237:639, 1987
41. Egan JE, Weber JL, Ballou WR, et al: Efficacy of murine malaria sporozoite vaccines: implications for human vaccine development. Science 236:453, 1987
42. Spitalny GL, Rivera-Ortiz C, Nussenzweig RS: *Plasmodium berghei:* the spleen in sporozoite-induced immunity to mouse malaria. Exp Parasitol 62:670, 1976
43. Verhave JP, Strickland GT, Jaffe HA, Ahmed A: Studies on the transfer of protective immunity with lymphoid cells from mice immune to malaria sporozoites. J Immunol 121:1031, 1978

44. Verhave JP, Meuwissen JH, Golenser J: Cell-mediated reactions and protection after immunization with sporozoites. Isr J Med Sci 14:611, 1978
45. Chen DH, Tigelaar RE, Weinbaum FI: Immunity to sporozoite-induced malaria infection in mice. I. The effect of immunization of T and B cell-deficient mice. J Immunol 118:1322, 1977
46. Ferreira A, Schofield L, Schellekens H, et al: Gamma interferon inhibits the development of exoerythrocytic forms of malaria parasites. Science 232:881, 1986
47. Hommel M, David PH, Oligino LD: Surface alterations of erythrocytes in *Plasmodium falciparum* malaria. Antigenic variation, antigenic diversity, and the role of the spleen. J Exp Med 157:1137, 1983
48. David PH, Hudson DE, Hadley TJ, et al: Immunization of monkeys with a 140 kilodalton merozoite surface protein of *Plasmodium knowlesi* malaria: appearance of alternate forms of this protein. J Immunol 134:4146, 1985
49. Barnwell JW, Howard RJ, Coon HA, Miller LH: Splenic requirement for antigenic variation and expression of the variant antigen on the erythrocyte membrane in clone *Plasmodium knowlesi* malaria. Infection 40:985, 1983
50. Klotz FW, Hudson DE, Coon HG, Miller LH: Vaccination induced variation in the 140 kD merozoite surface antigen of *Plasmodium knowlesi* malaria. J Exp Med 165:359, 1987
51. Weidanz WP: Malaria and alterations in immune reactivity. Br Med Bull 38:167, 1982
52. Orjih AU, Nussenzweig R: Plasmodium berghei suppression of antibody response to sporozoite stage by acute blood stage infection Clin Exp Immunol 38:1, 1979
53. Kemp DJ, Coppel RL, Cowman AF: Expression of *Plasmodium falciparum* blood-stage antigens in *Escherichia coli:* Detection with antibodies from immune sera. Proc Natl Acad Sci USA 80:3787, 1983
54. McCutchan TF, Hansen JL, Dame JB, Mullins JA: Mung bean nuclease cleaves *Plasmodium* genomic DNA at sites before and after genes. Science 224:625, 1984
55. Dame JB, Williams JL, McCutchan TF, et al: Structure of the gene encoding the immunodominant surface antigen in the sporozoite of the human malaria parasite *Plasmodium falciparum*. Science 225:593, 1984
56. Nussenzweig RS, Vanderberg JP, Most H, Orton C: Protective immunity produced by the injection of x-irradiated sporozoites of *Plasmodium berghei*. III. Specificity of the protection. Nature 222:488, 1969
57. Nussenzweig RS, Nussenzweig V: Development of sporozoite vaccines. Philos Trans R Soc London [Biol] 307:117, 1984
58. Nussenzweig RS, Vanderberg J, Most H: Protective immunity produced by the infection of x-irradiated sporozoites of *Plasmodium* berghei. IV. Dose response, specificity and humoral immunity. Milit Med 134:1176, 1969
59. Nussenzweig V, Nussenzweig RS: Circumsporozoite protein of malaria parasites. Cell 42:401, 1985
60. Nardin EH, Nussenzweig V, Nussenzweig RS, et al: Circumsporozoite proteins of human malaria parasites *Plasmodium falciparum* and *Plasmodium vivax*. J Exp Med 156:20, 1982
61. Ellis J, Ozaki LS, Govadz RW, et al: Cloning and expression in *E. coli* of the malaria sporozoite surface antigen gene from *Plasmodium knowlesi*. Nature 302:536, 1983
62. Ozaki LS, Svec P, Nussenzweig RS, et al: Structure of the *Plasmodium knowlesi* gene coding for the circumsporozoite protein. Cell 34:815, 1983
63. Enea V, Ellis J, Zavala F, et al: DNA cloning of *Plasmodium falciparum* circumsporozoite gene: amino acid sequence of repetitive epitope. Science 225:628, 1984

64. Zavala F, Cochrane AH, Nardin EH, et al: Circumsporozoite proteins of malaria parasites contain a single immunodominant region with two or more identical epitopes. J Exp Med 157:1947, 1983
65. Zavala F, Tam JP, Cochrane AH, et al: Rationale for development of a synthetic vaccine against *Plasmodium falciparum* malaria. Science 228:1436, 1985
66. Ballou WR, Rothbard J, Wirtz RA, et al: Immunogenicity of synthetic peptides from circumsporozoite protein of *Plasmodium falciparum*. Science 228:996, 1985
67. Mazier D, Mellouk S, Beaudoin RL, et al: Effect of antibodies to recombinant and synthetic peptides on *P. falciparum* sporozoites in vitro. Science 231:156, 1986
68. Hollingdale MR, Nardin EH, Savanat T: Inhibition of entry of *Plasmodium falciparum* and *P. vivax* sporozoites into cultured cells: an in vitro assay of protective antibodies. J Immunol 132:909, 1984
69. Ballou WR, Sherwood JA, Neva FA, et al: Safety and efficacy of a recombinant DNA *Plasmodium falciparum* sporozoite vaccine. Lancet 1:1277, 1987
70. Herrington DA, Clyde DF, Losonsky G, et al: Safety and immunogenicity in man of a synthetic peptide malaria vaccine against *Plasmodium falciparum* sporozoites. Nature 328:257, 1987
71. Young JF, Hockmeyer WT, Gross M, et al: Expression of *Plasmodium falciparum* circumsporozoite proteins in *Escherichia coli* for potential use in a human malaria vaccine. Science 228:958, 1985
72. Good MF, Berzofsky JA, Malay WL, et al: Genetic control of the immune response in mice to a *Plasmodium falciparum* sporozoite vaccine: widespread nonresponsiveness to single malaria T epitope in highly repetitive vaccine. J Exp Med 164:655, 1986
73. Good MF, Maloy WL, Lunde MN, et al: Construction of synthetic immunogen: use of new T-helper epitope on malaria circumsporozoite protein. Science 235:1059, 1987
74. Cochrane AH, Gwadz RW, Ojo-Amaize E, et al: Antigenic diversity of the circumsporozoite proteins in the *Plasmodium cynomolgi* complex. Mol Biochem Parasitol 14:111, 1985
75. Sharma S, Svec P, Mitchell GH, Godson GN: Diversity of circumsporozoite antigen genes from two strains of the malarial parasite *Plasmodium knowlesi*. Science 229:779, 1985
76. Sharma S, Gwadz RW, Schlesinger DH, Godson GN: Immunogenicity of the repetitive and nonrepetitive peptide regions of the divergent CS protein of *Plasmodium knowlesi*. J Immunol 137:357, 1986
77. Zavala F, Masuda A, Graves PM, et al: Ubiquity of the repetitive epitope of the CS protein in different isolates of human malaria parasites. J Immunol 135:2790, 1985
78. Weber JL, Hockmeyer WT: Structure of the circumsporozoite protein gene in 18 strains of *Plasmodium falciparum*. Mol Biochem Parasitol 15:305, 1985
79. Pirson PJ, Perkins M: Characterization with monoclonal antibodies of a surface antigen of *Plasmodium falciparum* merozoites. J Immunol 134:1946, 1985
80. Dvorak JA, Miller LH, Whitehouse WC, Shiroishi T: Invasion of erythrocytes by malaria parasites. Science 187:748, 1975
81. Hadley TJ, Klotz FW, Miller LH: Invasion of erythrocytes by malaria parasites: a cellular and molecular overview. Annu Rev Microbiol 40:451, 1986
82. Holder AA, Freeman RR: The three major antigens on the surface of *Plasmodium falciparum* merozoites are derived from a single high molecular weight precursor. J Exp Med 160:624, 1984
83. Holder AA, Freeman RR, Newbold CI: Serological cross-reaction between high

molecular weight proteins synthesized in blood schizonts of *Plasmodium yoelli, Plasmodium chabaudi* and *Plasmodium falciparum*. Mol Biochem Parasitol 14:293, 1983
84. Epstein N, Miller LH, Kaushel D, et al: Monoclonal antibodies against a specific surface determinant on malarial (*Plasmodium knowlesi*) merozoites block erythrocyte invasion. J Immunol 127:212, 1981
85. David PH, Hadley TJ, Aikawa M, Miller LH: Processing of a major surface glycoprotein occurs during the ultimate stages of differentiation in *Plasmodium knowlesi* malaria. Mol Biochem Parasitol 11:267, 1984
86. Holder AA, Freeman RR: Biosynthesis and processing of a *Plasmodium falciparum* schizont antigen recognized by immune serum and a monoclonal antibody. J Exp Med 156:1528, 1982
87. Lyon JA, Haynes JD: *Plasmodium falciparum* antigens synthesized by schizonts and stabilized at the merozoite surface when schizonts mature in the presence of protease inhibitors. J Immunol 136:2245, 1986
88. Lyon JA, Haynes, JD Diggs CL, et al: *Plasmodium falciparum* antigens synthesized and stabilized at the merozoite surface by antibodies when schizonts mature in the presence of growth inhibitory immune serum. J Immunol 136:2252, 1986
89. Majarian WR, Daly TM, Weidanz WP, Long CA: Passive immunization against murine malaria with an IgG3 monoclonal antibody. J Immunol 132:3131
90. Schmidt-Ullrich R, Brown J, Whittle H, Peck-Sun L: Human hybridomas secreting monoclonal antibodies to the Mr 195,000 *Plasmodium falciparum* blood stage antigen. J Exp Med 163:179, 1986
91. Holder AA, Freeman RR: Immunization against blood-stage rodent malaria using purified parasite antigens. Nature 294:361, 1981
92. Freeman RR, Holder AA: Characteristics of the protective responses of BALB/c mice immunized with a purified *Plasmodium yoelli* schizont antigen. Clin Exp Immunol 54:609, 1983
93. Perrin LH, Merkli B, Locke L, et al: Antimalarial immunity in Saimiri monkeys. Immunization with surface components of asexual blood stages. J Exp Med 160:441, 1984
94. Perrin LH, Loche M, Dedet JP, et al: Immunization against *Plasmodium falciparum* asexual blood stages using soluble antigens. Clin Exp Immunol 56:67, 1984
95. Dubois P, Dedet J-P, Fandur T et al: Protective immunization of the squirrel monkey against asexual blood stages of *Plasmodium falciparum* by use of parasite fractions. Proc Natl Acad Sci USA 81:229, 1984
96. Siddiqui WA, Tam LQ, Kramer KJ, et al: Merozoite surface coat precursor protein completely protects Aotus monkeys against *Plasmodium falciparum* malaria. Proc Natl Acad Sci USA 84:3014, 1987
97. Holder AA, Lockeyer MJ, Odink KG, et al: Primary structure of the precursor to the three major surface antigens of *Plasmodium falciparum* merozoites. Nature 317:270, 1985
98. Weber JL, Leininger WM, Lyon JA: Variation in the gene encoding a major merozoite surface antigen of the human malaria parasite *Plasmodium falciparum*. Nucleic Acids Res 14:3311, 1986
99. Perlman H, Berzins K, Wahlgren M, et al: Antibodies in malarial sera to parasite antigens in the membrane of erythrocytes infected with early asexual stages of *Plasmodium falciparum*. J Exp Med 159:1686, 1984
100. Brown GV, Culvenor JG, Crewther PE, et al: Localization of the ring-infected

erythrocyte surface antigen (RESA) of *Plasmodium falciparum* in merozoites and ring-infected erythrocytes. J Exp Med 162:774, 1985
101. Wahlin B, Wahlgren M, Perlman H, et al: Human antibodies to a Mr 155,000 Da *Plasmodium falciparum* antigen efficiently inhibit merozoite invasion. Proc Natl Acad Sci USA 81:7912, 1984
102. Coppel RL, Cowman AF, Anders RF, et al: A *Plasmodium falciparum* antigen present on the erythrocyte surface is composed of repeated amino acid sequences. Nature 310:789, 1984
103. Collins WE, Anders RF, Pappaioanou M, et al: Immunization of Aotus monkeys with recombinant proteins of an erythrocyte surface antigen of *Plasmodium falciparum*. Nature 323:259, 1986
104. Miller LH, Haynes JD, McAuliffe FM, et al: Evidence for differences in erythrocyte surface receptors for the malarial parasites, *Plasmodium falciparum* and *Plasmodium knowlesi*. J Exp Med 146:277, 1977
105. Pasvol G, Wainscot JS, Weatherall DJ: Erythrocytes deficient in glycophorin resist invasion by the malarial parasite *Plasmodium falciparum*. Nature 297:64, 1982
106. Perkins M: Surface proteins of *Plasmodium falciparum* merozoites binding to the erythrocyte receptor glycophorin. J Exp Med 160:788, 1984
107. Ravetch JV, Kochan J, Perkins M: Isolation of the gene for a glycophorin-binding protein implicated in erythrocyte invasion by a malaria parasite. Science 227:1593, 1985
108. Van Schravendijk MR, Wilson RJM, Newbold CI: Possible pitfalls in the identification of glycophorin-binding proteins of *Plasmodium falciparum*. J Exp Med 166:376, 1987
109. Jungery M, Boyle D, Patel T, et al: Lectin-like polypeptides of *Plasmodium falciparum* bind to red cell sialoglycoproteins. Nature 301:704, 1983
110. Camus D, Hadley, TJ: A *Plasmodium falciparum* antigen that binds to host erythrocytes and merozoites. Science 230:553, 1985
111. Haynes JD, Klotz FW, Miller LH: A 135 kilodalton receptor molecule from malaria binds to a human erythrocyte ligand associated with Duffy antigens and correlates with invasion. Clin Res 35:615A, 1987
112. Mitchell GH, Hadley TJ, Klotz FW, et al: Invasion of erythrocytes by *Plasmodium falciparum* malaria parasites: evidence for receptor heterogeneity and two receptors. Blood 67:1519, 1986
113. Hadley TJ, Klotz FW, Pasvol P, et al: *Falciparum malaria* parasites invade erythrocytes that lack glycophorin A and B (M^kM^k): strain differences indicate receptor heterogeneity and two pathways for invasion. J Clin Invest 80:1190, 1987
114. Campbell GH, Miller LH, Hufson D, et al: Monoclonal antibody characterization of *Plasmodium falciparum* antigens. Am J Trop Med Hyg 33:1051, 1984
115. Udeinya IJ, Schmidt JA, Aikawa M, et al: Falciparum malaria-infected erythrocytes specifically bind to cultured human endothelial cells. Science 213:555, 1981
116. Schmidt JA, Udeinya IJ, Leech JH, et al: *Plasmodium falciparum* malaria: an amelanotic melanoma cell line bears receptors for the knob ligand on infected erythrocytes. J Clin Invest 70:279, 1982
117. Rudzinska MA, Tager W: The fine structure of trophozoites and gametocytes in *Plasmodium coatneyi*. J Protozool 15:73, 1968
118. Luse SA, Miller LH: *Plasmodium falciparum* malaria. Ultrastructure of parasitized erythrocytes in cardiac vessels. Am J Trop Med Hyg 20:655, 1971

119. Udeinya IJ, Graves PM, Carter R, et al: *Plasmodium falciparum:* effect of time in continuous culture on binding to human endothelial cells and amelanotic melanoma cells. Exp Parasitol 56:207, 1983
120. Langreth SG, Reese RT: Antigenicity of the infected-erythrocyte and merozoite surfaces in falciparum malaria. J Exp Med 150:1241, 1979
121. Kilejian A, Abati A, Trager W: *Plasmodium falciparum* and *Plasmodium coatneyi:* immunogenicity of "knob-like" protrusions on infected erythrocyte membranes. Exp Parasitol 42:157, 1977
122. Kilejian A: Characterization of a protein correlated with the production of knob-like protrusions on membranes of erythrocytes infected with *Plasmodium falciparum.* Proc Natl Acad Sci USA 76:4650, 1979
123. Leech JH, Barnwell JW, Aikawa M, et al: *Plasmodium falciparum* malaria: association of knobs on the surface of infected erythrocytes with a histidine-rich protein and the erythrocyte skeleton. J Cell Biol 98:1256, 1984
124. Aley SB, Sherwood JA, Howard RJ: Knob-positive and knob-negative *Plasmodium falciparum* differ in expression of a strain-specific malarial antigen on the surface of infected erythrocytes. J Exp Med 160:1585, 1984
125. Barnwell JW, Ockenhouse CF, Knowles DM II: Monoclonal antibody OKM5 inhibits the in vitro binding of *Plasmodium falciparum*-infected erythrocytes to monocytes, endothelial and C32 melanoma cells. J Immunol 135:3494, 1985
126. Roberts DD, Sherwood JA, Spitalnik S, et al: Thrombospondin binds falciparum malaria parasitized erythrocytes and may mediate cytoadherence. Nature 318:64, 1985
127. Wilson RJM, McGregor, IA Hall P, et al: Antigens associated with *Plasmodium falciparum* infections in man. Lancet 2:201, 1969
128. Anders PF, Brown GV, Edwards A: Characterization of an S antigen synthesized by several isolates of *P. falciparum.* Proc Natl Acad Sci USA 80:6652, 1983
129. Winchell EJ, Ling I, Wilson RJM: Metabolic labelling and characterization of S-antigens, the heat stable strain-specific antigens of *Plasmodium falciparum.* Mol Biochem Parasitol 10:287, 1984
130. Coppel RL, Cowman AF, Lingelbach KR, et al: Isolate-specific S-antigen of *Plasmodium falciparum* contains a repeated sequence of eleven amino acids. Nature 306:751, 1983
131. Saul A, Cooper J, Ingram L, et al: Invasion of erythrocytes in vitro by *Plasmodium falciparum* can be inhibited by monoclonal antibody directed against an S-antigen. Parasite Immunol 7:587, 1985
132. Howard RJ, Uni S, Aikawa M, et al: Secretion of a malarial histidine-rich protein (Pf HRP II) from *Plasmodium falciparum* infected erythrocytes. J Cell Biol 103:1269, 1986
133. Carter R, Chen DH: Malaria transmission blocked by immunization with gametes of the malaria parasite. Nature 263:57, 1976
134. Carter R, Miller LH, Renner J et al: Target antigens in malaria transmission blocking immunity Phil Trans R Soc Lond [Biol] 307:201, 1984
135. Gwadz RW: Malaria: successful immunization against the sexual stages of *Plasmodium gallinaceum.* Science 193:1150, 1976
136. Gwadz RW, Koontz LC: *Plasmodium knowlesi:* persistence of transmission blocking immunity in monkeys immunized with gamete antigens. Infect Immun 44:137, 1984
137. Mendis KN, Munesinghe YD, de Silva YNY, et al: Malaria transmission blocking

immunity induced by natural infections of *Plasmodium vivax* in humans. Infect Immun 8:231, 1986
138. Miller LH, David PH, Hudson D, et al: Monoclonal antibodies to a 140,000-MW protein on *Plasmodium knowlesi* merozoites inhibit their invasion of rhesus erythrocytes. J Immunol 132:438, 1984
139. Collins FH, Sakai RK, Vernik KD, et al: Genetic selection of a *plasmodium*–refractory strain of the malaria vector *anopheles gambiae*. Science 234:607, 1986

18 Diagnosis, Treatment, and Prevention of Malaria Due to *Plasmodium falciparum*

Carolyn Petersen
James H. Leech

Plasmodium falciparum is the most important of the human malaria parasites because it causes the most morbidity and mortality and because it is resistant to many of the available antimalarial drugs. *Plasmodium vivax, Plasmodium ovale,* and *Plasmodium malariae* may cause considerable morbidity, but they rarely cause death and are usually sensitive to chloroquine, the most widely used antimalarial drug. In contrast, falciparum malaria in a nonimmune individual such as a traveler is a medical emergency, which demands prompt diagnosis, hospitalization, and treatment with appropriate drugs. In some imported cases of falciparum malaria, death has resulted from delayed diagnosis or improper treatment. Because of the clinical importance of *P. falciparum,* the focus of this chapter will be on the pathophysiology, clinical recognition, treatment, and prevention of falciparum malaria. The life cycle of malaria parasites is discussed in Chapter 17.

PATHOPHYSIOLOGY OF FALCIPARUM MALARIA

P. falciparum is the only malaria parasite that frequently kills its host. This fact has suggested to many observers that *P. falciparum* is an imperfect parasite since the death of the host is also harmful to the parasite. One potential explanation for the seemingly self-defeating virulence of *P. falciparum* is that it has only recently (in an evolutionary time frame) begun to infect humans and has not yet thoroughly adapted to its "new" host. There is now evidence to support this notion. Studies of the base composition and organization of DNA from various *Plasmodium* species showed that the less virulent *P. vivax* is closely related to malaria parasites of monkeys,[1] which suggests that *P. vivax* probably coevolved with humans (i.e., as humans evolved from lower primates, *P. vivax* evolved with them from a parasite of lower primates). In contrast, the DNA of *P. falciparum* is unlike that of other primate malaria parasites and is more like the DNA of a group of rodent and avian malaria parasites[1]. Thus, *P. falciparum* probably did not evolve from a malaria parasite of lower primates and may have infected humans much later in their evolutionary history, providing less time for the parasite to become adapted to its new host. Perhaps our species can look forward to a gradual decrease in the virulence of falciparum malaria.

The clinical manifestations of malaria are due to asexual blood-stage (erythrocytic) parasites. Sporozoites, exoerythrocytic (liver-stage) parasites, and gametocytes do not cause disease. The fundamental processes in the pathogenesis of falciparum malaria are:

1. The rupture of schizont-infected erythrocytes which destroys host erythrocytes and releases merozoites plus a multitude of parasite molecules into the bloodstream, some of which may be pyrogenic or toxic.
2. Cytoadherence between infected erythrocytes containing trophozoites and schizonts and the venular endothelium of the host, resulting in sequestration of infected erythrocytes within the postcapillary venules of several organs. Sequestration contributes to an increased survival of *P. falciparum* parasites, thereby causing higher parasitemias, and may cause obstruction of blood flow, alterations of the endothelium, or local metabolic derangements.
3. Host factors such as genetically determined resistance to malaria and acquired immunity.

Rupture of Schizont-Infected Erythrocytes

P. falciparum has a 48-hour life cycle within the host erythrocyte, during which the parasite develops from a small ring form into a larger, metabolically active trophozoite, divides asexually to produce a schizont, and finally ruptures the host erythrocyte, releasing 8 to 26 daughter merozoites, which invade erythrocytes and reinitiate the cycle. The principal consequences of the rupture of schizont-infected erythrocytes are production of fever and destruction of host erythrocytes. Fever is the classic manifestation of malaria and characteristically occurs as paroxysms separated by periods of normal temperature. The paroxysms of fever occur at the time of rupture and are probably caused by the release of unidentified pyrogens. The fever pattern is determined by the degree to which the parasites are synchronized. Occasionally, *P. falciparum* parasites are highly synchronized, rupture together, and produce a regular, intermittent fever every 48 hours. More commonly, however, *P. falciparum* infections are asynchronous, the parasites do not rupture together, and the fever pattern is irregular, daily, or continuous.

Hemolytic anemia is a common manifestation of falciparum malaria and is predominantly due to the destruction of host erythrocytes by rupturing schizonts. Indeed, a rapid fall in hematocrit is usually indicative of a high parasitemia. The severity of anemia, however, often appears to be disproportionate to the degree of parasitemia, and additional mechanisms may also contribute to anemia. It has been suggested that immune hemolysis has a role in the anemia of falciparum malaria,[2] but recent studies have not confirmed this and instead indicate that dyserythropoiesis during and immediately after acute malaria is more important.[3] Hemolysis may also be secondary to a Coombs-positive hemolytic anemia induced by quinine or to the administration of oxidant drugs such as primaquine to patients with glucose-6-phosphate dehydrogenase (G6PD) deficiency.

The intravascular destruction of erythrocytes may cause hemoglobinuria and renal failure (blackwater fever). However, acute tubular necrosis resulting from a variety of insults (shock, hemoconcentration, cortical anoxia) is probably a more common cause of renal failure in falciparum malaria.

Cytoadherence

The biology and immunology of cytoadherence are discussed in Chapter 17 in connection with the endothelial binding ligand. Briefly, erythrocytes containing trophozoite- and schizont-stage parasites develop surface protrusions (knobs) by which the infected erythrocytes adhere to the endothelium of postcapillary venules.[4] The mature parasites are thereby sequestered within the vasculature of host organs, especially the heart, brain, skeletal muscle, and intestine,[5] and avoid circulating through the spleen, which is a major site of parasite destruction in malaria.[6] By evading the spleen, *P. falciparum* parasites survive in greater numbers than other species of human malaria parasites and reach higher parasitemias. High parasitemias are associated with several complications of falciparum malaria, including severe anemia and renal failure, and one study[7] has reported that parasitemia is correlated with prognosis.

Besides aiding the survival of erythrocytic parasites, cytoadherence and sequestration have direct physiologic consequences on the host. The brain is the principal target organ, and the constellation of symptoms and signs is designated *cerebral malaria* and is the most common manifestation of severe falciparum malaria.[8] The symptoms of cerebral malaria are: (1) alterations in the level of consciousness, including coma; (2) focal nervous system disorders such as hemiparesis, movement disorders, and focal seizures; and (3) delirium or psychosis. These symptoms are usually reversible in patients who survive. The pathogenesis of cerebral malaria has not been clearly established. Pathologically, the cerebral venules are tightly packed with infected erythrocytes.[9] Studies in eastern Thailand demonstrated that the proportion of infected erythrocytes and the tightness of packing of these cells were higher in the vessels of the brain than in other organs where sequestration occurs.[9] Although infected erythrocytes have procoagulant activity,[10] platelets and intravascular thrombi were absent and there was no acute or chronic inflammation in the brains of patients dying with cerebral malaria.[9] Immune complexes were not identified.[9] Thus, the pathology of the brain in cerebral malaria is not consistent with intravascular coagulation, inflammatory mechanisms, or autoimmunity. In addition, the blood-brain barrier is intact,[11] and most patients do not have increased intracranial pressure.[12] One potential mechanism for the pathogenesis of cerebral malaria is a reduction in cerebral blood flow and decreased oxygen consumption by the brain secondary to the increased cerebral hematocrit caused by sequestration. Supporting this mechanism is the observation that comatose patients with cerebral malaria have cerebrospinal fluid lactic acidosis.[13] Other hypothesized mechanisms include damage to the endothelium caused by adherent infected erythrocytes; petechial hemorrhages proximal to sites of sequestration and obstruction; and localized hypoglycemia or lactic acidosis due to glycolytic metabolism by large numbers of sequestered parasites. The occurrence of cerebral malaria does not correlate with the level of parasitemia in the peripheral blood.

With high parasitemias, cytoadherence may also affect other organs. Diarrhea and malabsorption occasionally occur in falciparum malaria and may be caused by sequestration of infected erythrocytes within the venules of the small intestine.[14] Interestingly, there appear to be few if any cardiac manifestations of falciparum malaria despite the marked sequestration that occurs in the heart. Pulmonary edema does occur, often as a terminal event.[15] The pulmonary capillary wedge pressure is usually normal,[16] and there is evidence of injury to the endothelial cells of pulmonary capillaries,[15] the mechanism of which has not been determined.

Host Factors

It is generally assumed that acquired immunity (discussed in Ch. 17) protects against severe disease. Immunity is acquired slowly, may lapse after residence for several years outside of a malaria endemic area, and may be reduced during pregnancy, by treatment with corticosteroids or other immunosuppressive drugs, or by splenectomy. Iron deficiency may protect children from severe malaria, but the protective mechanism has not been established. Some patients who reside in endemic areas of Africa, Indonesia, and Papua New Guinea develop chronic massive splenomegaly and a lymphocytic infiltrate in the sinusoids of the liver (tropical splenomegaly).[17] Often, these patients have very high levels of antimalarial antibodies and no detectable parasites in their peripheral blood, but they may respond to treatment with antimalarials.[17] The pathogenesis of this syndrome is unknown.

Burkitt's lymphoma, a tumor of children in which B lymphocytes are infected with the Epstein-Barr virus (EBV), is common in areas of Africa where falciparum malaria is highly endemic. Although the reasons for this epidemiologic association between the two diseases are unknown, it has been shown that T-cell control of EBV-infected B cells is lost during infections with *P. falciparum,* leading to an abnormal proliferation of B cells and secretion of large amounts of antibody.[18] This observation may help explain the frequency of Burkitt's lymphoma and the high levels of antibody found in people living in areas where *P. falciparum* is endemic. Chronic malaria may prevent the host from having a normal immune response to antigenic challenges and thus cause a reduced response to certain antigens,[19] including vaccines,[20] and a greater chance of intercurrent infection during falciparum malaria.

Genetically determined resistance is one of the most interesting and poignant effects of malaria on mankind. Because *P. falciparum* is a common infection that kills children before they are able to reproduce, it has exerted an important selective pressure favoring mutant genes that confer some resistance to falciparum malaria. Many hemoglobinopathies, erythrocyte enzyme defects, and erythrocyte membrane defects occur predominantly in areas where malaria is endemic, suggesting that they have been selected because they provide some degree of protection against malaria.[21,22] The persistence of the gene for sickle hemoglobin as a balanced polymorphism among blacks of West African descent provides the best example of the selection of a mutant gene by an infectious disease.[22] Heterozygous sickle cell trait reduces the severity of falciparum malaria by inhibiting the intraerythrocytic parasites.[23] The thalassemias[24,25] and possibly G6PD deficiency[26,27] may exert a similar protective effect. Hereditary elliptocytosis reduces the deformability of the erythrocyte membrane[28] and inhibits the invasion of erythrocytes by merozoites.[29] The selection of these mutant genes is an important legacy of falciparum malaria that will continue to affect mankind for generations even if malaria is ultimately eradicated.

CLINICAL RECOGNITION OF FALCIPARUM MALARIA

Malaria is the most common severe acute febrile illness imported into the United States and should be the first diagnostic consideration in any ill traveler or immigrant who has been to or through an endemic area. Other causes of malaria in the United States include congenital malaria in the offspring of mothers from endemic areas; transfusion malaria from blood products or among intravenous drug users; and introduced cases in which anopheline mosquitoes become infected by feeding on a traveler or immigrant and proceed to infect other local residents. There was a major outbreak of introduced *P. vivax* malaria near San Diego, California in 1986.[30] The clinical manifestations and complications of falciparum malaria will be discussed first, followed by a suggested approach to the clinical recognition of falciparum malaria in travelers and immigrants.

Clinical Manifestations of Falciparum Malaria

Patients infected by mosquito bite usually have an incubation period of 8 to 25 days (average 12) before the onset of symptoms. However, chemoprophylaxis may prolong the incubation period to a month or more. The incubation period for transfusion malaria and congenital malaria is usually shorter since there is no exoerythrocytic stage. Before the onset of fever many patients have a prodrome of malaise, myalgia, headache, and cough, which is often mistaken for a viral illness. The most characteristic symptom is the paroxysm of a shaking chill followed by fever and then sweating. The fever of falciparum malaria is more often irregular than periodic, is frequently hectic, and in many patients is accompanied by nausea, vomiting, diarrhea, headache, abdominal pain, or delirium. Some patients may be remarkably asymptomatic between paroxysms. Although falciparum malaria in nonimmune individuals usually produces a profound, acute illness, individuals with some acquired immunity (such as immigrants from endemic areas) may have a more indolent course. In untreated or inadequately treated patients, *P. falciparum* usually persists for 100 to 200 days, although some infections have lasted for 3 to 4 years. During chronic infections the parasitemia may rise and fall periodically, and symptoms usually coincide with the increases. Exacerbations may be temporally related to intercurrent illness or surgery.

On physical examination many patients have splenomegaly and liver tenderness. Scleral icterus or jaundice may occur with severe hemolysis. Lymphadenopathy and rash are not caused by malaria. Patients usually have a normochromic, normocytic anemia, modest leukopenia, and thrombocytopenia; hyponatremia is common; and the urine may contain free hemoglobin. Transaminases may be elevated to three or four times the normal value, but higher levels should suggest another disease, such as hepatitis. The serum glucose should be checked since hypoglycemia is increasingly being recognized as a major complication of falciparum malaria,[31,32] especially in pregnancy.[33]

Complications of Falciparum Malaria

Cerebral malaria is the most important complication of falciparum malaria and probably accounts for 80 percent of malaria deaths.[8] The occurrence of cerebral malaria does not necessarily correlate with the degree of parasitemia, and some patients with low parasitemias have developed cerebral symptoms. As discussed above, patients may have an encephalopathy, seizures, or, less commonly, focal neurologic abnormalities. It must be emphasized that cerebral malaria is a diagnosis of exclusion, and other potential causes of cerebral symptoms, such as hypolgycemia, transient postictal coma, meningitis, brain abscess, and encephalitis must be excluded. Neck rigidity and photophobia are rare in cerebral malaria. Retinal hemorrhages have been identified in about 15 percent of cases,[34] but papilloedema is very rare[8] and should suggest another diagnosis, such as a brain abscess or other space-occupying lesion. Some patients have dysconjugate gaze, but pupillary, corneal, oculocephalic, and oculovestibular reflexes are normal.[8] Muscle tone and tendon reflexes are increased, and the Babinski response is usually extensor bilaterally.[8] The cerebrospinal fluid (CSF) opening pressure is usually normal.[12] The CSF may contain small numbers of lymphocytes and a slightly elevated protein concentration.[12] However, there is no compromise of the blood-brain barrier, and computed tomographic (CT) brain scanning has indicated that most patients have no evidence of cerebral edema.[35] Thus, there is no rationale for use of corticosteroids or osmotically active drugs such as mannitol in the treatment of cerebral malaria, and dexamethasone has been demonstrated to lack efficacy in these patients.[12] Of those who survive, fewer than 5 percent have neurologic sequelae.[8]

Patients with high parasitemias are at great risk of severe hemolytic anemia and renal failure. When renal failure occurs, uremia progresses very rapidly owing to the severely catabolic state of patients with falciparum malaria. Although jaundice is common in patients with hemolysis, hepatic failure is exceedingly rare. Hypoglycemia appears to be a very common complication of severe falciparum malaria[31–33]; in most adult patients its onset follows administration of quinine and is probably due to the release of insulin from the pancreas, which is stimulated by quinine,[31] but pregnant women and children may become hypoglycemic with low or normal insulin levels and without receiving quinine.[32,33] Some patients with falciparum malaria have malabsorption,[14] which may affect the efficacy of orally administered drugs.[36] Pulmonary edema is a terminal event in many patients.

Falciparum malaria in pregnancy increases the chances of stillbirth or a low-birth-weight infant, especially in primiparous women,[8] and is an important cause of maternal death in the tropics.[33]

Clinical Recognition and Diagnosis of Falciparum Malaria

Patients with malaria usually have fever or history of a fever, but occasionally they may present with flu-like symptoms, cough, diarrhea, or cerebral symptoms. As discussed previously, fever patterns of all kinds may be seen. The diagnosis of malaria requires the identification of malaria parasites on Giemsa-stained blood smears, which should be examined immediately and every 6 to 12 hours until the diagnosis is confirmed or rejected. Parasites may not be observed on some blood smears because nonimmune patients may have symptoms with very low parasitemias and because sequestration of *P. falciparum* parasites may produce marked fluctuations in the number of parasites in the peripheral circulation. Although thick smears permit more blood to be screened in less time, they require greater experience on the part of the microscopist. If falciparum malaria is suspected on clinical grounds (see below) but a competent microscopist is not available, the patient should be kept under observation until the blood smear can be reviewed.

Once the diagnosis of malaria has been suspected or confirmed, the next step is to identify the illness as falciparum malaria, since this influences management. Although the diagnosis of falciparum malaria ultimately requires microscopic identification of specific morphologic characteristics of the parasites (see below), it is possible for clinicians to identify patients with probable falciparum malaria on the basis of their history alone.

Travelers and immigrants with falciparum malaria usually come from countries in which *P. falciparum* is the predominant malaria parasite. Thus, approximately 75 percent of U.S. falciparum malaria patients are infected in sub-Saharan Africa,[37] and most of the others are infected in India, southeast Asia, and Haiti.[38] Although Papua New Guinea and the Amazon basin are less visited by American travelers, *P. falciparum* is common in both regions, and falciparum malaria should be strongly suspected in travelers or immigrants from these areas.

A second element of the patient's history that may suggest falciparum malaria is an interval of 6 weeks or less between arrival in the United States and the onset of symptoms. In 1985 approximately 90 percent of all patients with falciparum malaria had onset of symptoms within 4 weeks of arriving in the United States[38]; in contrast, malaria due to *P. vivax* had its onset throughout the first 12 months after arrival in the United States. Thus, an ill traveler or immigrant who has recently arrived from Africa, India, Haiti, Southeast Asia, Papua New Guinea, or the Amazon basin should be considered on clinical grounds to be at risk for falciparum malaria until the diagnosis can be excluded by a competent microscopist.

The morphologic characteristics of *P. falciparum* include: a predominance of ring-stage parasites on the peripheral blood smear, since the trophozoite- and schizont-infected erythrocytes are sequestered; appliqué forms in which the ring appears to lie adjacent to the periphery of the erythrocyte; double chromatin dots; multiply infected erythrocytes; and crescent-shaped gametocytes. Identification of *P. falciparum* parasites may be extremely difficult for inexperienced microscopists, and if falciparum malaria is suspected on clinical grounds, the diagnosis should be excluded only by a competent microscopist. DNA hybridization probes that recognize highly reiterated species-specific sequences of *P. falciparum* DNA have recently been developed.[39] These probes are highly sensitive and specific for identification of blood samples containing *P. falciparum* parasites.[40] Currently, their principal use is in epidemiologic studies, but as nonradioactive labeling reagents become available and clinical laboratories develop expertise with DNA hybridization technology, they may become available for the diagnosis of patients with acute malaria.

TREATMENT OF FALCIPARUM MALARIA

Patients with falciparum malaria should be admitted to a hospital and treatment should be started promptly. Once treatment has been initiated, it is important to follow patients closely for the possible occurrence of complications and to continue to examine blood smears to determine whether the parasites are being killed by the drugs. *P. falciparum* parasites are widely and increasingly resistant to many antimalarial drugs, and a clinical response cannot be taken for granted. There is an urgent need for the development of new antimalarials with different structures and different mechanisms of action.

Antimalarial Drugs

Antimalarial drugs (Table 18-1) are usually categorized according to the life cycle stage against which they are active and their rapidity of action. The treatment of patients with falciparum malaria relies primarily on three drugs, chloroquine (a 4-aminoquinoline) and the cinchona alkaloids quinine and quinidine, all of which rapidly kill erythrocytic parasites. Quinidine is a stereoisomer of quinine and is very effective against *P. falciparum*.[41] Resistance to

Table 18-1. Principal Antimalarial Drugs

Drug	Mechanism	Excretion[a]	Toxicity	Resistance
Chloroquine	Unknown	Metabolism and renal (weeks)	Itching (Africans) Retinitis (rare)	Worldwide
Quinine Quinidine	Unknown	Metabolism & renal (11 hours)	Cinchonism Hypotension Hypoglycemia Abortion Arrythmias	SE Asia
Fansidar (Pyrimethamine and sulfadoxine)	Anti-DHFR Antifolate	Renal (90–100 hours)	Skin reactions[b] TEN[c] Agranulocytosis Anemia Kernicterus	SE Asia S America E Africa
Tetracycline	Impairs protein synthesis	Renal (8 hours)	Photosensitivity	Unknown
Doxycycline	Like Tetracycline	Metabolism and fecal (18 hours)	Photosensitivity	Unknown
Proguanil	Anti-DHFR Inhibits exoerythrocytic parasites	Renal (<12 hours)	Rare	Locally in Malaysia, Papua New Guinea, E Africa

[a] Drug half-life is in parentheses.
[b] Including Stevens-Johnson syndrome.
[c] Toxic epidermal necrolysis.

chloroquine occurs throughout the world; recent studies indicate that this may be due to rapid efflux of the drug from resistant parasites,[42] a mechanism that is similar to the one responsible for multidrug resistance of some cancer cells. The calcium channel blocker verapamil has been shown to reverse chloroquine resistance in vitro.[43] It has been suggested that chloroquine resistance may persist even when drug pressure is removed, perhaps because chloroquine-resistant parasites have biologic advantages over wild-type parasites.[44] Modest resistance of *P. falciparum* to quinine has been observed in Thailand,[45] but the minimum inhibitory concentrations are still below the clinically achievable blood levels. The mechanism of resistance to quinine is unknown. Two new drugs, mefloquine (another quinoline derivative)[46] and qinghaosu (a sesquiterpene extracted from the Chinese medicinal herb *Artemisia annua*)[46] are promising antimalarials, but they are not yet available to practicing clinicians in the United States.

Additional drugs that are active against erythrocytic parasites include the sulfas, pyrimethamine, proguanil, tetracycline, erythromycin, and clindamycin. In general, these drugs kill erythrocytic parasites more slowly than chloroquine and quinine and should not be relied on as the primary drug for treating patients with falciparum malaria, especially if the malaria is severe. They may be very useful in combination with quinine or quinidine in achieving complete eradication of erythrocytic parasites. Resistance to the combination of pyrimethamine and sulfadoxine (Fansidar) appears to be increasing and has been reported in East Africa, Southeast Asia, and South America.[8] Resistance to pyrimethamine appears to be due to altered properties of the target enzyme dihydrofolate reductase (DHFR), which results in reduced affinity of the enzyme for the drug.[47]

Drug Regimens

Unfortunately, there is now no area of the world from which chloroquine-resistant *P. falciparum* has not been reported, and thus, the use of this drug in the treatment of falciparum malaria has become problematic. Many strains of *P. falciparum,* especially those acquired in West Africa, are still sensitive to chloroquine. However, in the treatment of nonimmune travelers the risks of using a potentially ineffective drug are considerable, since complications and death may occur rapidly. Therefore, it is our opinion that most patients with falciparum malaria should be treated with quinine or quinidine regardless of where the infection was acquired. All patients with transfusion or needle-stick falciparum malaria should also be treated with quinine or quinidine. The drugs can be given orally to patients with uncomplicated falciparum malaria but should be given by slow intravenous infusion to patients with severe cases (see below).

Patients with uncomplicated falciparum malaria should be treated with quinine sulfate plus tetracycline or quinidine plus tetracycline (Table 18-2). An alternative regimen is quinine or quinidine plus pyrimethamine and a sul-

Table 18-2. Drug Regimens for the Treatment of Falciparum Malaria

Clinical Setting	Drug Regimen
Uncomplicated falciparum malaria	Quinine 650 mg tid for 3 days plus tetracycline 250 mg qid for 10 days Quinidine may be substituted for quinine. Tetracycline should not be used in pregnant women or in children less than 8 years old. Alternative regimen: quinine 650 mg tid for 10 days plus pyrimethamine 25 mg bid for 3 days plus sulfadiazine or sulfasoxazole 500 mg qid for 5 days
Severe falciparum malaria (parasitemia > 5%; cerebral malaria; organ dysfunction; rapid fall in hematocrit)	Quinidine: loading dose of 15 mg/kg IV over 4 hours in intensive care unit with cardiac monitoring. Then, 7.5 mg/kg every 8 hours with each dose infused over 4 hours with cardiac monitoring. Tetracycline 500 mg every 6 hours when patient can swallow

fonamide, but, as discussed above, many falciparum malaria patients may have parasites that are resistant to these drugs. Quinine may produce symptoms resembling cinchonism (nausea, vomiting, tinnitus, and vertigo), but this is not an indication to alter or discontinue treatment. Rarely, quinine may produce a Coombs-positive hemolytic anemia or immune thrombocytopenia, requiring that the drug be stopped immediately. Patients receiving antimalarial doses of quinine or quinidine will usually have conduction changes on the electrocardiogram (prolongation of the Q-T interval by 25 to 40 percent),[41] which can be followed for evidence of drug absorption and potential toxicity.

Patients with severe falciparum malaria should be treated with intravenous quinine or quinidine in an intensive care unit (Table 18-2). Parenteral quinidine is usually more readily available than quinine. The criteria for diagnosing severe falciparum malaria include: high parasitemia (more than 100,000 parasites per cubic millimeter of blood); severe anemia or a rapid fall in hematocrit; cerebral malaria; renal failure; or pulmonary edema. A loading dose of quinine or quinidine should be given so that a therapeutic drug level is achieved rapidly.[45,48–50] Parenteral doses of these drugs must be infused slowly (over at least 4 hours) to prevent hypotension or acute cardiac toxicity. When the patient can take oral medication, tetracycline or pyrimethamine plus a sulfonamide should be added. Quinine and quinidine are excreted by the kidneys, and the dose should be reduced in patients with renal failure.

Ancillary measures in the treatment of falciparum malaria include antipyretics to lower the temperature, especially in pregnant women, since high fever may cause fetal distress. Patients with cerebral malaria and seizures or febrile convulsions can be treated with diazepam or phenobarbital. Corticosteroids should not be given to patients with severe malaria since dexamethasone has been shown to be deleterious in a double blind trial in patients with cerebral malaria.[12] All patients with cerebral symptoms should have a blood sample drawn for glucose assay, and 100 ml of 50 percent dextrose should be administered immediately. Fluid requirements must be assessed individually, but circulatory overload must be avoided because of the potential for pulmonary edema. In patients with renal failure uremia may progress rapidly, and it may be necessary to begin dialysis emergently. Hypotension should be treated initially with volume expansion and pressors if necessary, and broad-spectrum antimicrobial therapy should be started.

Numerous anecdotal reports have described the successful use of exchange transfusion in patients with severe falciparum malaria.[51] An exchange transfusion may reduce the parasite burden and remove circulating toxins more rapidly than chemotherapy alone. Although it is difficult to make concrete recommendations about the use and timing of exchange transfusions in malaria, we suggest that this mode of therapy be strongly considered in patients with very high parasitemias (more than 10 percent of erythrocytes infected) or organ failure (cerebral malaria, renal failure, pulmonary edema). Chemotherapy with quinine or quinidine should be initiated rapidly regardless of whether or not an exchange transfusion is performed.

Patients with falciparum malaria should be followed closely even after the initiation of chemotherapy since complications or drug resistance may occur. Parasitemia is usually resolved in 2 to 3 days, and the patient should be afebrile within 2 to 4 days. Gametocytes are not affected by most antimalarial drugs, and their continued presence in the blood is not indicative of treatment failure. Patients who were exposed to *P. vivax* or *P. ovale* should be treated with primaquine to eradicate the persistent liver stages. The G6PD level should be checked first.

PREVENTION OF MALARIA IN TRAVELERS

Physicians who advise travelers can provide information and recommend prophylactic drugs to their patients. Of these two services, the information they provide is probably the more important. First and most important, patients traveling to malaria endemic areas should be advised that they may develop malaria during or after their trip despite use of chemoprophylactic drugs and precautions against mosquitoes. They should be informed that malaria may occur as long as 1 year or more after their return home. Second, patients can be advised of the risk of infection in the area they intend to visit. This risk will be greater in areas where transmission is intense, such as Africa, rural areas of Southeast Asia, and Papua New Guinea. Transmission in some areas is seasonal. The risk is usually substantially less in urban areas. Third, patients should be informed that they can reduce their contact with mosquitoes by wearing long sleeves and long pants in the evening, using an insect repellant that contains diethyl-*m*-toluamide (DEET), and by either sleeping inside screened buildings or using mosquito netting at night. Careful attention to these measures can reduce the risk of infection 10-fold or more.[52]

The chemoprophylaxis of malaria is imperfect because of resistance on the part of the parasites and the toxicity of some of the available drugs. Travelers to all malaria endemic areas should take chloroquine phosphate, 500 mg weekly, beginning 2 weeks before the trip, weekly during the trip and for 6 weeks after returning home. If there has been exposure to *P. vivax* or *P. ovale,* primaquine, 26.3 mg daily for 14 days, should be taken to prevent relapses. For travelers visiting most areas with *P. falciparum* malaria, it is our view that the combination of chloroquine 500 mg weekly and proguanil 200 mg daily provides the best combination of safety and efficacy. Proguanil is an inhibitor of DHFR and is active against liver-stage parasites. The drug can therefore block infection before the blood stage is reached. Proguanil as well as chloroquine must be taken for 6 weeks after the traveler returns home. This regimen is also recommended by many British malariologists[8]. Unfortunately, proguanil is not available in the United States, but it may be purchased in many countries where malaria is endemic. *P. falciparum* malaria resistant to this combination has been reported.[53]

The U. S. Centers for Disease Control makes a different recommendation. Individuals traveling for less than 3 weeks to areas with chloroquine resistant *P. falciparum* are advised to take along three Fansidar tablets, to be taken orally as a single dose in case of a febrile illness where medical care is not available.[54] For longer-term visits to areas with intense transmission of resistant parasites, weekly Fansidar is recommended.[54] However, Fansidar has proved to have significant toxicity (Stevens-Johnson syndrome and toxic epidermal necrolysis in approximately one patient per 5,000 to 8,000), and resistance to Fansidar is increasing.

Finally, doxycycline taken as a daily dose of 100 mg has been shown to reduce the number of malaria cases among a group of Thai children.[55] Doxycycline is contraindicated in pregnancy and should not be given to children less than 8 years old. Its principal toxicity is sun sensitivity. Widespread use of prophylactic doxycycline in endemic areas will almost certainly be followed by emergence of resistant parasites.

REFERENCES

1. McCutchan TF, Dame JB, Miller LH, Barnwell JB: Evolutionary relatedness of *Plasmodium* species as determined by the structure of DNA. Science 225:808, 1984
2. Facer CA: Direct Coombs antiglobulin reactions in Gambian children with *Plasmodium falciparum* malaria. II. Specificity of erythrocyte-bound IgG. Clin Exp Immunol 39:279, 1980
3. Phillips RE, Looareesuwan S, Warrell DA, et al: The importance of anemia in cerebral and uncomplicated falciparum malaria: role of complications, dyserythropoiesis and iron sequestration. Q J Med 58:305, 1986
4. Luse S, Miller LH: *Plasmodium falciparum* malaria: ultrastructure of parasitized erythrocytes in cardiac vessels. Am J Trop Med Hyg 20:660, 1971
5. Miller LH: Distribution of mature trophozites and schizonts of *Plasmodium falciparum* in the organs of *Aotus trivirgatus,* the night monkey. Am J Trop Med Hyg 18:860, 1969
6. Wyler DJ, Oster CN, Quinn TC: The role of the spleen in malaria infections. p. 183.

In: The Role of the Spleen in Immunology of Parasite Diseases. Trop Dis Res Ser No. 1. Schabe & Co., Basel, Switzerland, 1979
7. Field JW, Niven JC: A note on prognosis in relation to parasite counts in acute subtertian malaria. Trans R Soc Trop Med Hyg 30:569, 1937
8. Bradley DJ, Newbold CI, Warrell DA: Malaria. p. 54744. In: Oxford Textbook of Medicine. Oxford University Press, 1987
9. MacPherson GG, Warrell MJ, White NJ, et al: Human cerebral malaria. A quantitative ultrastructural analysis of parasitized erythrocyte sequestration. Am J Pathol 119:385, 1985
10. Udeinya IJ, Miller LH: *Plasmodium falciparum:* effect of infected erythrocytes on clotting time of plasma. Am J Trop Med Hyg 37:246, 1987
11. Warrell DA, Looareesuwan S, Phillips RE, et al: Function of the blood-cerebrospinal barrier in human cerebral malaria: rejection of the permeability hypothesis. Am J Trop Med Hyg 35:882, 1986
12. Warrell DA, Looareesuwan S, Warrell MJ, et al: Dexamethasone proves deleterious in cerebral malaria. A double-blind trial in 100 comatose patients. N Engl J Med 306:313, 1982
13. White NJ, Warrell DA, Looareesuwan S, et al: Pathophysiological and prognostic significance of cerebrospinal-fluid lactate in cerebral malaria. Lancet 1:776, 1985
14. Karney WW, Tong MJ: Malabsorption in *Plasmodium falciparum* malaria. Am J Trop Med Hyg 21:1, 1972
15. Brooks MH, Kiel FW, Sheehy TW, Barry KG: Acute pulmonary edema in falciparum malaria. N Engl J Med 279:732, 1968
16. James MFM: Pulmonary damage associated with falciparum malaria: a report of ten cases. Ann Trop Med Parasitol 79:123, 1985
17. Pitney WR: The tropical splenomegaly syndrome. Trans R Soc Trop Med Hyg 62:717, 1968
18. Whittle HC, Brown J, Marsh K, et al: T-cell control of Epstein-Barr virus-infected B cells is lost during *P. falciparum* malaria. Nature 312:449, 1984
19. Ho M, Webster K, Looareesuwan S, et al: Antigen-specific immunosuppression in human malaria due to *Plasmodium falciparum.* J Infect Dis 153:763, 1986
20. Williamson WA, Greenwood BM: Impairment of the immune response to vaccination after acute malaria. Lancet 1:1328, 1978
21. Allison AC: Protection by the sickle-cell trait against subtertian malarial infection. Br Med J 1:290, 1954
22. Allison AC: Polymorphism and natural selection in human populations. Cold Spring Harbor Symp on Quantitative Biology 29:137, 1964
23. Friedman MJ, Roth EF, Nagel RL, Trager W: *Plasmodium falciparum:* physiological interactions with the human sickle cell. Exp Parasitol 47:73, 1979
24. Flint J, Hill AVS, Bowden DK, et al: High frequencies of alpha-thalassemia are the result of natural selection by malaria. Nature 321:744, 1986
25. Brockelman CR, Wongsattayanont B, Tan-Ariya P, et al. Thalassemic erythrocytes inhibit in vitro growth of *Plasmodium falciparum.* J Clin Microbiol 25:56, 1987
26. Martin SK, Miller LH, Alling D, et al: Severe malaria and glucose-6-phosphate dehydrogenase deficiency: a reappraisal of the malaria/G6PD hypothesis. Lancet 1:524, 526, 1979
27. Usanga EA, Luzzatto L: Adaptation of *Plasmodium falciparum* to glucose-6-phosphate dehydrogenase-deficient host red cells by production of parasite-encoded enzyme. Nature 313:793, 1985

28. Mohandas N, Lie-Injo LE, Friedman M, Mak JW: Rigid membranes of Malayan ovalocytes: likely genetic barrier against malaria. Blood 63:1385, 1984
29. Hadley T, Saul A, Lamont G, Hudson DE: Resistance of Melanesian elliptocytes (ovalocytes) to invasion by *Plasmodium knowlesi* and *Plasmodium falciparum* malaria parasites in vitro. J Clin Invest 71:780, 1983
30. *Plasmodium vivax* malaria–San Diego County, California, 1986. MMWR 35:679, 1986
31. White NJ, Warrell DA, Chanthavanich P, et al: Severe hypoglycemia and hyperinsulinemia in falciparum malaria. N Engl J Med 309:61, 1983
32. White NJ, Miller KD, Marsh K, et al: Hypoglycemia in African children with severe malaria. Lancet 1:708, 1987
33. Looareesuwan S, Phillips RE, White NJ, et al: Quinine and severe falciparum malaria in late pregnancy. Lancet 2:4, 1985
34. Looareesuwan S, Warrell DA, White NJ, et al: Retinal hemorrhage: a common sign of prognostic significance in cerebral malaria. Am J Trop Med Hyg 32:911, 1983
35. Looareesuwan S, Warrell DA, White NJ, et al: Do patients with cerebral malaria have cerebral edema? Lancet 1:434, 1983
36. Herzog C, Ellis CJ, Innes JA, Fletcher KA: Possible role of drug malabsorption in recrudescence of falciparum malaria. Lancet 2:1157, 1982
37. Lobel HO, Campbell CC, Schwartz IK, Roberts JM: Recent trends in the importation of malaria caused by *Plasmodium falciparum* into the United States from Africa. J Infect Dis 152:613, 1985
38. Malaria Surveillance—Annual Summary for 1985. Centers for Disease Control, Sept. 1986
39. Barker RH, Suebsaeng L, Rooney W, et al: Specific DNA probe for the diagnosis of *Plasmodium falciparum* malaria. Science 231:1434, 1986
40. McLaughlin GL, Ruth JL, Jablonski E, et al: Use of enzyme-linked synthetic DNA in diagnosis of falciparum malaria. Lancet 1:714, 1987
41. Phillips RE, Warrell DA, White NJ, et al: Intravenous quinidine for the treatment of severe falciparum malaria. N Engl J Med 312:1273, 1985
42. Krogstad DJ, Gluzman IY, Kyle DE, et al: Efflux of chloroquine from *Plasmodium falciparum:* mechanism of chloroquine resistance. (Abstr.) 27th Interscience Conf. on Antimicrobial Agents & Chemotherapy, 1987
43. Martin SK, Odoula AMJ, Milhous WK: Reversal of chloroquine resistance in *Plasmodium falciparum* by verapamil. Science 235:899, 1987
44. Rosario VE: Genetics of chloroquine resistance in malaria parasites. Nature 261:585, 1976
45. White NJ, Looareesuwan S, Warrell DA, et al: Quinine loading dose in cerebral malaria. Am J Trop Med Hyg 32:1, 1983
46. Li G, Arnold K, Guo X, et al: Randomised comparative study of mefloquine, qinghaosu, and pyrimethamine-sulfadoxine in patients with falciparum malaria. Lancet 2:1360, 1984
47. McCutchan TF, Welsh JA, Dame JB, et al: Mechanism of pyrimethamine resistance in recent isolates of *Plasmodium falciparum*. Antimicrob Agents Chemother 26:656, 1984
48. White NJ, Looareesuwan S, Warrell DA, et al: Quinine pharmacokinetics and toxicity in cerebral and uncomplicated falciparum malaria. Am J Med 73:564, 1982
49. Silamut K, White NJ, Looareesuwan S, et al: Binding of quinine to plasma proteins in falciparum malaria. Am J Trop Med Hyg 43:681, 1985

50. Nielsen RL, Kohler RB, Chin W, et al: The use of exchange transfusions: a potentially useful adjunct in the treatment of fulminant falciparum malaria. Am J Med Sci 277:325, 1979
51. Peto TEA, Gilks CF: Strategies for the prevention of malaria in travelers: comparison of regimens by means of a risk-benefit analysis. Lancet 1:1256, 1986
52. Henderson A, Simon JW, Melia W: Failure of malaria chemoprophylaxis with proguanil-chloroquine combination in Papua New Guinea. Trans R Soc Trop Med Hyg 80:838, 1986
53. Revised recommendations for preventing malaria travelers to areas with chloroquine-resistant Plasmodium falciparum. MMWR 34:186, 1985
54. Pang LW, Boudreau EF, Limsomwong N, Singharaj P: Doxycycline prophylaxis for falciparum malaria. Lancet 1:1161, 1987 (See also critical letters that followed in issue of 6/27/87.)

19 Recent Advances in the Treatment of Helminthic Infections: Ivermectin, Albendazole, and Praziquantel

Robert S. Goldsmith

The past two decades have seen an extraordinary development of safe and effective new drugs for the treatment of many helminthic infections. Several major chemotherapeutic problems remain, however, including satisfactory treatment in onchocerchiasis, cysticercosis, and echinococcosis and the need to develop a broad-spectrum anthelmintic effective as a single-dose treatment in the four intestinal nematode infections: ascariasis, trichuriasis, strongyloidiasis, and hookworm disease. Some potential solutions for these problems have recently appeared. Ivermectin appears to be a significant advance over older drugs for treatment of onchocerciasis; mebendazole and albendazole are the first chemotherapeutic agents for treatment of echinococcosis; and praziquantel is the first agent to treat cysticercosis and the first safe and effective agent to treat clonorchiasis and opisthorchiasis. Albendazole has a broad spectrum of action against the intestinal nematodes, whereas praziquantel has a broad spectrum of action against most cestode and trematode infections.

Table 19-1 presents current methods of treatment for the major helminthic disorders, including drug(s) of choice and alternative drugs. Comments follow on the use of ivermectin in onchocerciasis, albendazole in the treatment of the soil-transmitted helminthic diseases and in hydatid disease, and praziquantel as an anticestode and antitrematode agent. The chapter concludes with summaries of clinical pharmacologic data on the three drugs.

IVERMECTIN IN THE TREATMENT OF ONCHOCERCIASIS

Onchocerchiasis is one of the major causes of blindness in the developing world (see Ch. 2). An estimated 20 million to 40 million persons are infected in parts of sub-Saharan Africa, the Americas (southern Mexico, Guatemala, Venezuela, Brazil, Colombia, and Ecuador), and the Arabian peninsula. Of these, about 10 million have serious eye damage and impaired vision, and an estimated 1 million have been blinded by the condition. A large proportion of infected persons also have skin involvement, leading to marked pruritus and skin disfigurement. Although both adult worms and microfilariae are found in the human host, only the microfilariae are responsible for the eye and skin pathology.

Treatment of onchocerciasis is unsatisfactory. The standard approach for many years has been to administer diethylcarbamazine to reduce the number of microfilariae and thus prevent progression of the disease and suramin to kill the adult worms. As both drugs have significant toxicity and require close medical supervision, they are difficult to administer to individual patients and are impractical for mass treatment. Diethylcarbamazine, which facilitates rapid destruction of the microfilariae by the host's cellular immune system, may initiate the Mazzotti reaction, with fever, prostration, hypotension, photophobia, and iridocyclitis. Death of microfilariae in the tissues of the eye may result in new punctate keratitic lesions, optic neuritis, chorioretinitis, and permanent visual field losses. Serious side effects of suramin therapy include peripheral neuropathy, nephrotoxicity, exfoliative dermatitis, and (rarely) death.

Several studies indicate that ivermectin is at least as effective as diethylcarbamazine in reducing the number of microfilariae in the skin and anterior chamber but has fewer systemic and ocular side effects. The reduction in microfilariae occurs more slowly in the skin (by several weeks) and more slowly in the anterior chamber (by several months). The reduction in microfilariae also persists longer, probably up to 1 year. Very limited information is available, however, to confirm that ivermectin also protects against the posterior chamber toxicity of diethylcarbamazine. Additional studies are needed to establish the optimal dose, the precise mechanism of action against the parasite, and the degree of safety in persons of all ages, particularly those with advanced ocular disease. Thus, although ivermectin does not kill the adult worms, it may be possible with repeated treatments at 6- to 12-month intervals to protect against progression of the disease.

Table 19–1. Drugs for the Treatment of Helminthic Infections (*Table continues.*)

Infecting Organism	Drug of Choice	Alternative Drugs
Roundworms (nematodes)		
Ascaris lumbricoides (roundworm)	Pyrantel pamoate	Piperazine, mebendazole, levamisole,[a] bephenium,[1] or albendazole[a,b]
Trichuris trichiura (whipworm)	Mebendazole	Oxantel-pyrantel pamoate[a] or albendazole[a,b,d]
Necator americanus (hookworm) *Ancylostoma duodenale* (hookworm)	Pyrantel pamoate[c] or mebendazole	Bephenium,[a] tetrachloroethylene,[a] levamisole,[a] or albendazole[a,b,d]
Combined infection with *Ascaris, Trichuris,* and hookworm	Mebendazole or oxantel-pyrantel pamoate[a]	Albendazole[a,b,d]
Combined infection with *Ascaris* and hookworm	Mebendazole or oxantel-pyrantel pamoate[a]	Bephenium[a] or albendazole[a,b,d]
Strongyloides stercoralis (threadworm)	Thiabendazole	Albendazole,[a,b,d] mebendazole,[c,d] or cambendazole[a,b,d]
Enterobius vermicularis (pinworm)	Mebendazole or pyrantel pamoate	Pyrvinium pamoate or albendazole[a]
Trichinella spiralis (trichinosis)	ACTH, corticosteroids, and thiabendazole[d] or mebendazole[c,d]	None
Trichostrongylus species	Pyrantel pamoate[c] or mebendazole[c]	Bephenium[a] or levamisole[a]
Cutaneous larva migrans (creeping eruption)	Thiabendazole	Diethylcarbamazine[d,e] or albendazole[a,b,d]
Visceral larva migrans	Thiabendazole[c,d] or mebendazole[c,d]	Diethylcarbamazine[c,d,e]
Angiostrongylus cantonensis	Levamisole[a,d]	None
Wuchereria bancrofti (filariasis) *Brugia malayi* (filariasis) Tropical eosinophilia *Loa loa* (loiasis)	Diethylcarbamazine[e]	None
Onchocerca volvulus (onchocerciasis)	Ivermectin[a,b]	Diethylcarbamazine[e] plus suramin[f]
Dracunculus medinensis (guinea worm)	Metronidazole[c]	Thiabendazole[c] or mebendazole[c]
Intestinal capillariasis	Mebendazole[3]	Thiabendazole[c]

Of additional importance in ivermectin usage is its potential to interrupt transmission when administered once or twice yearly in mass treatment programs, either alone or in combination with vector control measures.[1] Experimental findings show that during the period of drug-induced reduction in skin levels of microfilariae, treated patients are unable to infect the blackfly vector.

ALBENDAZOLE IN THE TREATMENT OF THE SOIL-TRANSMITTED HELMINTHIC INFECTIONS

Four intestinal nematode infections, also known as the soil-transmitted helminthiases—ascariasis, trichuriasis, strongyloidiasis, and hookworm infec-

Table 19–1. Drugs for the Treatment of Helminthic Infections (*Continued*).

Infecting Organism	Drug of Choice	Alternative Drugs
Flukes (trematodes)		
Schistosoma haematobium (bilharziasis)	Praziquantel	Metrifonate[a]
Schistosoma mansoni	Praziquantel	Oxamniquine
Schistosoma japonicum	Praziquantel	
Clonorchis sinensis (liver fluke)	Praziquantel[c]	Mebendazole[c,d] or albendazole[a,b,d]
Opisthorchis species		
Paragonimus westermani (lung fluke)	Praziquantel[c]	Bithionol[f]
Fasciola hepatica (sheep liver fluke)	Bithionol[f]	Emetine, dehydroemetine,[f] or praziquantel[c,d]
Fasciolopsis buski (large intestinal fluke)	Praziquantel[c] or niclosamide[c]	Dichlorophen,[a,d] tetrachloroethylene,[a] or bephenium[a]
Heterophyes heterophyes and *Metagonimus yokogawai* (small intestinal flukes)	Praziquantel[c] or niclosamide[c]	Bephenium[a] or tetrachloroethylene[a]
Tapeworms (cestodes)		
Taenia saginata (beef tapeworm)	Niclosamide	Praziquantel,[c] dichlorophen,[a] paromomycin,[c] or mebendazole[c,d]
Diphyllobothrium latum (fish tapeworm)	Niclosamide	Praziquantel,[c] dichlorophen,[1] or paromomycin[e]
Taenia solium (pork tapeworm)	Niclosamide[c]	Praziquantel[c] or mebendazole[c,d]
Cysticercosis (pork tapeworm larval stage)	Praziquantel[b,c]	Albendazole[a,b,d]
Hymenolepis nana (dwarf tapeworm)	Praziquantel[c]	Niclosamide or paromomycin[c]
Hymenolepis diminuta (rat tapeworm)	Niclosamide[c]	Praziquantel[c,d]
Dipylidium caninum		
Echinococcus granulosus (hydatid disease)	Albendazole[a,b,d]	Mebendazole[b,c,d]
Echinococcus multilocularis		

[a] Not available in the United States; available in some other countries.
[b] Undergoing clinical investigation.
[c] Available in the United States but not labeled for this indication.
[d] Effectiveness not established or not at a high level.
[e] Available in the United States from Lederle Laboratories. Telephone (914) 735-5000.
[f] Available in the United States only from the Parasitic Disease Drug Service, Parasitic Diseases Branch, Centers for Disease Control, Atlanta 30333. Telephone (404) 639-3670 during the day, (404) 639-2888 nights, weekends, and holidays (emergencies only).

(Reproduced, with permission, from Katzung BG (ed): *Basic & Clinical Pharmacology*, 3rd ed. Appleton & Lange, East Norwalk, CT, 1987.)

tion—continue to be major public health problems in the developing world. The most important of these infections is hookworm disease, in which the parasites contribute to diarrhea but have as their greatest impact blood loss and accompanying protein loss. The iron deficiency anemia can be severe, with blood hemoglobin levels as low as 1 to 2 g percent, and has important consequences with regard to growth and development in children and their susceptibility to infections. Trichuriasis and strongyloidiasis also contribute to diarrhea. When these infections are severe, anemia and prolapse of the rectum may be seen in trichuriasis, whereas in strongyloidiasis marked systemic spread may lead to overwhelming infection and death. Severe consequences of ascariasis result from the tendency of the worms to migrate and from intususception or volvulus due to masses of the worms.

Since the late 1960s it has become possible to treat these infections with new, more effective, and safer drugs, particularly mebendazole, pyrantel pamoate, oxantel pamoate, thiabendazole, levamisole, and albendazole.[2] Piperazine and bephenium hydroxynaphthoate have a somewhat longer history of use. All these drugs except thiabendazole are free from significant side effects and are moderately to highly effective against one or more of the parasites. Thus, treatment needs for individual patients have been nearly met. However, the search for a broad-spectrum anthelmintic for mass chemotherapy in the developing world continues.

An *ideal* drug for mass application, particularly in children, would have the following features: (1) effectiveness against all four of the parasites; (2) effectiveness against both adult and larval stages; (3) effectiveness as single-dose therapy; (4) suitability for oral administration and palatability; (5) safety, even in small children and in pregnancy; (6) absence of adverse side effects, (if present, side effects should be infrequent, mild, and transient); (7) stability at ambient temperatures; and (8) sufficiently low cost to permit mass usage.[3] Table 19-2 summarizes experience with seven drugs developed since the late 1960s with regard to their potential to meet some of these criteria. Dithiazanine iodide and thiabendazole have some effectiveness against all four parasites.

Table 19-2. Adequacy of Broad-Spectrum Anthelmintics to Treat Ascariasis, Trichuriasis, Strongyloidiasis, and Hookworm Infections[a]

Drug	Ascariasis	Trichuriasis	Strongyloidiasis	Hookworm	Days Medicated	Toxicity
Dithiazanine iodide	+	+	+	±	5–21	4+
Thiabendazole	+	±	+	±	2	2+
Pyrantel pamoate	+	0	0	+[b]	1	
Oxantel/pyrantel pamoate	+	+[c]	0	+[b]	1	
Levamisole	+	0	0	+	1	1+
Mebendazole	+	+	0	+	3	
Albendazole[d]	+	+	+[e]	+	1	

[a] + = moderately to highly effective; ± = low order of effectiveness; 0 = not effective.
[b] Heavy necatoriasis requires a 3-day course of treatment.
[c] Requires a 2-day course.
[d] Heavy ascariasis, trichuriasis, and necatoriasis require more than 1 day of treatment.
[e] Requires a 3-day course.

Dithiazanine had to be withdrawn, however, when idiosyncratic absorption led to some deaths in children. Thiabendazole requires a 2-day course of treatment, is not highly active against hookworms or trichurids, and causes gastrointestinal and other side effects in up to one-third of patients. Rarely, these side effects are severe and require discontinuation of treatment. Two deaths have occurred in children from Stevens-Johnson syndrome. Pyrantel pamoate is effective only against ascarids and hookworms; its congenor, oxantel pamoate, is effective only against trichurids. A preparation that combines pyrantel and oxantel is available in some parts of the world; although it is active against the three parasites, more than 1 day of treatment is required for *Trichuris* and *Necator* infections. Mebendazole is also effective against the three parasites but requires twice daily treatment for 3 days. Except for thiabendazole, none of these drugs is effective in strongyloidiasis.

Albendazole is active against the four parasites, is safe to use (except in pregnancy), and nearly meets the criteria of a single-dose treatment. Its limitations are that in strongyloidiasis even a 3-day course achieves only about an 80 percent cure rate and in heavy ascariasis, trichuriasis, and hookworm infection due to necatoriasis, treatment must continue for more than 1 day to achieve high cure rates. Nevertheless, a single-dose does markedly reduce worm burdens in ascariasis, trichuriasis, and both types of hookworm infection. A single dose also is highly effective in the treatment of pinworm infection. Further testing is necessary to confirm that albendazole can serve as an alternative drug, albeit less effective than praziquantel, in the treatment of opisthorchiasis, clonorchiasis, and infections by the large tapeworms. A single report indicates potential for the drug in the treatment of cysticercosis.

ALBENDAZOLE IN THE TREATMENT OF HYDATID DISEASE

Two larval forms of *Echinococcus* are of serious public health importance in humans, namely, *E. granulosus,* the cause of cystic echinococcosis or hydatid disease, and *E. multilocularis,* responsible for alveolar echinococcosis.[4,5] Cystic disease is mainly a problem in regions of intensive sheep husbandry, where transmission is from dog to sheep to dog. In humans the cysts, which are the larval stage of the infection, can reach almost any anatomic site but are found principally in the liver and less often in the lungs and bone. The cysts continue to enlarge slowly for many years, producing symptoms either because of their mass or occasionally because they become infected or rupture, which may lead to allergic symptoms that are sometimes severe. Until recently, surgical removal of cysts, when feasible, was the only approach to therapy. Under the best conditions, however, surgical mortality is 4 percent, postoperative problems are not uncommon, and recurrence of disease occurs in 10 percent of cases (Morris, 83).

The first drug to show a chemotherapeutic effect in hydatid disease was mebendazole.[6] Results, however, were unpredictable. Cures were obtained in some patients, but in others the drug either inhibited growth without killing cysts or had no effect. Other deficiencies of the drug were its infrequent serious side effects (agranulocytosis, cyst rupture with allergic reactions, glomerulonephritis) and the need to administer high doses for long periods (e.g., 50 mg/kg—approximately 35 tablets—daily for 3 months).

Albendazole is the most recently introduced drug for treatment of hydatid disease. Although the drug shows promise, it is very difficult to evaluate critically the results of medical treatment for hydatid disease. As only approximately 135 patients treated with albendazole have been reported in the literature,[7–11] and as they have not been followed for a sufficient time (up to about 30 months), conclusions can not be drawn. However, albendazole is much more readily absorbed than mebendazole, which permits a substantially lower dosage of albendazole to be used, yet its active metabolite, the sulfoxide, reaches effective concentrations in cyst wall and fluid. A current regimen is four tablets (800 mg) daily over 2 to 3 months. Some patients show complete disappearance of cysts; others show reduction in cyst size. As with mebendazole, however, treatment failures also occur, and liver and bone cysts may be more difficult to cure than lung cysts. Drug side effects include fever, cyst leakage, and leukopenia; none were life-threatening.

PRAZIQUANTEL IN THE TREATMENT OF TREMATODE AND CESTODE INFECTIONS

Praziquantel, introduced and evaluated in the past decade, has the unique characteristic of being an effective broad-spectrum drug against most of the human trematodes and cestode infections. Other attributes include oral administration, a short course (1 to 2 days), and freedom from toxicity. Although praziquantel has frequent side effects (e.g., dizziness, headache, drowsiness), they are generally mild and transient.

In the treatment of trematode infections, praziquantel is the first highly effective drug against clonorchiasis and opisthorchiasis, and it is the first oral drug to be effective against all five schistosome species that infect humans. Praziquantel appears to be equally active against the other trematode infections, except for fascioliasis, in which its effectiveness is of a low order. The drug is also promising as a potential single-dose oral medication for mass treatment of schistosomiasis, paragonimiasis, and opisthorchiasis.

As to the mature cestode infections, a single dose of praziquantel is highly effective against the large tapeworms and in the treatment of *Hymenolepis nana* infections. With respect to larval cestode infections, however, the drug has not been useful in the treatment of hydatid disease, although several in vitro studies show activity against protoscolices. Of considerable importance has been the recognition of praziquantel as the first drug to be effective in the treatment of neurocysticercosis.[12–15] The drug appears to be most effective in parenchymal disease, and less so in the presence of meningeal involvement or cerebral hypertension. Some continuing problems with praziquantel treatment are optimum dose, duration of therapy, and selection of patients likely to respond. Lack of controlled studies, however, continues to make these evaluations difficult. Therapeutic decisions in cysticercosis require considerable clinical judgment, and consultation with a physician experienced in the treatment of this disease is recommended.

CLINICAL PHARMOCOLOGY OF IVERMECTIN, ALBENDAZOLE, AND PRAZIQUANTEL[2]

Ivermectin

Ivermectin, a recently introduced drug in veterinary medicine, is being tested in humans for its efficacy in onchocerciasis.[16–20] Although in veterinary medicine the drug has a wide spectrum of action against many nematodes and ectoparasites, sufficient data are not yet available in humans to assess ivermectin's potential for the treatment of other parasitic infections.[21]

Chemistry

Ivermectin, a semisynthetic macrocylic lactone derivative of avermectin B, is 22,23-dihydroavermectin B_1. The avermectin family of compounds is produced by fermentation of the soil actinomycete *Streptomyces avermitilis*.

Absorption, Metabolism, and Excretion

Ivermectin is given only orally to humans, but in animals it is also given parenterally. There is little published information on the pharmacokinetics of the drug in humans; the half-life appears to be 10 to 12 hours.

In animals high concentrations are maintained in the tissues for prolonged periods. In sheep, after intravenous administration of 200 μg/kg, the half-life was 7.4 days. Radiolabeled drug residues, highest in liver and fat, were found up to 21 to 28 days. Excretion is mainly in feces, with less than 2 percent appearing in the urine. The drug does not cross the blood-brain barrier.

Pharmacologic Effects and Anthelmintic Actions

Anthelmintic Actions. Gamma-aminobutyric acid (GABA) is a neurotransmitter in both vertebrates and invertebrates. Whereas in mammals it is only found in the central nervous system, in nematodes and arthropods it regulates peripheral muscles. The proposed mechanism of action for the avermectins, including ivermectin, is that they paralyze nematodes and arthropods by disrupting GABA-mediated transmission of signals in peripheral nerves. It is not clear whether ivermectin (1) acts as a GABA agonist, (2) stimulates the release of GABA from presynaptic nerve endings, or (3) increases GABA binding at postsynaptic receptors.[20] The end result, however, is irreversible blocking of transmission from interneurons to excitatory motorneurons; for many nematode and arthropod species this results in paralysis and death.

In onchocerciasis, ivermectin acts both against microfilariae in the tissues (perhaps not in the eye) and on embryogenesis in female worms. The adult worms are not otherwise affected. The drug's precise mode of action on microfilariae is unknown; apparently it paralyzes them, which may facilitate their removal by the reticuloendothelial system before they can degenerate and release toxic material.[22] Observations on female worms indicate that intrauterine microfilariae are damaged and degenerate and are reduced in numbers.

Animal experimental data indicate that ivermectin potency is remarkably high, and that small doses, typically less than 300 μg/kg, are effective.

Pharmacologic Action in Humans. As GABA-regulated transmission in mammals occurs only in the central nervous system and ivermectin does not readily cross the blood-brain barrier, ivermectin has no paralytic action in mammals. Based on animals studies, the drug appears to have a wide margin of safety with regard to crossing the blood-brain barrier; it is estimated that 50 to 100 times the therapeutic dose is needed before toxic effects occur.

Though ivermectin is free of mutagenic effects, teratogenic effects have been observed in mice at doses above 0.2 mg/kg/day.[22] Occasional unexplained maternal deaths have also occurred at this dosage. Embryotoxicity has not been observed, however, except at dosages that were near or at maternotoxic levels.

Clinical Uses

Onchocerciasis. In double blind studies conducted in Ghana, Senegal, Liberia, and Mali, 150 patients with high skin microfilarial concentrations and (in most cases) ocular involvement were treated for 7 days with either diethylcarbamazine (total dose 1,100 mg), a single dose of ivermectin (200 μg/kg) and placebo, or placebo.[1,22–28] Ivermectin was as effective as or more so than diethylcarbamazine in reducing the number of microfilariae in the skin and anterior chamber but did so more slowly and with significant reduction in systemic and ocular reactions. The reduction in microfilariae also persisted longer. The skin microfilariae density decreased to near zero within a month, remained low for about 6 months, and then gradually increased to 2 to 10 percent of the pretreatment level by 12 months post-treatment. By comparison, the microfilariae density in diethylcarbamazine-treated patients reached near zero about a week after the start of treatment and increased to 10 to 45 percent by 12 months. Microfilariae counts in the anterior chamber in ivermectin-treated patients showed an increase in the first week, followed by a gradual fall to near zero 3 months post-treatment. Diethylcarbamazine caused greater systemic reactions than ivermectin. Also, the following eye changes were seen in diethylcarbamazine-treated but not in ivermectin-treated patients: anterior chamber changes (punctate keratitis and limbitis) in a few patients and posterior chamber changes (chorioretinitis and optic nerve atrophy) in two.[22]

Other Parasites. Although ivermectin is effective against a wide range of intestinal nematodes in domestic animals, the drug has not been shown to be effective against human bowel nematodes. Animal studies suggest possible usefulness in human strongyloidiasis, controversial usefulness in trichuriasis, and no effect in *Necator americanus* infections.[21] In humans, the drug has shown some effectiveness in *Wuchereria bancrofti* filariasis.

Adverse Reactions

Side effects after a single oral dose of 50 to 200 μg/kg appear to be mild, well tolerated, and of short duration; these include fever, headache, rash, increased pruritus, joint and muscle pain, lymph gland pain and tenderness, hypotension, and tachycardia. In several patients, dizziness persisted for 48 hours; in others, intermittent fever continued for several days. Symptoms were usually controlled with antihistamines and antipyretics, but steroid treatment for several days was necessary in rare instances. Some nonspecific electrocardiographic changes were noted in patients who received 200 μg/kg.

Toxic overdoses of ivermectin appear to cause nausea, vomiting, abdominal cramps, tachycardia, hypotension, hypothermia, and urticaria.

Cautions and Contraindications

As ivermectin enhances GABA activity, it is probably best to avoid concomitant use of other drugs that enhance GABA activity, such as barbiturates, benzodiazepines, and valproic acid. The drug should not be used in pregnancy.

Preparations and Dosage

The minimum effective dose remains to be determined. The 100 μg/kg dose may be as effective as higher doses and may be associated with fewer adverse reactions than the 200 μg/kg dose.[29]

Albendazole (Zental)

Albendazole, introduced in 1979 as a broad-spectrum oral anthelmintic, has had extensive clinical trials.[30–34] The drug is used in ascariasis, trichuriasis, strongyloidasis, and for hookworm and pinworm infections, but effectiveness varies by species. Few comparative studies with other anthelmintics have been reported.

Albendazole is in early clinical trials for the treatment of hydatid disease. A single report recently described its efficacy in cysticerocosis.

Chemistry

Albendazole, a synthetic benzimidazole carbamate, is methyl-(5-propylthio)-1-H-benzimidazol-2-yl) carbamate. The compound is nearly insoluble in water.

Absorption, Metabolism, and Excretion

After oral administration, albendazole is rapidly absorbed and metabolized mainly to albendazole sulfoxide and, to a lesser extent, to other metabolites. After a 400-mg oral dose, the sulfoxide attains a maximum plasma concentration of 40 to 550 ng/ml in 1 to 3 hours; its half-life is 8 to 9 hours. Variations in plasma concentration between individuals are attributed to differences in absorption. Concurrent ingestion of fat may increase absorption, but this is not established. The metabolites are mainly excreted in the urine; only a small amount is excreted in the feces.

Pharmacologic Effects and Anthelmintic Actions

Anthelmintic Actions. Albendazole blocks glucose uptake by larval and adult stages of susceptible parasites, depleting their glycogen stores and decreasing formation of ATP. Morphologically there is disintegration of microtubules in the syncytial tegument. As a result, the parasite is immobilized and dies. The drug has larvicidal effects in *Necator americanus* infections and ovicidal effects in ascariasis, ancylostomiasis, and trichuriasis.

Pharmacologic Effects. Based on experimental animal studies, albendazole is not expected to have pharmacologic effects in humans at therapeutic oral doses (5 mg/kg). In dogs, however, a high intravenous dose of 1 mg/kg resulted in marked hypotension and decreased ventricular contractility. In long-term (30 days) toxicity studies in rats and dogs, diarrhea, anemia, weight loss, leukopenia, and elevation of alkaline phosphatase were observed in some animals given 48 mg/kg/day. Some sheep treated for 6 weeks with 10 to 20 mg/kg showed bone marrow depression. In pregnant rabbits and rats treated with 30 mg/kg/day, the drug was teratogenic and embryotoxic.

Clinical Uses

Pinworm Infections. Cure rates of 100 percent were achieved with a single 400-mg dose.

Other Intestinal Nematode Infections. In multiple studies, albendazole given as a single dose of 400 mg (sometimes 200 mg twice for one day) showed the following cure rates: light ascariasis (96 to 100 percent), heavy ascariasis (85 to 89 percent), *Ancylostoma duodenale* (86 to 95 percent), *Necator ameri-*

canus (33 to 90 percent); and *Trichuris trichuria* (30 to 83 percent). In those not cured, egg counts were markedly reduced. To achieve higher cure rates in heavy ascariasis and satisfactory reduction in worm burden in moderate to heavy necatoriasis and trichuriasis will probably require repeated treatment for 2 to 3 days or a higher initial single dose. Optimal dosages remain to be determined.

Strongyloidiasis. A 400-mg dose daily for 3 days resulted in cure rates of 48 to 81 percent.

Hydatid Disease. Two studies[7,35] confirmed that following a course of albendazole (10 mg/kg/day for 10 to 30 days), sulfoxide levels of 53 to 1,235 ng/ml are reached in cyst fluid. In published reports of treated patients, about 135 persons were followed for up to 30 months after receiving a course of about 10 mg/kg daily for 1 to 3 months. Some persons showed improvement with shrinkage or disappearance of cysts. Failures in others were evident by continued growth of cysts, viable protoscolices found postoperatively, or severe drug side effects. Lung cysts appear to be easiest to treat; liver and bone cysts are more refractory. In multicenter WHO-coordinated clinical trials, albendazole was successful in three of four lung cysts, 21 percent of liver cysts, and 17 percent of cysts in other locations.[36] Current indications for use of albendazole are inoperable lesions, disseminated disease, and possibly as a pre- or postoperative course to kill the parasite, thus reducing the risk of recurrence due to operative spillage.[9]

Cysticercosis. A single report[37] described marked reduction in number of cysts and good tolerance of the drug when seven patients were treated for 1 month with a daily dose of 15 mg/kg.

Other Infections. A 400-mg dose daily for 3 days achieved marked egg reductions in *Opisthorchis viverrini* and *Clonorchis sinensis* infections,[38] and about 80 percent cure rates in *Taenia saginata* infections; 400 mg daily for 5 days can be tried in cutaneous larva migrans infections.[39]

Adverse Reactions

When used for 1 to 3 days, albendazole appears to be nearly devoid of significant side effects. Mild transient epigastric distress, diarrhea, headache, nausea, dizziness, lassitude, and insomnia have been attributed to the drug in about 6 percent of patients, but in two placebo-controlled studies, the incidence of side effects was similar in treatment and control groups. When albendazole was used for 30 days or longer in the treatment of hydatid disease in three studies totaling approximately 100 patients, the following findings were reported[8–10]: fever in 5 patients; reversible leukopenia in 2 patients; alopecia in 3 patients; reversible low-grade transaminase elevations in 16 (high in one patient, with severe hepatitis on liver biopsy); and cyst leakage in 2 patients, one with an anaphylactic reaction.

Contraindications and Cautions

The safety of albendazole has not been established in children under 2 years of age. Because the drug is teratogenic and embryotoxic in some animal species, it should not be used in pregnancy. It may also be contraindicated in the presence of cirrhosis.

Preparations and Dosage

Albendazole (Zental) is available as 200-mg tablets and as a flavored suspension (100 mg/5 ml). For pinworm infections, ascariasis, ancylostomiasis, or light necatoriasis or trichuriasis, the treatment for adults and children over 2 years is a single dose of 400 mg orally with meals. This dose for light necatoriasis or trichuriasis usually reduces the worm burden to satisfactory levels. In pinworm infection, the recommendation here is that the dose be repeated in 2 weeks. The dosage to achieve high cure rates in heavy ascariasis or satisfactory reduction in worm burden in moderate to heavy necatoriasis or trichuriasis has not yet been determined, but 400 mg daily for 2 days may be adequate. In the treatment of strongyloidiasis, 400 mg is given daily for 3 days. When necessary, treatment for any of the infections can be repeated after 2 weeks.

Dosages for the treatment of hydatid disease are not established. A current treatment program is 800 mg daily for 30 days, the course to be repeated two to three times, with 2-week intervals between courses. Blood levels of albendazole sulfoxide should be monitored.

Albendazole is not available in the United States but can be obtained for treatment of selected cases of hydatid disease. An investigational new drug number must be obtained from the FDA prior to contacting the distributor of the drug.

Praziquantel

Chemistry, Absorption, Metabolism, and Excretion

Praziquantel is a synthetic isoquinoline-pyrazine derivative and is slightly soluble in water. It is rapidly absorbed (about 80 percent) after oral administration. Peak serum concentrations of 1 μg/ml are reached 1 to 2 hours after an oral dose of 50 mg/kg. Praziquantel passes the blood-brain barrier, which results in cerebrospinal fluid concentrations of 14 to 20 percent of the drug's plasma concentration. The concentration in bile (in dogs) is nearly three times that in venous blood. Most of the drug is rapidly metabolized to mono- and polyhydroxylated products after a first pass in the liver; the half-life of the drug is 1 to 1.5 hours, while that of its metabolites is 4 to 6 hours. Excretion, principally as metabolites, is mostly via the kidney; 80 to 85 percent of radioactively labeled praziquantel is excreted within 4 days, 90 percent of this in the first day.

Pharmacologic Effects

In humans, no major alterations in biochemical or hematologic tests have been described, and the drug has not caused reactions in patients with glucose-6-phosphate dehydrogenase deficiencies or hemoglobinopathies. Transient elevations in liver function tests may occur and, rarely, minor electrocardiographic changes, but no significant damage to vital organs has been reported.

In experimental animals, no effects are seen until doses approximately 100 times the human therapeutic range are reached; signs of cerebral toxicity are then noted.

In a wide variety of mutagenicity studies, no abnormalities have been found. Tests for carcinogenicity, embryotoxicity, and teratogenicity have also been negative. Several reports suggest that praziquantel acts as a comutagen in *Salmonella typhimurium* and mammalian cell test systems; the significance of these findings has not been determined. Mutagenic urinary metabolites of praziquantel have been reported by one group of investigators.

Anthelmintic Actions

In spite of its short half-life, praziquantel is the active agent; its metabolites are inactive.

The threshold serum concentration of praziquantel for therapeutic effect is about 0.3 μg/ml. Praziquantel's in vitro action on all platyhelminths appears to be the same—the drug increases cell membrane permeability to calcium, resulting in marked contraction, followed by paralysis of worm musculature. Vacuolization and disintegration of the tegmen occur, and parasite death follows. In cestodes the sites of vacuolization are restricted to the neck of the strobila, but in trematodes, vacuoles occur in numerous areas over the entire surface. Only a slight reaction occurs with *Paragonimus westermani*. Although *Fasciola hepatica* does absorb the drug, no reaction occurs. In vitro studies with *Hymenolepis diminuta* and with schistosomes have shown that praziquantel also inhibits glucose uptake under anaerobic and aerobic conditions; however, this effect is thought to be secondary.

In schistosome infections of animals, praziquantel is effective against adult worms of both sexes and against the immature stages; adult worms residing in terminal venules are rapidly immobilized and then passively shift to the liver. In addition, when a single high dose of praziquantel is given concurrently with an infecting dose of cercariae, all immature forms are killed; thus, praziquantel has a prophylactic effect.

Clinical Uses

Schistosomiasis. Praziquantel is a drug of choice for all forms of schistosomiasis.[36,40] It is effective in adults and children and is well tolerated by patients in the hepatosplenic stage of advanced disease.[41] At various 1-day dosage schedules, high cure rates (80 to 95 percent) are achieved at 3 to 6 months, with marked reduction of egg counts in those not cured.

Studies that compared praziquantel and oxamniquine in the treatment of *Schistosoma mansoni* infections showed no significant differences in efficacy or side effects. A comparison of praziquantel with metrifonate in the treatment of *Schistosoma haematobium* infections showed no important differences in side effects, but praziquantel was more effective.[42] No schistosomal drug resistance is known for praziquantel.

Clonorchiasis and Opisthorchiasis. In multiple studies of *Clonorchis* infections, cure rates (disappearance of eggs) at 2 months post-treatment ranged from 86 to 100 percent of patients after a 1-day course of 25 mg/kg three times daily.[43–45] In a long-term follow-up, some patients failed to be cured when reexamined at 1 year, though no failures occurred among an equivalent group treated for 2 days.

Praziquantel may be more effective against *Opisthorchis* infections, for at 2 months the 1-day course resulted in 98 to 100 percent cure rates.

Paragonimiasis. When treated with 25 mg/kg three times for 1 day only, 71 to 75 percent of patients with pulmonary disease were cured; treatment for 2 to 3 days increased cure rates to 89 to 100 percent.[46]

Taeniasis and Diphyllobothriasis. Single-dose therapy (10 mg/kg) is curative in 97 to 100 percent of cases.[47]

Neurocysticercosis and Subcutaneous Cysticercosis. Praziquantel continues under clinical investigation for use in neurocysticercosis, which is infection by the larval stage of *Taenia solium*.[14,15,48–50] Live cysts are killed in subcutaneous tissue, muscle, and brain, but the drug does not appear to affect calcified cysts. In subcutaneous cysticercosis, initial changes start at 2 weeks; thereafter, the cysts tend to diminish in size, biopsies show degenerative changes, and the majority of cysts disappear after about 3 months.

In neurocysticercosis, therapy in some patients may result in apparent cure, with resolution of symptoms, changes in cysts by cerebral tomograms (disappearance, reduction in size, or calcification of lesions), and clearance of abnormal cerebrospinal fluid findings. In other patients there may be a remarkable improvement in findings, including reduction in cerebral hypertension and amelioration of seizures. Another category of patients, however, shows no change or continued progression of the disease leading to death.

Hymenolepiasis nana. Praziquantel is the drug of choice and the first drug to be highly effective.[51,52] Retreatment may be required.

Other Parasites. Limited trials indicate a high order of effectiveness of praziquantel against fasciolopsiasis, metagonimiasis, and other forms of heterophyiasis. However, in fascioliasis, praziquantel had only a low order of effectiveness at dosages as high as 25 mg/kg three times daily for 3 to 5 days. Two studies have shown that praziquantel adversely affects protoscolices of *Echinococcus granulosa* in vitro, although it does not affect the germinal membrane in vivo.

Adverse Reactions

Mild and transient side effects directly attributable to the drug are common. They begin within several hours after ingestion and may persist for hours to 1 day. Most frequent are headache, dizziness, drowsiness, and lassitude; others include nausea, vomiting, anorexia, abdominal pain (epigastric or generalized), loose to mushy stools, pruritus, urticaria, arthralgia, myalgia, and low-grade fever. Low-grade fever, pruritus, and skin rashes (macular and urticarial), sometimes associated with augmented eosinophilia, may also appear several days after starting the medication and are more likely to be due to the release of foreign proteins from dying worms than to a direct action of the drug. In intestinal schistosomiasis, bloody diarrhea may occur following treatment, particularly in patients with a history of prior episodes.

Praziquantel appears to be better tolerated in children than in adults. Side effects may be more frequent in heavily infected patients. The intensity and frequency of side effects also increase with dosage: they are mild and infrequent at dosages of 10 mg/kg given once but may occur in up to 50 percent of patients who receive 25 mg/kg three times in 1 day.

In neurocysticercosis, adverse reactions are of two types: (1) those characteristic of praziquantel usage at high dosage and (2) exacerbations of old symptoms or occurrence of new neurologic symptoms (often accompanied by increasing cerebrospinal fluid pleocytosis) due to inflammatory reactions around dying parasites. Administration of corticosteroids lessens these symptoms. In a few patients who received high doses, a benign hyperglycemia was seen, which was reversible with discontinuation of treatment.

Contraindications and Cautions

The only specific contraindication is ocular cysticercosis; parasite destruction in the eye may cause irreparable eye damage. The drug can be used in the presence of liver impairment due to parasitic infection. Safety of the drug in children under 4 years is not established.

Because the drug induces dizziness and drowsiness, patients should not drive and should be so warned if their work requires physical coordination or alertness.

The drug should preferably not be taken during pregnancy; an increase in abortion rate was found in rats treated with three times the human dose. In lactating women, although praziquantel appears in milk at about one-fourth plasma levels, the drug may be given to the mother provided the infant is not nursed on the day of treatment and for three subsequent days.

Preparations and Dosages

Praziquantel (Biltricide, Ceneride, Cesol, Cysticide) is prepared in various strengths by different manufacturers—150-mg, 500-mg, and 600-mg tablets. The tablets are taken with liquid after a meal; they should be swallowed immediately and not be chewed because their bitter taste can induce retching and vomiting. If the drug is taken more than once on the same day, the interval between doses should be not less than 4 nor more than 6 hours.

Optimal dosage schedules are still being determined for some parasites.

Schistosomiasis. One dosage for all forms of schistosomiasis is 20 mg/kg three times daily for 1 day. Lower dosages are also recommended: *S. haematobium* and *S. mansoni* (40 mg/kg, once); heavy *S. mansoni* (25 to 30 mg/kg twice in one day); *S. japonicum* (30 mg/kg, twice in one day).

***Clonorchis sinensis, Opisthorchis* spp., and *Paragonimus* spp.** A 2-day course of treatment of 25 mg/kg three times daily is recommended.

***Taenia saginata* and *D. latum*.** A single does of 10 mg/kg has been used successfully for *T. saginata* infections and 25 mg/kg for *D. latum* infections. Within 24 to 48 hours after treatment, a disintegrating worm is usually passed by normal peristalsis. Pre- and post-treatment purges are not necessary. If the scolex is searched for but not found—or is not searched for—cure can be presumed only if regenerated segments have not reappeared 3 to 5 months after treatment.

***Taenia solium*.** Give a single dose of 10 mg/kg. At present, it is recommended that an effective purge (such as magnesium sulfate, 15 to 30 g) be given 2 hours after treatment to eliminate all mature segments before eggs can be released from disintegrating segments. Since praziquantel does not kill the eggs, it is theoretically possible that larvae released from eggs in the large bowel could penetrate the intestinal wall and give rise to cysticercosis. This hazard is probably minimal. Experimental evidence suggests that peptic digestion (i.e., regurgitation of segments into the stomach) is necessary before hatching is possible.

Neurocysticercosis. This disorder should be treated in the hospital by a specialist. Current suggested treatment is 50 mg/kg/day in two or three divided doses for 15 days. To decrease or block cerebral and meningeal tissue inflammatory reactions and edema that result from dying parasites, steroids (4 to 16 mg/day in divided doses of dexamethasone or equivalent) should be administered concurrently and for about 3 days afterward and then gradually reduced.

***Hymenolepis nana*.** *H. nana* infections are treated with a single 25 mg/kg dose of praziquantel.

REFERENCES

1. Aziz MA: Chemotherapeutic approach to control of onchocerciasis (Editorial). Rev Infect Dis 8:500, 1986
2. Goldsmith RS: Clinical pharmacology of the anthelmintic drugs. In Katzung BG (ed): Basic and Clinical Pharmacology. 3rd ed. Appleton & Lange, East Norwalk, CT, 1987
3. Janssens PG, De Muynck A: Mass treatment. In Vandeu Bossche H, Thienpont D, Janssens PG (eds): Chemotherapy of Gastrointestinal Helminths. Springer-Verlag, Berlin, 1985
4. Pawlowski ZS: Epidemiological basis for chemotherapy of human echinococcosis. Int J Clin Pharmacol Res 5:75, 1985
5. Matossian RM, Rickard MD, Smyth JD: Hydatidosis: a global problem of increasing importance. Bull WHO 55:499, 1977
6. Bryceson ADM, Cowie AGA, MacLeod C, et al: Experience with mebendazole in the treatment of inoperable hydatid disease in England. Trans R Soc Trop Med Hyg 76:510, 1982
7. Saimot AG, Cremieux AC, Hay JM, et al: Albendazole as a potential treatment for human hydatidosis. Lancet 2:652, 1983
8. Davis A, Pawlowski ZS, Dixon H: Multicentre clinical trials of benzimidazolecarbamates in human echinococcosis. Bull WHO 64:383, 1986
9. Morris DL, Dykes PW, Marriner S, et al: Albendazole—objective evidence of response in human hydatid disease. JAMA 253:2053, 1985
10. Chevrel B: Hydatidose. Deuxième Congrès International de Médicine Tropicale de Langue Française, Sousse, 10/14–16/85. Med Chir Dig 15:38, 1986
11. Okelo GBA: Hydatid disease: research and control in Turkana. III. Albendazole in the treatment of inoperable hydatid disease in Kenya—a report on 12 cases. Trans R Soc Trop Med Hyg 80:193, 1986
12. Groll EW: Chemotherapy of human cysticercosis with praziquantel. In Flisser A (Ed): Cysticercosis: Present State of Knowledge and Perspectives. Academic Press, Orlando, FL 1982
13. Nash TE, Neva FA: Recent advances in the diagnosis and treatment of cerebral cysticercosis. N Engl J Med 311:1492, 1984
14. Sotelo J, Escobedo F, Rodriguez-Carbajal J, et al: Therapy of parenchymal brain cysticercosis with praziquantel. N Engl J Med 310:1001, 1984
15. Robles C, Sedano AM, Vargas-Tentori N, Galindo-Virgen S, et al: Long-term results of praziquantel therapy in neurocysticercosis. J Neurosurg 66:359, 1987
16. Campbell WC, Fisher MH, Stapley EO, et al: Ivermectin: A potent new antiparasitic agent. Science 221:823, 1983
17. Campbell WC: Ivermectin: An update. Parasitology Today 1:10, 1985
18. Koch H: Ivermectin: novel systemic antiparasitic agent. Pharmacy Int 2: 55, 1984
19. Editorial: Ivermectin in onchocerciasis. Lancet 2:1021, 1984
20. Bennett DG: Clinical pharmacology of ivermectin. JAVMA 189:100, 1986
21. Rajasekariah GR, Deb BN, Dhage KR, Bose S: Response of laboratory-adapted human hookworm and other nematodes to ivermectin. Ann Trop Med Parasitol 80:615, 1986
22. Aziz MA: Ivermectin vs. onchocerciasis. Parasitology Today 2:233, 1986
23. Diallo S, Aziz MA, Lariviere M, et al: A double-blind comparison of the efficacy and safety of ivermectin and diethylcarbamazine in a placebo controlled study of Senegalese patients with onchocerciasis. Trans R Soc Trop Med Hyg 80:927, 1986

24. Dadzie KY, Bird AC, Awadzi K, et al: Ocular findings in double-blind study of ivermectin versus diethylcarbamazine versus placebo in the treatment of onchocerciasis. Br J Ophthamol 71:78, 1987
25. Greene BM, Taylor HR, Cupp EW, et al: Comparison of ivermectin and diethylcarbamazine in the treatment of onchocerciasis. N Engl J Med 313:133, 1985
26. Taylor HR, Murphy RP, Newland HS, et al: Treatment of onchocerciasis. The ocular effects of ivermectin and diethylcarbamazine. Arch Ophthalmol 104:863, 1986
27. Awadzi K, Dadzie KY, Schulz-Key H, et al: The chemotherapy of onchocerciasis. XI. A double-blind comparative study of ivermectin, diethylcarbamazine and placebo in human onchocerciasis in northern Ghana. Ann Trop Med Parasitol 80:433, 1986
28. Lariviere M, Aziz M, Weimann D, et al: Double-blind study of ivermectin and diethylcarbamazine in African onchocerciasis patients with ocular involvement. Lancet 2:174, 1985
29. White AT, Newland HS, Taylor HR, et al: Controlled trial and dose finding study of ivermectin for treatment of onchocerciasis. Proceedings from the Wellcome Filariasis Seminar 1985. Trop Med Parasitol 37:96, 1986
30. Firth M (ed): Symposium on albendazole in helminthiasis. Royal Society Medicine International Congress and Symposium Series, No. 57. Royal Society of Medicine, Academic Press, and Grune & Stratton, 1983
31. Rossignol JF, Maisonneuve H: Albendazole: a new concept in the control of intestinal helminthiasis. Gastroenterol Clin Biol 8:569, 1984
32. Marriner SE, Morris DL, Dickson B, Bogan JA: Pharmacokinetics of albendazole in man. Eur J Clin Pharmacol 30:705, 1986
33. Coulaud JP, Rossignol JF: Albendazole: a new single dose anthelmintic. Study in 1455 patients. Acta Trop (Basel) 41:87, 1984
34. Pene P, Mojon M, Garin JP, et al: Albendazole: a new broad spectrum anthelmintic. Double-blind multicenter clinical trial. Am J Trop Med Hyg 31:263, 1982
35. Morris DL: Chemotherapy of hydatid disease. J Antimicrob Chemother 11:494, 1983
36. Davis A, Wegner DHG: Multicentre trials of praziquantel in human schistosomiasis: design and techniques. Bull WHO 57:767, 1979
37. Escobedo F, Penagos P, Rodriguez J, Sotelo J: Albendazole therapy for neurocysticercosis. Arch Intern Med 147:738, 1987
38. Pungpark S, Bunnag D, Harinasuta T: Albendazole in the treatment of opisthorchiasis and concomitant intestinal helminthic infections. Southeast Asian J Trop Med Public Health 15:44, 1984
39. Coulaud JP, Binet D, Voyer C, et al: Treatment of cutaneous larva migrans "Larbish" with albendazole: report of 18 cases. Bull Soc Pathol Exotique Filiales 75:534, 1982
40. Chen MG, Hua XJ, Wang MJ, et al: Dose finding double-blind clinical trial with praziquantel in schistosomiasis japonica patients. Southeast Asian J Trop Med Public Health 16:228, 1985
41. Katz N, Rocha RS: Double-blind clinical trial comparing praziquantel with oxamniquine in schistosomiasis mansoni. Rev Inst Med Trop Sao Paulo 24:310, 1982
42. Mahmoud AA: Praziquantel for the treatment of helminthic infections. Adv Intern Med 32:193, 1987
43. Bunnag D, et al: *Opisthorchis viverrini:* clinical experience with praziquantel in hospital for tropical diseases. Arzneimittel-Forschung 34:1173, 1984

44. Chen C-Y, Hsieh W-C: Clinical investigation of praziquantel in the treatment of clonorchiasis sinensis. J Formosan Med Assoc 81:1434, 1982
45. Jong EC, et al: Praziquantel for the treatment of Clonorchis/Opisthorchis infections: report of a double-blind, placebo-controlled trial. J Infect Dis 152:637, 1985
46. Johnson RJ, Jong EC, Dunning SB, et al: Paragonimiasis: diagnosis and the use of praziquantel in treatment. Rev Infect Dis 7:200, 1985
47. Fan PC, Chung WC, Chan CH, Chen FY: Studies on taeniasis in Taiwan. V. Field trial on evaluation of therapeutic efficacy of mebendazole and praziquantel against taeniasis. Southeast Asian J Trop Med Public Health 17:82, 1986
48. Bell DR: Cysticercosis: a new hope. Br Med J 289:857, 1984
49. Robles C (ed): International Symposium on the Medical Treatment of Neurocysticercosis, Mexico, 9/10-11/82 [Symposium Internacional sobre Tratamiento Médico de la Neurocisticercosis]. Salud Publica Mexico 24:605, 1982
50. Sotelo J, Torres B, Rubio-Donnadieu F, et al: Praziquantel in the treatment of neurocysticercosis: Long-term follow-up. Neurology 35:752, 1985
51. Campos R, Bressnan MCRV, Evangelista MGBF: Activity of praziquantel against *Hymenolepis nana,* a different development state, in experimentally infected mice. Rev Inst Med Trop Sao Paulo 26:334, 1984
52. Farid Z, Ayad El-Masry N, Wallace CK: Treatment of *Hymenolepis nana* with a single oral dose of praziquantel. Trans R Soc Trop Med Hyg 78:280, 1984

SUGGESTED READINGS

Campbell WC: The chemotherapy of parasitic infections. J Parasit 72:45, 1986

Campbell WC, Rew RS: The chemotherapy of parasitic diseases. Plenum Press, New York, 1986

Classen HG, Schramm V (eds): Praziquantel (Embay 8440, Biltricide). Biltricide Symposium on African Schistosomiasis, Nairobi, Kenya, 2/24–26/80. Drug Res 31:535, 1981

Classen HG, Schramm V (eds): Int Symp Human Trematode Infections in Southeast and East Asia, Kyongju, Republic of Korea, 10/19–21/83. Drug Res 34:1115, 1984

Editorial: Albendazole: worms and hydatid disease. Lancet 2:675, 1984

Groll EW: Praziquantel. Adv Pharmacol Chemother 20:219, 1984

Isaacs RD: Hydatid disease. An approach in 1986. Curr Ther 49, 1986

James DM, Gilles HM: Human antiparasitic drugs: pharmacology and usage. John Wiley, Chichester, 1985

Knobloch J, Delgado E, Alvarez A, et al: Human fascioliasis in Cajamarca/Peru. I. Diagnostic methods and treatment with praziquantel. Trop Med Parasitol 36:88, 1985

Mansfield JM: Parasitic diseases: the chemotherapy. Vol. 2. Marcel Dekker, New York, 1984

McMahon JE: A comparative trial of praziquantel, metrifonate and niridazole against *Schistosoma haematobium*. Ann Trop Med Parasitol 77:139, 1983

Mott KE, Dixon H, Osei-Tutu E, et al: Effect of praziquantel on hematuria and proteinuria in urinary schistosomiasis. Am J Trop Med Hyg 34:1119, 1985

Ramalingam S, Sinniah B, Krishnan U: Albendazole, an effective single dose, broad spectrum anthelmintic drug. Am J Trop Med Hyg 32:984, 1983

Rim HJ: The current pathobiology and chemotherapy of clonorchiasis. Korean J Parasitol suppl., Monogr Ser 3, 24, 1986

Rossignol JF, Maisonneuve H: Albendazole: placebo-controlled study in 870 patients with intestinal helminthiasis. Trans R Soc Trop Med Hyg 77:707, 1983

Ruenwongsa P, Thamavit W: Increased efficacy of liposomes-encapsulated praziquantel in treatment of opisthorchiasis in hamsters. Southeast Asian J Trop Med Public Health 14:501, 1983

Schantz PM: Effective medical treatment for hydatid disease? JAMA 253:2095, 1985

Symposium on albendazole. Compend Invest Clin Latino-am 1; suppl. 1, 1981

Symposium on albendazole. Medicine d'Afrique Noire; suppl., special number July 1982

Taraschewaki H, Mahborn H, Bunnag D, et al: Effects of praziquantel on human intestinal flukes (*Fasciolopsis buski* and *Heterophyes heterophyes*). Zentralbl Bakteriol [A] 262:542, 1986

Vanden Bossche H: Pharmacology of anthelmintics. In Vanden Bossche H, Thienpoint D, Janssens PG (eds): Chemotherapy of gastrointestinal helminths. Springer-Verlag, Berlin, 1985

Viravan C, Bunnag D, Harina Suta T, et al: Clinical field trial of praziquantel in opisthorchiasis in Nong Ranya village, Kohn Kaen Province, Thailand. Southeast Asian J Trop Med Public Health 17:63, 1986

Webbe G: Medical treatment of human hydatidosis. Med Chir Dig 15:41, 1986

Zhejiang Clinical Cooperative Research Group for Praziquantel: clinical evaluation of praziquantel in treatment of schistosomiasis japonicum. Chin Med J [Engl] 93:375, 1980

Index

Page numbers followed by *f* represent figures; those followed by *t* represent tables.